THE LUNG

PHYSIOLOGIC BASIS OF PULMONARY FUNCTION TESTS

THIRD EDITION

THE LUNG

PHYSIOLOGIC BASIS OF PULMONARY FUNCTION TESTS

THIRD EDITION

Robert E. Forster II, M.D.

Isaac Ott Professor and Chairman
Department of Physiology
University of Pennsylvania School of Medicine
Philadelphia, Pennsylvania

Arthur B. DuBois, M.D.

Professor of Epidemiology and Physiology
Yale University School of Medicine
Director, John B. Pierce Foundation Laboratory
New Haven, Connecticut

William A. Briscoe, M.D.

Professor of Medicine
Cornell University Medical College
Attending Physician
The New York Hospital
New York, New York,

Aron B. Fisher, M.D.

Professor of Physiology and Medicine
Director, Institute for Environmental Medicine
University of Pennsylvania School of Medicine
Philadelphia, Pennsylvania

YEAR BOOK MEDICAL PUBLISHERS, INC.

CHICAGO • LONDON

1 2 3 4 5 6 7 8 9 KC 89 88 86

Library of Congress Cataloging-in-Publication Data

The Lung: physiologic basis of pulmonary function tests.

Includes bibliographies and index.
1. Pulmonary function tests. 2. Lungs—Diseases—Diagnosis. I. Forster, Robert E., 1919– .
[DNLM: 1. Lung—physiology. 2. Respiratory Function Tests. WF 600 L963]
RC734.P84L86 1986 616.2′4075 86-5624
ISBN 0-8151-1822-8

Sponsoring Editors: Stephany S. Scott/Kevin M. Kelly
Manager, Copyediting Services: Frances M. Perveiler
Production Project Manager: Max Perez
Proofroom Supervisor: Shirley E. Taylor

In memory of
Julius H. Comroe, Jr., M.D. (1911–1984)
and
William Alexander Briscoe, M.D. (1918–1985)
in whose happy company *The Lung* was written

Preface to the First Edition

Pulmonary physiologists understand pulmonary physiology reasonably well. Many doctors and medical students do not. One reason is that most pulmonary physiologists, in their original and review articles, write for other pulmonary physiologists and not for doctors or medical students. This is *not* a book for pulmonary physiologists; it is written for doctors and medical students. Like the Beaumont Lecture* upon which it is based, it has only one purpose—to explain in simple words and diagrams, those aspects of pulmonary physiology that are important to clinical medicine.

A few words of explanation:

1. This is not an illustrated book but a monograph constructed largely around illustrations. Most of the illustrations are schematic; artistic license has been used freely to achieve clarity.
2. Our monograph strives for understanding of physiological principles and broad concepts more than for technical completeness. Details of procedures have been presented in an earlier publication (*Methods in Medical Research* [Chicago: Year Book Publishers, Inc., 1950], Vol. 2).
3. Pulmonary physiology can be explained in words, pictures, or equations. Most physicians shudder at equations; therefore words and pictures predominate and the occasional equation is accompanied by a verbal explanation and full apology. However, all important equa-

* "The Physiological Diagnosis of Pulmonary Disease," delivered by J. H. Comroe, Jr., to the Wayne County Medical Society, Detroit, February 1, 1954.

tions are presented in an Appendix for the enjoyment of those who have difficulty with words and pictures.

4. There are no references in the text. This is not because we wish to slight pulmonary physiologists (including ourselves) but because documentation often breaks the continuity of thought. Selected references are given in the Appendix, but even these represent only a small fraction of important articles that have been written on this subject.
5. The case reports (Part II) have been presented deliberately with minimal clinical detail, and the reader is asked to accept that the diagnoses have been based on adequate clinical study.
6. This is not a primer; a primer would not enable the physician to cope with some of the more baffling concepts such as ventilation/blood flow ratios, diffusing capacity, physiological dead space, distribution, compliance, alveolar ventilation, or transpulmonary pressure. On the other hand, this is not an encyclopedia, and no attempt has been made to include all contributions in this small volume.

J. H. COMROE, JR.
R. E. FORSTER, II
A. B. DUBOIS
W. A. BRISCOE
E. CARLSEN

Preface to the Third Edition

The first edition of *The Lung: Clinical Physiology and Pulmonary Function Tests* served as a text of pulmonary function testing and clinical physiology, as its subtitle indicated, and also as a textbook of pulmonary physiology and even of pathophysiology, for medical students, clinicians, and auxilliary medical professionals. We expanded the pathophysiology in the second edition, adding illustrative clinical cases and five chapters on pulmonary evaluation for several clinical specialities.

In considering the content of the third edition we concluded that *The Lung* should return to its origin as a monograph constructed largely on illustrations and focus on the scientific basis of pulmonary function tests. In the 30 years of *The Lung's* existence there has been an explosive expansion of interest in pulmonary function testing. There are excellent small texts on pulmonary function tests, clinical physiology, and pulmonary physiology, and there are several comprehensive textbooks on clinical pulmonary disease that include synopses of pulmonary function testing. The manufacture of pulmonary test equipment has evolved into a major industry.

Clearly, *The Lung* cannot fulfill all of the roles it appeared to fill in the past. Therefore, we eliminated the clinical material and reduced the size of the third edition. We added new illustrations and rewrote the entire text. We are grateful to many for their helpful criticism and hope that this volume will be as useful as the previous editions to clinicians and medical students.

ROBERT E. FORSTER II, M.D.
ARTHUR B. DUBOIS, M.D.
WILLIAM A. BRISCOE, M.D.
ARON B. FISHER, M.D.

Contents

PART TWO

PART ONE

1

Introduction to Pulmonary Physiology

The major function of the cardiovascular and respiratory systems is to provide an adequate amount of *arterialized* blood at each moment to all of the tissues of the body. The lungs alone cannot acccomplish this. Several processes are involved: First, mixed venous blood, low in O_2 and high in CO_2, is returned to the right atrium and ventricle to be pumped through the pulmonary circulation. Second, the mixed venous blood flowing through the pulmonary capillaries is arterialized, i.e., receives O_2 from the alveolar gas and gives off excess CO_2. Third, the arterialized blood is distributed to all of the tissues of the body according to their needs. Fourth, exchange of O_2 and CO_2 occurs between the blood in the tissue capillaries and the tissue cells themselves. The first, third, and fourth of these processes are the major function of the cardiovascular system. The second process, the loading of mixed venous blood with enough O_2 at a high enough pressure and the unloading of excess CO_2, is the primary function of the lung; this book discusses only *pulmonary* function.

A large number of physiologic tests has been developed for the qualitative and quantitative evaluation of pulmonary function in patients with suspected abnormalities of the cardiopulmonary system. These are as important to the practice of medicine as are tests of hepatic, renal, cardiovascular, and neuromuscular function. Tests of pulmonary function are of definite value both in diagnosis and in guiding therapy of patients with cardiopulmonary disorders. They have led to a better understanding of pulmonary physiology in healthy men and women of all age groups and to more precise knowledge of the pathologic physiology and natural course of pulmonary disease. They can aid in the early detection of pulmonary dysfunction and can assist in differential diagnosis in patients. They can be used for the objective evaluation of therapeutic measures and so can contribute to the development of more rational measures of treatment. Various tests are used in screening populations, in outpatient clinics, on hospitalized patients, and in intensive care units. Finally, they can provide objective data in patients who may or may not have pulmonary disability, and thereby help to determine, during the lifetime of the patient, if a specific function of the lung has been impaired.

The use of physiologic tests does not supplant other diagnostic procedures. Physiologic tests indicate only how disease has altered function; they cannot make a pathologic diagnosis. For example, function tests may reveal the existence of a right-to-left shunt but in themselves cannot locate it anatomically as being intracardiac or intrapulmonic. Furthermore, they do not reveal alterations in all types of pulmonary disease, but do so only when the lesion disturbs function and disturbs it sufficiently that present tests can recognize with certainty the deviation from normal values. In general, they cannot detect slight reduction in functioning pulmonary tissue or the presence of small regions in the lungs that have neither ventilation nor blood flow. Results of physiologic tests may be normal in the presence of lesions such as fibrotic cavities, cysts, or carcinomatous nodules unless these lesions occupy so much space that they reduce the lung volume well below normal limits or are located so strategically that they disturb pulmonary function. Pulmonary function studies will not tell where the lesion is, what the lesion is, or even that a lesion exists, if it does not interfere with the function of the lung. Therefore, they supplement and do not replace a good history and physical examination and radiologic, bacteriologic, bronchoscopic, and pathologic studies.

As in the case of physiologic tests of other systems, no single pulmonary function test yields all the information desired in any single patient. The primary function of the lung is, as already stated, to arterialize the mixed venous blood. This involves the addition of adequate amounts of O_2 and the elimination of proper quantities of CO_2. This is achieved by pulmonary gas exchange, which involves a number of processes (Fig 1). The first of these is VENTILATION; this includes both volume and distribution of the air ventilating the alveoli. A large enough volume of inspired air must reach the alveoli each minute, and this air must be distributed evenly to the hundreds of millions of alveoli

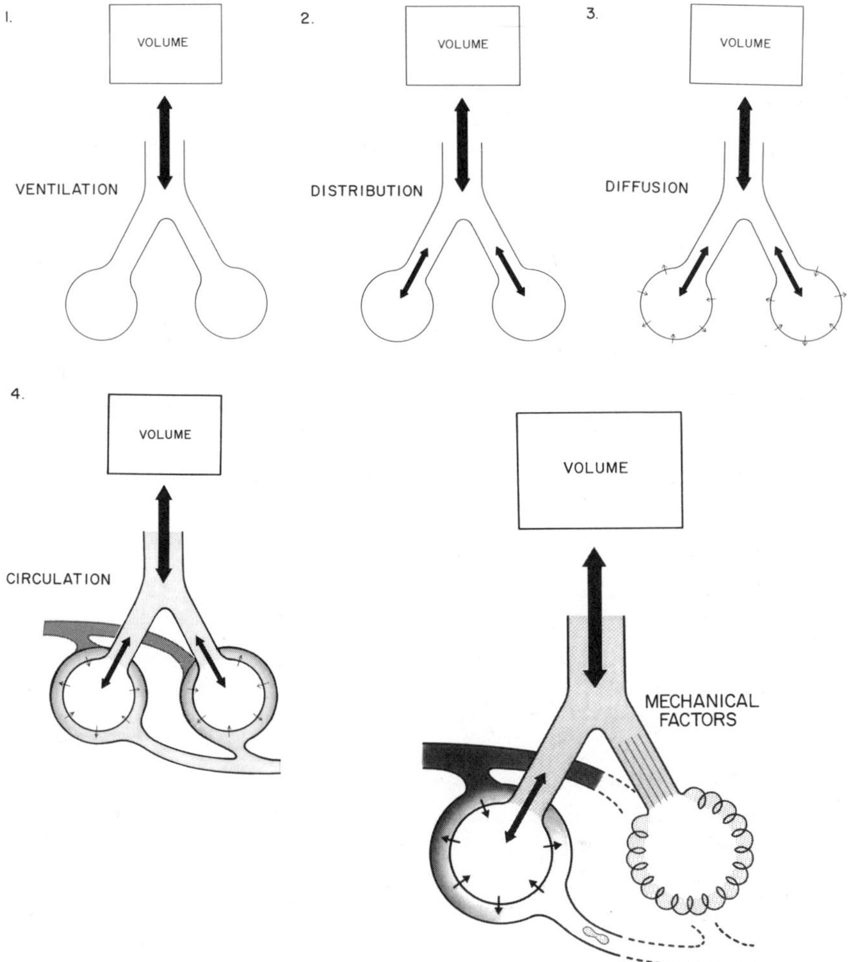

Fig 1.—Processes involved in pulmonary gas exchange. The alveoli, where rapid gas exchange occurs, are represented by rounded areas; leading into these are tubes depicting the conducting airways or anatomic dead space *(light gray in 5)* in which no effective gas exchange occurs. Rectangular blocks indicate the minute volume of breathing. The two arrows entering the alveoli show distribution of total inspired gas *(large arrow)* to various alveoli. In *3* and *4,* small arrows crossing alveolar walls designate the process of diffusion of O_2 out of the alveoli into the blood and of CO_2 from the blood into the alveoli. The shaded channel surrounding the alveoli in 4 represents pulmonary blood flow; it enters the capillary bed as mixed venous blood *(dark)* and emerges as arterialized blood *(light).* In *5,* the left side is a summary of the processes of ventilation, diffusion, and circulation. The right side represents the pulmonary "tissues" responsible for the mechanical properties of the lung: parallel lines in the conducting airways represent the fine airways responsible for airway resistance; the springlike coil surrounding the alveoli represents the elastic tissues of the lung; and stippled areas in the coil are the nonelastic tissues (see chapter 4).

in the lungs; i.e., the volume of air going to each alveolus should be in proportion to the volume of that alveolus. The second of these is the process of DIFFUSION, by which O_2 and CO_2 pass across the alveolocapillary membranes. The third is PULMONARY CAPILLARY BLOOD FLOW; this must be adequate in volume and all of the mixed venous blood must be distributed evenly to all the ventilated alveoli.

This gas exchange should be achieved with a minimal expenditure of energy by the respiratory and circulatory systems. The MECHANICAL FACTORS in ventilation are of great importance, because in some patients adequate pulmonary gas exchange may be achieved only by a considerable increase in the work of the respiratory muscles; indeed, in patients with advanced pulmonary disease, the crucial factor in survival may be whether the maximal effort available can produce adequate ventilation. The work required of the right ventricle in pumping blood through a restricted pulmonary vascular bed may also be of critical importance in survival.

The process of ventilation is controlled through the central and peripheral nervous systems, which coordinate the activity of the muscles involved in inspiration and expiration. The control of respiration therefore merits separate consideration.

Finally, the lung is not just an organ for gas exchange. In fact, it contains more different cell types than any other organ in the body. Recently, several tests of nonrespiratory functions of the lung have been described and are included in this book. Lung cell biology represents a rapidly expanding field of study, and it seems likely that the number of tests available for this area will soon increase.

The quantitative measurement of these processes of lung function requires a large number of physiologic tests. Not all of these are required in the management of each patient. Some of the tests are very simple and may be carried out in a physician's office; others require expensive apparatus or considerable technical experience and are normally carried out in a hospital pulmonary function laboratory; still others are research procedures and at present are available only in a few medical centers. However, some tests should be performed on every patient with known or suspected pulmonary disease, just as an electrocardiogram (ECG) or other physiologic tests are performed on patients with suspected heart disease.

This book is divided into two parts. The first of these considers separately each of the components of pulmonary function (lung volumes, ventilation, pulmonary blood flow, diffusion, control of ventilation, and the mechanics of breathing). The goal of this part is to present the scientific basis for understanding the rationale and limitations of tests of pulmonary function. The second part, the Appendix, includes information basic to the development of some tests of pulmonary function but not essential to their understanding, and lists tables of normal values.

2

The Lung Volumes

The first measurements used to test pulmonary function were those of the lung volumes (Fig 2). Actually, these do not evaluate *function* since they are essentially anatomic measurements. Changes in the lung volumes, however, are often caused by alterations in physiologic processes, and for this reason it is important to know normal values and how to interpret deviations from these.

By standard nomenclature, the total lung volume is subdivided into "volumes" and "capacities" (Table 1).

Subdivisions of lung volume named *volume* (such as tidal volume) are not further divisible into component parts, whereas *capacities* (such as functional residual capacity) consist of more than one volume (e.g., expiratory reserve volume plus residual volume).

Normal values for lung volumes and subdivisions in men and women are given in Table 2. The standard deviations from the mean show that there is considerable variation even in a homogeneous group; consequently, deviations from "normal" must be large to be significant in diagnosis.

A. VITAL CAPACITY AND ITS SUBDIVISIONS

The vital capacity and its subdivisions (inspiratory reserve volume, expiratory reserve volume, and tidal volume) can be measured directly by the use of simple volume recorders such as bellows or spirometers. Ap-

TABLE 1.—THE LUNG VOLUMES AND CAPACITIES

VOLUMES.—There are four primary volumes that do not overlap (Fig 2):

1. *Tidal volume,* or the depth of breathing, is the volume of gas inspired or expired during each respiratory cycle.
2. *Inspiratory reserve volume* is the maximal amount of gas that can be inspired from the end-inspiratory position.
3. *Expiratory reserve volume* is the maximal volume of gas that can be expired from the end-expiratory level.
4. *Residual volume* (formerly residual capacity or residual air) is the volume of gas remaining in the lungs at the end of a maximal expiration.

CAPACITIES.—There are four capacities, each of which includes two or more of the primary *volumes* (Fig 2):

1. *Total lung capacity* is the amount of gas contained in the lung at the end of a maximal inspiration.
2. *Vital capacity* is the maximal volume of gas that can be *expelled* from the lungs by forceful effort following a maximal inspiration.
3. *Inspiratory capacity* is the maximal volume of gas that can be inspired from the resting expiratory level.
4. *Functional residual capacity* is the volume of gas remaining in the lungs at the resting expiratory level. The resting *end-expiratory* position is used here as a base line because it varies less from breath to breath on a spirometer tracing than the end-inspiratory position.

proximate values are given in Table 2. The standard test is performed by asking the patient to inspire maximally and then expire completely into a bellows or spirometer.* In this test, no time limit is imposed on the patient, who may expire as quickly or as slowly as desired. (Measurement of the *rate* of his complete, forced expiration is important in assessing the mechanical factors in expiration and is discussed on p. 107.) The vital capacity can also be estimated as the sum of the separately measured inspiratory capacity and expiratory reserve volume, or as the maximal volume inspired after a complete expiration. However, these may give different values in some patients with lung disease.

Significance of Changes in Vital Capacity

Physically, the vital capacity test measures a volume of gas, the maximum that can be expelled from the lungs by forceful effort after a

*Some investigators also measure *(a)* the maximal volume *inspired* after a complete expiration or *(b)* the sum of the separately performed inspiratory capacity and expiratory reserve volume, and compare these with the standard measurement of vital capacity. Since some air may be "trapped" in alveoli by forced expiration beginning from the position of maximal inspiration, the test performed in the standard manner may yield lower values than *(a)* and *(b)* in patients with emphysema (see p. 105).

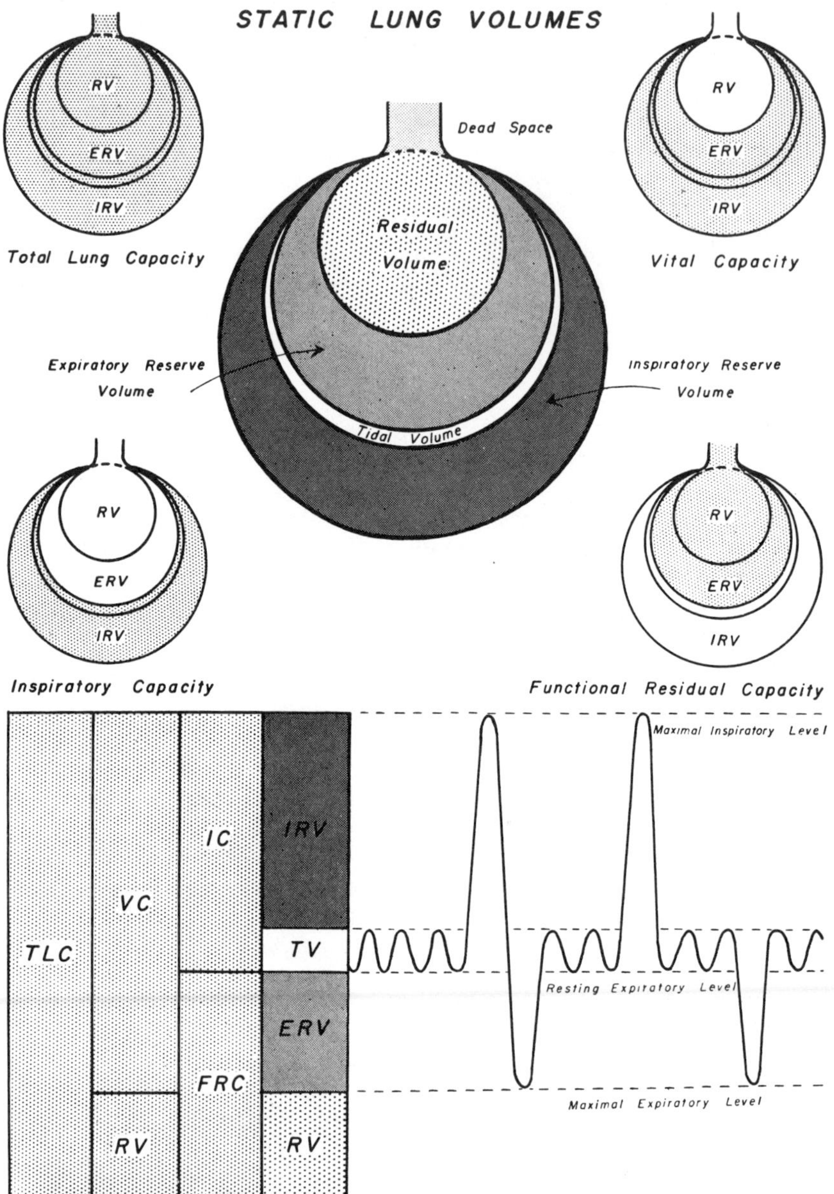

Fig 2.—*Above,* the large central diagram illustrates the four primary lung *volumes* and approximate magnitude. The outermost line indicates the greatest size to which the lung can expand; the innermost circle *(residual volume),* the volume that remains after all

TABLE 2.—TYPICAL LUNG VOLUMES IN HEALTHY SEATED SUBJECTS (APPROXIMATE VALUES, IN ML)

	MALE AGED 20–30 YR, 1.7 SQ M	MALE AGED 50–60 YR, 1.7 SQ M	FEMALE AGED 20–30 YR, 1.6 SQ M
Inspiratory capacity	3,200	2,600	2,200
Expiratory reserve volume	1,600	1,000	1,000
Vital capacity	4,800	3,600	3,200
Residual volume (RV)	1,600	2,400	1,000
Functional residual capacity	3,100	3,400	1,800
Total lung capacity (TLC)	6,300	6,000	4,200
RV/TLC × 100	25%	40%	24%

maximum inspiration. The physician wishes to know whether this volume is normal for a particular patient. The values in Table 2 are only *typical* figures for a healthy subject. The physician must compare the measured vital capacity in his or her patient with tabulated normal values in which surface area, height, weight, sex, and age are taken into consideration. (Formulae for predicting normal values are included in the Appendix.)

The physician must still bear in mind several points: (1) The vital capacity of healthy individuals, even though they be of the same sex, height, weight, and age, may vary as much as 20% from the average values. (2) The vital capacity may vary from time to time even in the same individual. For example, if the same individual were to repeat the same procedure a number of times, the vital capacity might vary as much as ± 200 ml from the mean value. When the individual is lying down, the vital capacity may be 300 ml less than when standing, partly because of an increase in pulmonary blood volume and partly because of a shift headward in the position of the diaphragm.

For these reasons, a "low" vital capacity obtained during the first examination of a patient cannot be regarded as subnormal with certainty unless it is 20% less than the average or predicted value. Further, even a "normal" vital capacity may be low for a particular patient if

---

air has been voluntarily squeezed out of the lungs. Surrounding the central diagram are four smaller diagrams; shaded areas in these represent the four lung *capacities*. The volume of dead space gas is included in residual volume, functional residual capacity, and total lung capacity when these are measured by routine techniques. *Below,* lung volumes as they appear on a spirographic tracing; shading in vertical bar next to tracing corresponds to that in central diagram above.

before the onset of disease it was much greater than the average predicted for his age and height. *Changes* in vital capacity are often helpful in diagnosis. If daily or weekly measurements are made in the same patient, a change of only 250 ml or more is meaningful if the patient is cooperative, always performs the test in the same position, and repeats the test several times.

Although we consider the mean of several trials to be most useful in detecting variations in data, the measurement most often used for the vital capacity is the maximum of several trials. Furthermore, the most widely used tables or predictive formulae of normal values deal with the maximum value, not the mean value.

Several examples illustrate these points. One patient's predicted vital capacity was 4,500 ml and his actual measured vital capacity was 3,800 ml. His measured vital capacity was, therefore, about 15% below the group average and could not on this basis be considered to be low. However, following bronchodilator therapy, the vital capacity increased to 4,200 ml. It is apparent that the initial value was actually low for this particular patient. Another patient, with a diffuse pneumonia, had a predicted vital capacity of 2,900 ml, but her actual vital capacity was 3,100 ml; two months later, after recovery, vital capacity was 4,030 ml, or 39% greater than the predicted "normal" value. The physician can, by making serial measurements, follow the course of some cardiopulmonary or respiratory diseases.

Reduction in vital capacity may occur in so many diseases that it is not pathognomonic of any single disorder and indeed does not necessarily signify pulmonary disease at all. On the other hand, it is possible that a patient may have pulmonary disability even though his vital capacity is in the normal range; this is commonly observed in emphysema.

Changes in Vital Capacity Caused By Disease

Vital capacity may be reduced by factors that affect the lung itself, *pulmonary factors,* or by *extrapulmonary* factors arising outside the lung.

Pulmonary Factors

Absolute Reduction in Distensible Lung Tissue.—Examples of this are pneumonectomy, pulmonary alveolar edema, pneumonia, and atelectasis.

Increases in Lung Stiffness that Limit Expansion.—Such as infiltrative interstitial lung diseases, pulmonary congestion with interstitial edema, and abnormalities of lung surfactant (respiratory distress syndrome [RDS]).

Increase in Residual Volume.—Owing to inability to empty the gas. Examples are lung cysts, emphysema, or airway obstruction, such as in asthma.

Extrapulmonary Factors

Limitation to Thoracic Expansion.—By tight strapping of the chest, thoracic deformities (such as kyphoscoliosis), or pleural fibrosis.

Limitation to Descent of the Diaphragm.—Owing to pregnancy or ascites.

Nervous or Muscular Dysfunction.—Such as thoracic pain (caused by fracture of a rib or by thoracic or upper abdominal incisions), muscular weakness (as caused by malnutrition), diffuse neuromuscular disease (such as Guillain-Barré syndrome), or lack of cooperation.

Significance of Changes in Inspiratory Capacity and Expiratory Reserve Volume

As an approximate guide, in the seated patient the inspiratory capacity normally is two thirds of the vital capacity and the expiratory reserve volume one third. The expiratory reserve volume characteristically is subject to considerable variability even among members of a homogeneous group and indeed in the same individual. Position is an important factor; the expiratory reserve may decrease 600 to 900 ml on change from the erect to the supine position largely because of the elevation of the diaphragm. In the supine position, inspiratory capacity is 75% and expiratory reserve volume 25% of vital capacity. In general, changes in the expiratory reserve volume are difficult to interpret and are not diagnostically useful.

B. RESIDUAL VOLUME AND FUNCTIONAL RESIDUAL CAPACITY

These two divisions of lung gas will be considered together since they are usually measured together. The residual volume, the volume of gas that remains in the lung at the end of a complete expiration, is the only one of the four lung volumes that cannot be measured by direct spirometry and must be determined by indirect means. (Normal values are given in Table 2.)

Residual volume and functional residual capacity are usually measured by either an open- or a closed-circuit method that estimates the volume of gas in the lungs in communication with the major airways at the time of the test. Each method requires that the measurements be made with relatively insoluble gases, i.e., gases that do not leave the alveolar gas readily to dissolve in blood or lung tissue.

The *open-circuit* method is based on the following principle (Fig 3). The *volume* of gas in the patient's lungs is unknown. It *is* known, however, when the patient is breathing air, that this gas contains about 80% N_2. If the *amount* of N_2 in his lungs could be determined, the total volume of alveolar gas could be calculated easily. The amount of N_2 is determined by washing all the N_2 out of the lungs and measuring it. This is achieved by having the patient *inspire* O_2 (N_2-free) and then *expire* into a spirometer (previously flushed with O_2 so that it is N_2-free). This continues for some minutes. The expired gas is collected in the spirometer so that its volume and N_2 concentration can be measured.

At the beginning of the test all of the N_2 in the lung-spirometer system is in the lungs; at the end it is all in the spirometer (Fig 3). In the example shown in Figure 3, at the end of the test the spirometer contains 40,000 ml of gas. The N_2 concentration of this gas is found to be 5%. Therefore, the spirometer contains $0.05 \times 40{,}000 = 2{,}000$ ml N_2, all of which came from the lungs; the other 38,000 ml of gas in the spirometer is mainly O_2, used to rinse the N_2 out of the lungs, plus some CO_2. since the 2,000 ml of N_2 existed in the lungs as 80% N_2, then the total alveolar gas volume, at the moment at which the N_2 washout began, was $2{,}000 \text{ ml} \times {}^{100}/_{80} = 2{,}500$ ml. Corrections must be made for small amounts of N_2 contained in "pure O_2" and for the amount of blood and tissue N_2 washed out as a result of lowering the alveolar P_{N_2}.†

In healthy young subjects, the alveolar N_2 is washed out almost completely after O_2 has been breathed for about 2 minutes. However, in patients with asthma or emphysema, parts of whose lungs may be very poorly ventilated, a longer period of breathing O_2 (frequently more than 7 minutes) is required; when there is a cyst that communi-

†P_{N_2}, P_{O_2}, P_{CO_2}, P_{H_2O}, and P_{CO} are symbols used to denote the *partial pressures* of N_2, O_2, CO_2, H_2O, and CO, respectively. For a complete list of symbols used by pulmonary physiologists, see the Appendix, C.

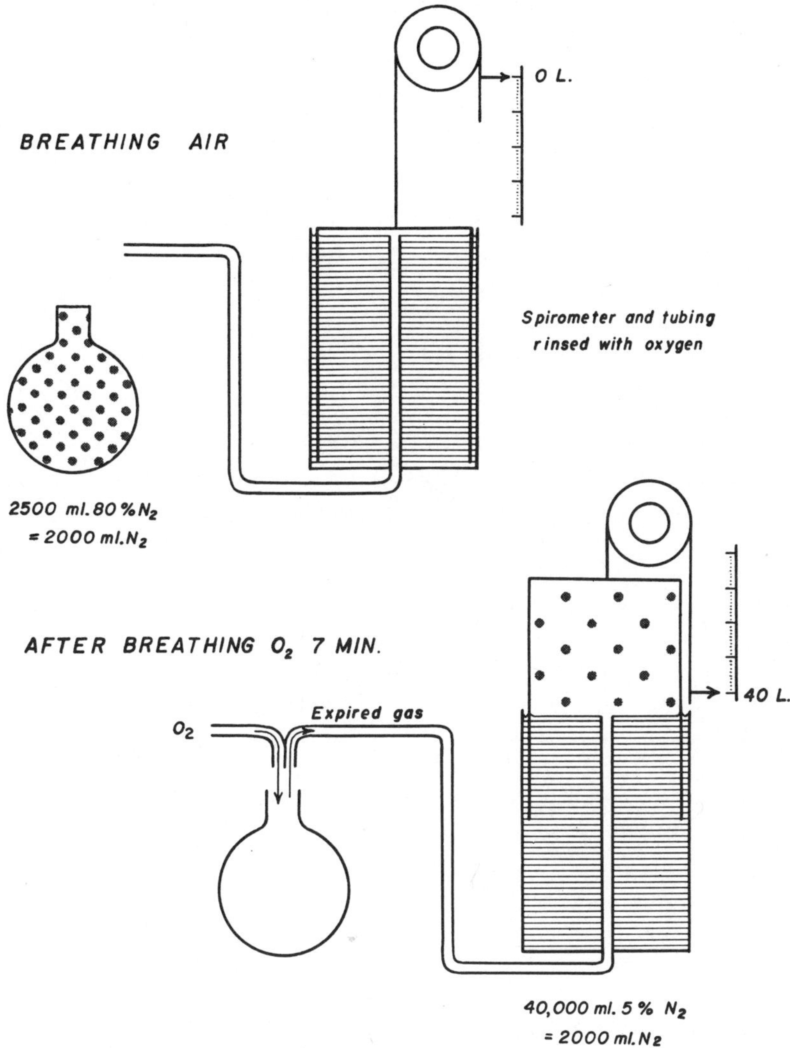

MEASUREMENT OF FUNCTIONAL RESIDUAL CAPACITY
OPEN CIRCUIT METHOD

Fig 3.—Dots represent molecules of N_2. Initially, all are in the lungs (as 80% N_2). During the breathing of O_2 (N_2-free), the N_2 molecules are washed out of the lungs and, with the O_2, are collected as expired gas in the spirometer. The total amount of O_2 that was in the lungs is calculated from measurement of the volume and N_2 concentration of the expired gas.

cates poorly with the airway or very poorly ventilated regions (as in emphysematous lungs) up to 45 minutes may be required.

The principle of the closed-circuit method is shown in Figure 4. The bellows represents a spirometer, bellows, or bag in the closed circuit. Helium (He) is usually used as the test gas. The initial concentration of He in the lungs is 0% and in the bellows is precisely known, in this case to be 10% (a known volume of He having been added to the bellows before starting the test). The initial volume of gas in the bellows is known; the initial volume of gas in the lungs is unknown. The subject then rebreathes from the bellows‡ until mixing is complete; i.e., the concentration of He is the same in both the lung and the bellows (see Fig 19). The initial volume of gas in the lung can then be computed.

The principle is the same as in the open-circuit method, i.e., the number of molecules of He is the same in the lung-bellows system at the end of the test as at the beginning (Fig 4).

If the bellows at the beginning of the test contains 2,000 ml of gas and its He concentration is 10% and if the lung contains no He, then the total amount of He present at the beginning of the test is 10% of 2,000, or 200 ml (volume × concentration = amount). The same amount of He, 200 ml, must be present in the mixed lung-bellows gas at the end of the test (assuming that an insignificant amount of the poorly soluble He enters tissues and blood). The equation and sample calculation (based on a final concentration of 5% He in both the lungs and bellows) are given in the tabulation.

In the open-circuit method, the volume of alveolar gas that is measured as the functional residual capacity (in a patient with unobstructed airways) is the volume contained in the lungs at the beginning of the

CALCULATION OF FUNCTIONAL RESIDUAL CAPACITY
HELIUM CLOSED-CIRCUIT METHOD

AT BEGINNING OF TEST (BEFORE REBREATHING)		AT END OF TEST (AFTER REBREATHING)
Amt. He in lungs + Amt. He in bellows	=	Amt. He in lungs + bellows
$V_L F_L + V_B F_B$	=	$(V_L + V_B)$ $(F_L \text{ or }_B)$
$0 + (2{,}000 \times 0.10)$	=	$(V_L + 2{,}000)$ (0.05)
200	=	$0.05\ V_L + 100$
2,000	=	V_L

V_L = Volume of gas in lungs

V_B = Volume of gas in bellows

F_L = Fractional concentration of He in lungs

F_B = Fractional concentration of He in bellows

‡O_2 is added and CO_2 is absorbed so that asphyxia does not develop.

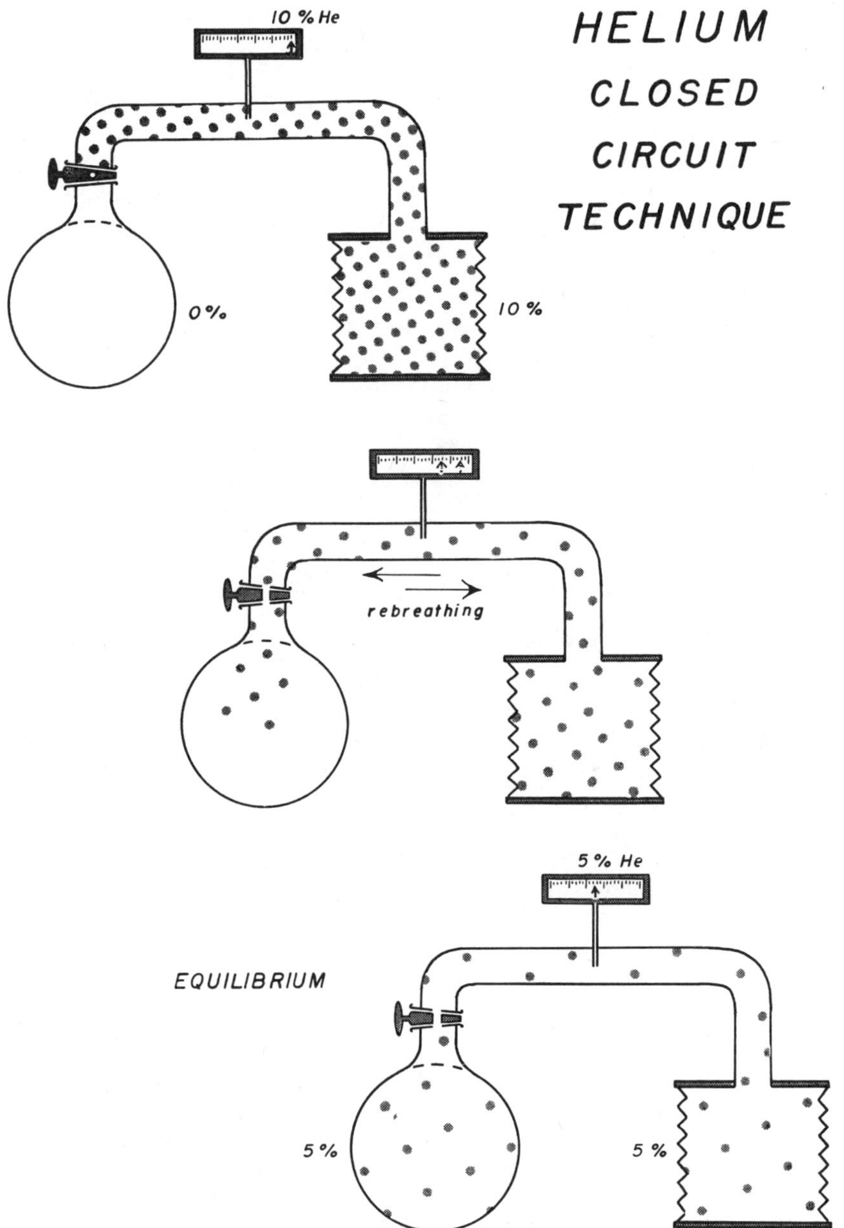

Fig 4.—Dots indicate molecules of helium. Initially, all are in the bellows (as 10% helium) and none in the lungs. Rebreathing results in their redistribution until equilibrium occurs, at which time lung volume can be calculated (see text).

test.* If the test began precisely at the moment of *complete expiration,* the residual volume is measured. If it began at *full inspiration,* total lung capacity is measured. If it began at the *end of a normal expiration,* the functional residual capacity is measured. The last is the preferred starting point because the resting expiratory level is more constant than the point of either complete inspiration or complete expiration; the expiratory reserve volume is then measured and subtracted from the functional residual capacity to obtain the residual volume. However, the resting expiratory level may fluctuate more than 100 ml, especially in patients with severe lung disease. Since changes in this level lead to corresponding changes in functional residual capacity, duplicate determinations cannot be expected to agree precisely. Day-by-day variations also occur; these may amount to $\pm 5\%$ for residual volume in healthy individuals and more in some patients with pulmonary disease.

If gas in all of the alveoli were in free communication with the major airways and if all alveoli were reasonably well ventilated, the open- and closed-circuit methods just described would provide fairly accurate values for functional residual capacity and residual volume. However, in certain patients with pulmonary disease, some areas of the lungs are very poorly ventilated and some, at least at the time of the test, act as though they were almost totally obstructed.† If the rebreathing period is extended up to 45 minutes the method will generally give the same value as the plethysmographic (body-box) method except if there is gas in the lungs not in free communication with the airways. This will be measured by the body-box method but not by the seven-minute equilibration methods.

To obtain a true value for the volume of all of the gas in the lungs, whether well-ventilated, poorly ventilated, or "nonventilated," another method of measurement may be used—the body plethysmographic (body-box) method.

*The functional residual capacity may change during the test. This does not affect the value obtained by the open-circuit method, but the closed-circuit method measures the volume of alveolar gas at the end of the test; allowance can be made for change in volume, since this is recorded on the spirometer record. The breathing circuit contains a CO_2 absorbent to prevent the buildup of this gas during the measurement, so the gas volume in the circuit diminishes as O_2 is consumed. To replace this loss, O_2 is added so as to keep the spirometer tracing at a constant level at the end of each breath, matching the metabolic rate of consumption (about 200 ml/min).

†No gas-containing space in the lung can remain indefinitely if it is not ventilated because the gas will be absorbed by the blood flowing around it, that is, they are really very poorly, not nonventilated. Obviously, "nonventilated" areas with "trapped" gas must be replenished with inspired gas from time to time.

Principle of Body Plethysmograph Method

This measures the volume of gas in the thorax whether in free communication with the airways or not, that is, THORACIC GAS VOLUME. The principle of its measurement in the body plethysmograph is based on Boyle's law, PV = P′V′, which states the relationship between changes in pressure and volume of a gas, if its temperature remains constant. The patient sits within the body plethysmograph while the door is closed airtight and breathes the air in the plethysmograph through a mouthpiece. At the desired point in the respiratory cycle (usually end-expiration, to measure functional residual capacity) the mouthpiece is occluded by an electrically controlled shutter; the patient continues to breathe against this obstruction. Figure 5 shows schematically the events that occur before and during an inspiration. At end-expiration *(left)*, we know that alveolar pressure, P, is equal to atmo-

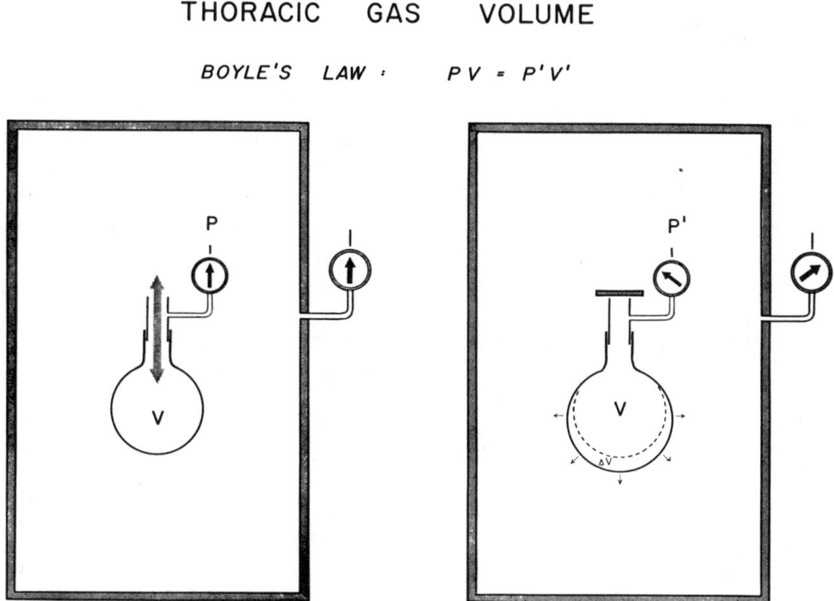

Fig 5.—Measurement of thoracic gas volume: Body plethysmograph technique. The rectangle represents the air-tight body plethysmograph. The patient is represented simply by his alveoli and conducting airway; *V* is the gas volume to be measured, and *ΔV* (right side) is the increase of volume when the patient inspires with airway occluded. The two circles with pointers represent pressure gauges—one measuring airway pressure and the other, plethysmographic pressure (see text). *P′* is the pressure corresponding to the new volume, *V′*, which is *V* + *ΔV*.

spheric pressure, because there is no gas flow; V, or thoracic gas volume, is unknown. The airway is then occluded. During the succeeding inspiration *(right),* the thorax enlarges and so decompresses the intrathoracic gas; this creates a new thoracic gas volume (V, original volume, plus ΔV, the increase in volume caused by decompression) and a new pressure, P′. The new pressure, P′, is measured by the gauge in the airway between the patient's mouth and the occluded airway; under conditions of no flow, mouth pressure is assumed to equal alveolar gas pressure. The increase in thoracic gas volume (ΔV) is determined by noting the rise in plethysmographic pressure that is detected by a very sensitive electrical gauge (enlargement of the thorax compresses the air around the patient). Knowing P, P′, and ΔV, we can solve the equation of Boyle's law (since $V + \Delta V = V'$) and can calculate the unknown, V, the original thoracic gas volume (see Appendix).

The plethysmographic method is much more rapid than other methods used to measure functional residual capacity; five determinations can easily be made on one individual in 5 minutes; another major clinical usefulness is in the determination of the true total lung capacity and of "nonventilated" lung volume. Functional residual capacity measured by the plethysmograph is the same as that measured by dilution methods in healthy individuals in whom there are no poorly or nonventilated areas. Thoracic gas volume, however, exceeds functional residual capacity, measured by 7-minute gas dilution methods, in obstructed patients, and the difference between them provides a quantitative measure of "nonventilated" lung volume.

Significance of Increase in Functional Residual Capacity

This represents *hyperinflation,* which may result from (1) *pulmonary factors* such as *(a)* structural changes reducing the elasticity of the lung such as occur in emphysema,* whether this be due to a disease or to a natural process of aging, or *(b)* partial obstruction to the airway predominantly expiratory, as in asthma or peribronchiolar fibrosis (see Fig 30); or (2) *extrapulmonary factors* increasing the size of the thorax, such as deformity of the thorax or acromegaly.

Functional residual capacity may be increased locally, such as in one lung or in one region of the lungs. This can be determined approximately by x-ray, by bronchospirometry, or by measurement of the

*The term emphysema will be used in this monograph to describe a pathologic condition of the lung characterized by reduction or loss of elastic fibers, ruptured alveolar septa and decrease in the pulmonary capillary bed, regardless of etiologic factors.

distribution of inspired radioactive gases. An example would be the compensatory overinflation of the remaining lung following surgical removal of lung tissue.

Hyperinflation of the lung generally indicates disease but does not in itself produce pulmonary disability. Individuals with an increased functional residual capacity may have little or no pulmonary incapacity. This is simply because the *ventilation* of the lung (see chapter 3) is more important to good function than the alveolar *volume.* To ensure adequate oxygenation of the blood, the alveolar P_{O_2} must be maintained at the proper level, usually about 100 mm Hg. This depends only upon whether ventilation supplies as much O_2 each minute to the alveoli as the pulmonary capillary blood removes. If the pulmonary capillary blood removes 250 ml of O_2 per minute, only 250 ml of O_2 must be added to alveolar gas by the process of ventilation; this is true whether the functional residual capacity is 2,000 ml or 4,000 ml.

An analogy may be helpful here: If 250 ml of O_2 was absorbed chemically each minute in a *small* air-tight box containing air, and simultaneously 250 ml of O_2 was piped into the box each minute, the O_2 concentration in the box would remain constant; if 250 ml of O_2 was absorbed chemically each minute in a *large* air-tight room containing air, and simultaneously 250 ml of O_2 was piped into the room, the O_2 concentration of the large room would again remain constant. Assuming rapid and uniform distribution in both the small box and the large room, the volume of the container therefore is unimportant in determining the O_2 concentration and partial pressure.

Actually, a *very small* functional residual capacity would be disadvantageous because alveolar P_{O_2} would fluctuate widely throughout the respiratory cycle, coming closer to mixed venous P_{O_2} during expiration (since expiration is, in a sense, equivalent to breath-holding) and closer to the inspired P_{O_2} during inspiration (see Fig 6, p. 27). This would lead to uneven ventilation and to slight anoxemia.

On the other hand, though a large functional residual capacity acts as a buffer against wide fluctuations in alveolar P_{O_2} and P_{CO_2}, it is a disadvantage when a rapid *change* in alveolar gas *composition* is necessary. For example, if a patient is given 100% O_2 to breathe instead of air, he will achieve a high alveolar O_2 concentration more slowly if his functional residual capacity is large than if this capacity is small, alveolar ventilation being held constant. Again, if it is desired to anesthetize a patient with a volatile anesthetic, or to cause hyperpnea by inhalation of 10% CO_2, it will take longer to achieve the desired alveolar concentration of the gas if the functional residual capacity is large (other things being equal).

An increase in functional residual capacity is also a disadvantage because the thorax is always larger than normal; because of this abnormal position, some muscular inefficiency and mechanical disadvantage may result. Certainly, a great enlargement of the functional residual capacity must lead to a reduction in inspiratory capacity (if the total lung capacity is not enlarged), and this usually limits the patients' ability to increase their ventilation on demand. The anatomic (respiratory) dead space is also larger when the lungs are hyperinflated. The *mechanical* factors that result in an enlarged functional residual capacity were discussed on page 20.

Significance of Changes in Residual Volume

An increase in functional residual capacity means that the lung is hyperinflated during quiet breathing. An increase in residual volume means that the lung is still hyperinflated even after *maximal* expiratory effort, i.e., the patient cannot, by voluntary effort, force his thorax and lungs to as small a volume as a normal person. This signifies that certain changes have developed in the thoracic cage, in the respiratory muscles, in the pulmonary tissues, or inside the conducting airways; these changes may be reversible in certain patients with partial bronchial obstruction, as in young asthmatics, but appear to be irreversible in patients with emphysema with loss of elasticity of alveolar or airway tissues.

Residual volume and functional residual capacity usually increase together. In some instances, residual volume may be increased without increase in functional residual capacity (if expiratory reserve volume decreases). An increase in residual volume occurring without increase in total lung capacity must mean that the vital capacity is reduced. However, the ability to *ventilate* is not necessarily reduced on this account, since the full vital capacity is rarely used even for maximal ventilation.

Residual volume may be decreased in some diffuse pulmonary restrictive diseases and in some diseases in which alveoli are occluded in many portions of the lung producing atelectasis.

The ratio, residual volume/total lung capacity, in healthy adults increases with age. It approximates 20% for the age group 15 to 34 years, 25% for 35 to 49 years, and 35% for the group over 50 years. This variation with age must be taken into account in interpretation. Use of the ratio alone tends to obscure the actual values for these lung volumes.

C. TOTAL LUNG CAPACITY

Typical figures for normal individuals are presented in Table 2. Total lung capacity is usually determined by measuring the functional residual capacity and adding the inspiratory capacity. Normal values can be calculated from a predicted value of normal vital capacity by dividing vital capacity by 0.8 for young adults, by 0.75 for middle-aged persons, and by 0.65 for those over 50. Since the total lung capacity equals the vital capacity plus residual volume, these factors are derived from the values of residual volume/total lung capacity in the paragraph above. Total capacity may vary from the estimated normal by ± 15% to 20% in healthy subjects.

Radiologists have been able to measure residual lung volume and total lung capacity from planimetric tracings of posterior-anterior and lateral films of the chest. Reasonable approximations may be obtained, since radiologic chest volume (minus lung tissue volume, blood vessel volume, and cardiac volume) is closely related to the pulmonary gas volume, although it has little value for routine use.

The total lung capacity is decreased in patients who have a net decrease in the sum of vital capacity and residual volume. The mechanisms or causes of these decreases are described under the headings for vital capacity and residual volume. Most often it is a decrease in the vital capacity that is most important. In emphysema there is an increase in residual volume that may decrease the vital capacity, particularly as the disease becomes more severe. The result is a normal or a moderately increased total lung capacity. Therefore, normal or increased total lung capacity does not imply that ventilation is normal or that the total lung surface for diffusion is normal in quantity or in its properties.

D. SUMMARY

The vital capacity, inspiratory capacity, and expiratory reserve volume are relatively easy to measure by using simple volume recorders. Since there is always a residual volume of gas in the lungs that cannot be expelled by maximal expiration, this volume (and also the functional residual capacity and total lung capacity, which include the residual volume) must be measured indirectly. Gas dilution methods measure the volume of the lung with open airways, and the body plethysmograph method measures all gas in the lung whether it is in well-ventilated, poorly ventilated, or "nonventilated" regions.

The interpretation of measured lung volumes requires basic knowledge of pulmonary physiopathology because (1) there may be no changes in lung volume in certain types of serious lung disease; (2) the variation in a homogeneous healthy group is so great that the interpretation of small changes is difficult; (3) even marked changes may be caused by extrapulmonary disorders; and (4) changes in lung volumes usually have less significance with respect to function than do changes in ventilation, diffusion, and circulation.

Nevertheless, routine serial determinations of the lung volumes, particularly the vital capacity, can help the physician in many problems related to diagnosis, therapy, and progression of pulmonary disease.

3

Pulmonary Ventilation

The major function of the *cardiovascular system* is to supply to the capillary bed of each tissue of the body a *volume* of blood that is adequate at each moment for the metabolic needs of each tissue. The cardiovascular system is well designed to increase or decrease *total* blood flow, according to overall demands, and to distribute more blood to metabolically active tissues and less to relatively inactive tissues. However, it has no control over the *composition* of the blood—how much glucose, amino acids, hormones, O_2, or CO_2 the blood contains.

The major function of the *respiratory system* is to maintain at optimal levels the partial pressure of O_2 and CO_2 in the pulmonary alveoli and in the arterial blood. This it does by *ventilation,* a cyclic process of inspiration and expiration (Fig 6) in which fresh air enters the alveoli and then an equal volume* of alveolar gas leaves them.

So far, we have discussed only the *static* lung volumes (chapter 2). Ventilation is a *dynamic* process. During inspiration, active muscular contraction enlarges the thorax; this further lowers intrathoracic pressure (normally subatmospheric at end-expiration) and causes pulmonary or alveolar gas pressure (normally atmospheric at end-expiration)

*This statement is only approximately true. As a rule, more O_2 is *absorbed* from the alveoli than CO_2 is *added;* for example, O_2 uptake may be 250 ml/min and CO_2 elimination only 200 ml/min. In this case, the alveolar gas volume "shrinks" by 50 ml/min, or at normal breathing rate 3 to 5 ml/breath. Thus, whenever the CO_2 output/O_2 uptake ratio (respiratory exchange ratio, R) is less than 1.0, the *expired* tidal volume is slightly less than the *inspired* tidal volume; the difference between these two volumes leaves the alveoli by way of the blood instead of through the bronchioles.

to become subatmospheric. Fresh air, at atmospheric pressure, then enters the airway and alveoli, where the pressure is lower.

Certain principles are fundamental to an understanding of this cyclic process of ventilation:

1. Let us begin at end-expiration. The partial pressures of O_2 and CO_2 in alveolar gas of a healthy individual are approximately equal to those in pulmonary capillary blood (P_{O_2}, 100 mm Hg; P_{CO_2}, 40 mm Hg). If a patient were to inspire gas of precisely the same chemical composition as that of his alveolar gas, this inspired tidal volume would enlarge his functional residual capacity, but it would not raise the alveolar P_{O_2} nor lower the alveolar P_{CO_2} (see Fig 6). Oxygen uptake would not stop on this account (any more than it would during breath-holding) because alveolar gas, even though not enriched by additional O_2, would still have a higher P_{O_2} than *mixed venous blood.* Continued removal of O_2 by the pulmonary capillary blood each minute without the addition of an equal amount of O_2 to the alveoli would result in arterial anoxemia. Simultaneously there would be CO_2 retention and respiratory acidosis.

2. The respiratory tract is composed of the conducting airway (nose, mouth, pharynx, larynx, trachea, bronchi, and bronchioles) and the alveoli. Rapid exchange of O_2 and CO_2 between gas and blood occurs only in the alveoli, and not in the conducting airway.

Fig 6.—During *inspiration,* one would expect that alveolar P_{O_2} would rise because fresh air (P_{O_2} = 149 mm Hg when saturated with water vapor at 37 ° C) is added to the alveolar gas (P_{O_2} = 98.5 mm Hg at end-expiration). During *expiration,* one would expect that alveolar P_{O_2} would decrease and alveolar P_{CO_2} would increase; this is because expiration is essentially breath-holding (with lung volume decreasing throughout the expiration), and blood continues to flow through the pulmonary capillaries and continues to remove O_2 and add CO_2.

NOTE: At the beginning of inspiration, alveolar P_{O_2} continues to fall (instead of rising) and alveolar P_{CO_2} continues to rise (instead of falling). This is because the first gas to enter the alveoli during inspiration is alveolar gas that filled the anatomic dead space at the end of the previous expiration; it does not alter the composition of gas in the alveoli, and exchange of O_2 and CO_2 continues as it did during expiration. After the dead space gas is drawn in, alveolar P_{O_2} rises sharply because *fresh inspired air* now adds O_2 to the alveoli far more rapidly than it is absorbed.

The top graph shows the variation in R values throughout the cycle; R is the gas exchange ratio and equals $\frac{CO_2 \text{ eliminated}}{O_2 \text{ absorbed}}$ at any moment.

It is obvious that a "spot sample" of expired alveolar gas is not representative of alveolar gas at all times during the respiratory cycle.

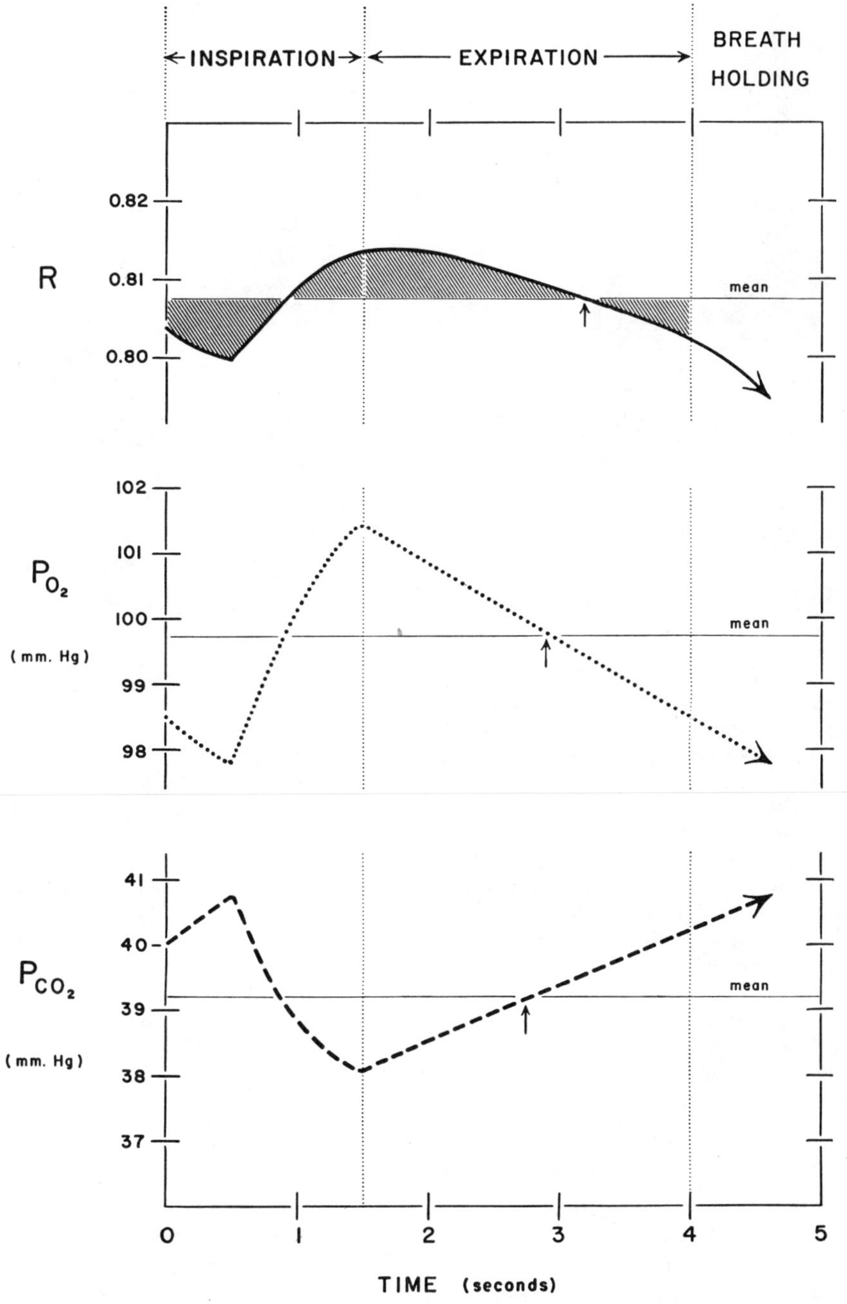

INSPIRATION
EXPIRATION
BREATH HOLDING

R
0.82
0.81
0.80
mean

P_{O_2}
(mm. Hg)
102
101
100
99
98
mean

P_{CO_2}
(mm. Hg)
41
40
39
38
37
mean

0 1 2 3 4 5

TIME (seconds)

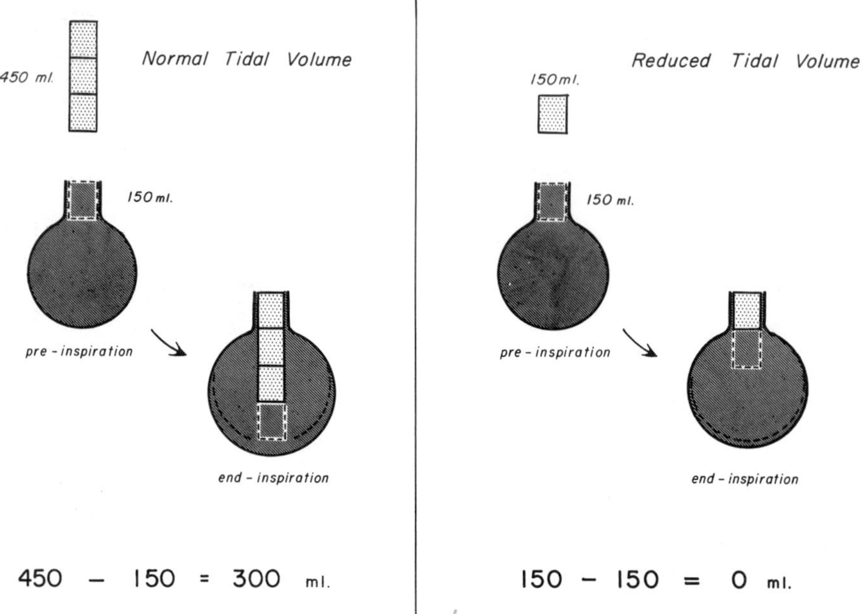

Fig 7.—Relation of tidal volume, anatomic dead space, and alveolar ventilation/breath. Circular part represents the alveoli, where rapid exchange of O_2 and CO_2 occurs, the tube leading to the alveoli represents all of the conducting airways.

(Left) Normal tidal volume: At the end of a normal expiration (preinspiration), the dead space is filled with 150 ml of alveolar gas. In this example, tidal volume during inspiration will be 450 ml (three blocks of 150 ml each). During inspiration, 450 ml of gas enters the alveoli (dotted line indicates preinspiratory alveolar volume). However, 150 ml is alveolar gas that had filled the dead space at the end of the last expiration; this, having the same *composition* as alveolar gas, does not raise alveolar P_{O_2} or lower alveolar P_{CO_2}. Two blocks (300 ml) of the *inspired* gas do reach the alveoli and do raise alveolar P_{O_2} and lower alveolar P_{CO_2}. The remaining block of inspired gas (150 ml) is left in the dead space at end-inspiration and is flushed out on the next expiration, thus never entering into gas exchange.

(Right) Reduced tidal volume: During inspiration, 150 ml of dead space gas enters the alveoli and the 150 ml of inspired air remains in the dead space, so that alveolar ventilation/breath should be zero. This schematic representation is, however, theoretical and particularly inaccurate when tidal volume is low.

The conducting airway, at the end of a normal expiration (preinspiration), is filled with *alveolar* gas (Fig 7). This alveolar gas is drawn back into the alveoli during the early part of the next inspiration. It does not raise alveolar P_{O_2} nor lower alveolar P_{CO_2}. Only the fresh air that goes beyond the conducting airway into the alveoli raises alveolar

P_{O_2} and lowers alveolar P_{CO_2}. In Figure 7, at end-inspiration only 300 ml of 450 ml of inspired fresh air has entered alveoli; the remainder (150 ml) has stayed in the conducting airway and is washed out during the next expiration (see also Fig 13, p. 40). This latter portion of the tidal volume is wasted, useless or ineffective as far as alveolar ventilation is concerned and is called "dead space" ventilation.

In this particular breath:

Tidal volume (V_T)	=	450 ml
Anatomic dead space ventilation (V_D)	=	150 ml
Alveolar ventilation ($V_T - V_D$)	=	300 ml

Alveolar ventilation then refers not to the volume of *gas* entering the alveoli, but the volume of *fresh air* entering them.

3. Deep breathing causes a greater fraction of the tidal volume of fresh air to enter the alveoli; shallow breathing causes a smaller fraction of the tidal volume to enter the alveoli. Figure 8 illustrates this. Assume that the volume of the conducting airway is 150 ml. In *A*, (250 − 150)/250 or 0.4 of the tidal volume of fresh air enters the alveoli; in *B*, (500 − 150)/500 or 0.7 of the tidal volume enters the alveoli; in *C*, (1,000 − 150)/1,000 or 0.85 of the tidal volume enters the alveoli.

4. In *high-frequency ventilation* small pump strokes (about 50 ml) of a ventilator attached to the airway, when repeated at frequencies of 10 to 20 cycles per second, have been found to produce enough alveolar ventilation to sustain life, even in some adults. From Figure 7 we would conclude that, when the tidal volume was decreased so that it exactly equals the volume of the conducting airway, alveolar ventilation would become zero. However, this is not true because inspired gas travels through the airways, not as a block with a square front (as pictured in Figure 9,A) but rather with a spike or cone front (as pictured in Figure 9,B), the tip of which enters the alveolar gas, where mixing can only take place by diffusion. In addition, bulk air flow from the pump presumably churns up and mixes the air in the trachea and main bronchi, which amplifies the effect of the extension of the cone through the dead space. Even under static conditions a few milliliters of inspired gas enter the alveoli when the tidal volume is only 60 to 70 ml and the volume of the conducting airway is 150 ml. The equation (alveolar ventilation/breath = tidal volume − anatomic dead space) therefore is not accurate when the tidal volume is low.

5. Since the major function of ventilation is to arterialize the mixed venous blood, it must supply each minute to the alveoli and pulmonary

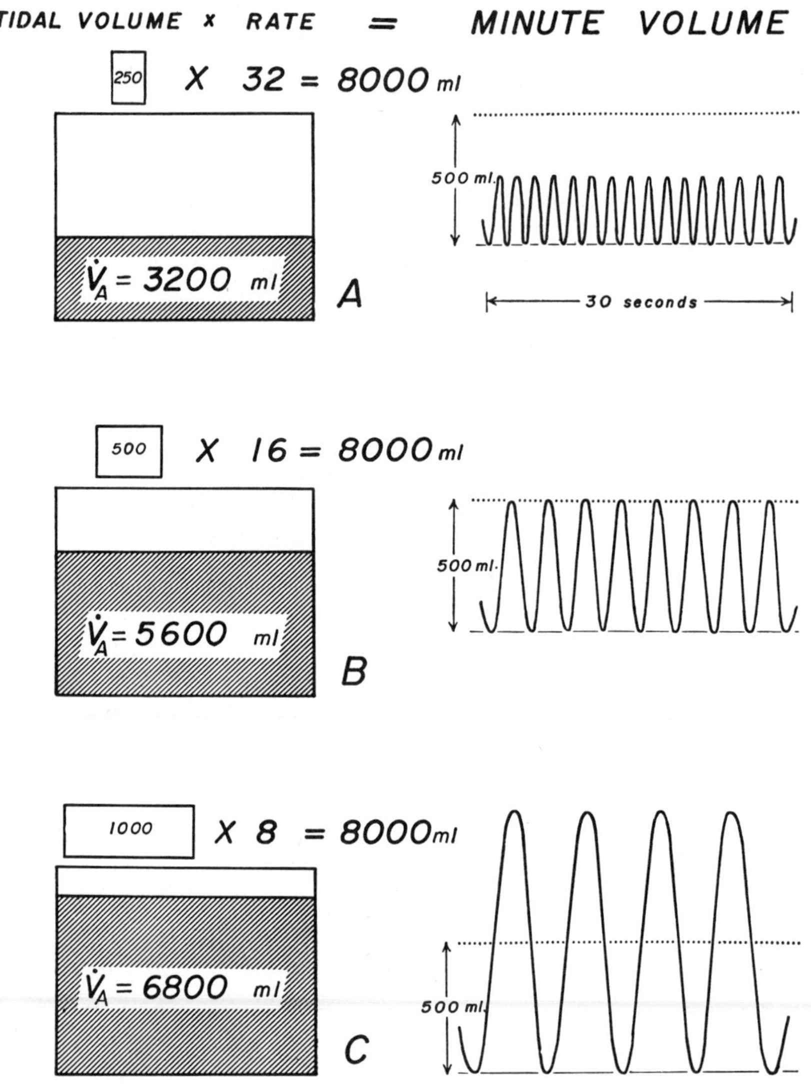

Fig 8.—Area of each small block represents tidal volume (250, 500, or 1,000 ml). Total area of each large block (shaded + unshaded areas) equals *minute* volume of ventilation; in each case it is 8,000 ml. Shaded area of each block represents volume of *alveolar* ventilation per minute; this varies in each case since Alveolar Ventilation/min = (Tidal Volume − Dead Space) × Frequency. A dead space of 150 ml is assumed in each case, although actually the dead space would increase somewhat with increasing tidal volume. *Right,* spirographic tracings.

capillary blood a volume of O_2 equal to that used by the body and must remove a volume of CO_2 approximately equal to that formed by the metabolic activity of tissues. The *supply* of O_2 each minute must equal the *requirements* each minute. Therefore, *minute* ventilation or *minute* volume of ventilation is a more important measurement than tidal volume or rate. However, *minute alveolar* ventilation is far more important than the overall minute volume of breathing since the latter includes the amount of ventilation of the anatomic dead space. Figure 8 shows that for equal, *un*corrected minute volumes of breathing, *alveolar* ventilation may be excessive *(A)*, adequate *(B)* or inadequate *(C)*.

Therefore, one cannot give precise "normal values" for *minute volume* of breathing because the useful part of this (the alveolar ventilation) depends on the pattern of breathing (tidal volume and frequency of respiration) and on the volume of the conducting airway. (See pp. 254 and 256 for approximate predicted values.)

6. "Normal" values for *alveolar* ventilation per minute must be related to the metabolic activity of the patient. If he is exercising or if he has fever or hyperthyroidism, "normal" values for alveolar ventilation will be higher than if he were basal, hypothermic, or hypothyroid.

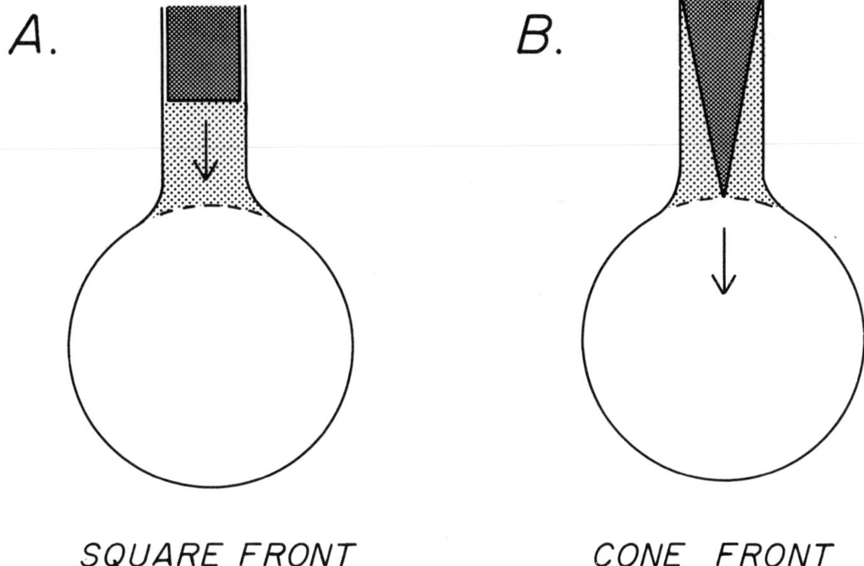

Fig 9.—Movement of inspired air through conducting airways. Gas moves through the conducting airways as a cone front *(B)*, not as a square front *(A)*. Movement into the gas of the terminal exchange unit (beyond the dashed line) is by diffusion, not convection.

In a healthy basal 150-lb adult male with a CO_2 output of 200 ml/min, under 4 L of *alveolar* ventilation per minute is adequate to arterialize his mixed venous blood. Alveolar *hypo*ventilation occurs when ventilation is too little; alveolar *hyper*ventilation, when it is too great (see pp. 44 and 46).

In the remainder of this section we shall assume, unless specified otherwise, *that alveolar ventilation and pulmonary capillary blood flow are uniform and that the diffusing capacity is normal;* i.e., we shall consider only the volume of alveolar ventilation and its component parts (frequency, tidal volume, and anatomic dead space volume) and discuss *(a)* how to measure these, and *(b)* the causes and effects of alveolar hypoventilation.

I. VOLUME OF PULMONARY VENTILATION

A. MINUTE VENTILATION

Frequency (Rate) of Breathing

This is the only respiratory measurement made routinely in most hospitals. The average frequency of breathing is about 11 to 14 respirations per minute in healthy individuals under basal conditions. Deviations from the normal rate are helpful clinically in calling attention to respiratory or pulmonary disorders. However, the rate of breathing is not very valuable as an index of useful ventilation because either rapid or slow rates may be associated with either hyperventilation or hypoventilation, depending on other factors (see Fig 8).

Tidal Volume (Depth of Breathing)

There are two basic ways to measure tidal volume: either (1) measure the volumes of individual breaths, inspired or expired, or (2) measure the total inspired or expired volume over a period of time and divide by the number of breaths, giving an average tidal volume. Individual breaths can be measured by a spirometer, or by integrating air flow. Multiple breaths can be collected in a Tissot spirometer or large plastic bag.

Average values for tidal volume in healthy basal males are approximately 450 to 600 ml, but there is considerable deviation from these figures. Considered alone, tidal volume is not useful as an index of alveolar ventilation because either increased or decreased tidal volume may be associated with hyperventilation or hypoventilation, depending on frequency and dead space volume (Fig 8).

B. RESPIRATORY DEAD SPACE

The fundamental concept of dead space is that a portion of lung ventilation is wasted and dead space volume or ventilation is a measure of the extent of this waste. While one straightforward mechanism of waste is the to-and-fro movement of gas in the conducting airways, as illustrated in Figure 7, others are nonuniformity of alveolar ventilation/alveolar capillary blood flow and right-to-left shunts across the pulmonary capillary bed. Because there are three types of wasted ventilation, this has given rise to different definitions of respiratory dead space of which the most important are ANATOMIC and PHYSIOLOGIC.

Anatomic Dead Space

The term means simply the internal volume of the conducting airway from the nose and mouth down to the alveoli. Its estimation during life must be based on the concept of a conducting airway (where *no* gas exchange occurs) leading abruptly to gas sacs or alveoli (where *rapid* gas exchange occurs). The simplest method of measurement is to fill the airways with a gas at a different concentration than in the alveoli and then measure the volume of this gas swept out the conducting airways. The measurement requires a continuous, rapid gas analyzer and a flow meter or spirometer.

Figure 10 illustrates the procedure and the principle involved. A N_2 analyzer or mass spectrometer is used for the continuous and almost instantaneous analysis of the N_2 concentration of gas entering or leaving the subject's mouth. The subject, who previously had been breathing room air, inspires a single breath of pure O_2; a N_2 analyzer records 0% N_2 (pure O_2) during inspiration. At end-inspiration, the dead space is filled with O_2 that has just been inspired. At the beginning of expiration, the first gas to issue from the mouth is pure O_2 (Fig 10, phase I) which has entered and left the dead space without *any* mixture with alveolar gas; therefore, the N_2 analyzer continues to record 0% N_2. Toward midexpiration, pure alveolar gas is exhaled, uncontaminated with dead space gas (phase III); its concentration here is recorded as 40% N_2, indicating that the inspired O_2 diluted the alveolar N_2 to half of its original concentration. (The actual concentration depends on the volume of O_2 inspired and the volume of the functional residual capacity just before inspiration). Between phases I and III is phase II. In this phase, the N_2 concentration of the expired gas rises rapidly; this represents the remainder of the dead space gas (pure

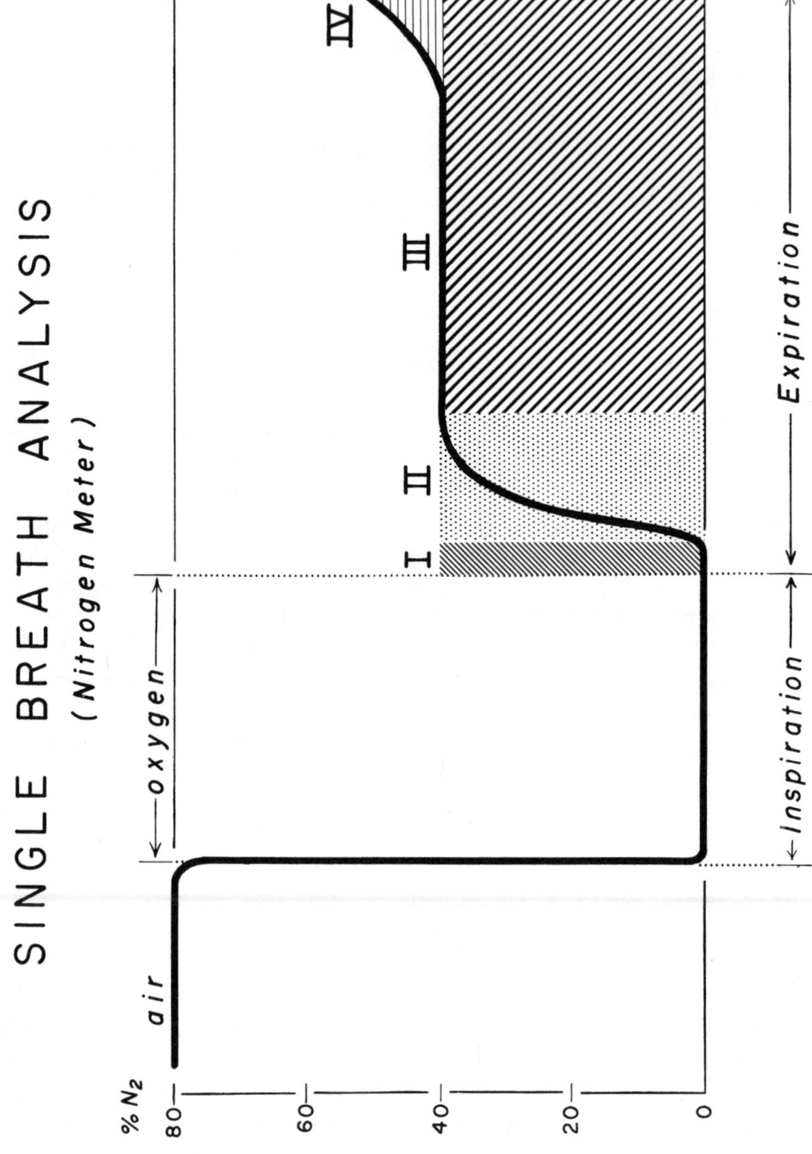
SINGLE BREATH ANALYSIS
(Nitrogen Meter)
air
oxygen
I
II
III
IV
% N2
80
60
40
20
0
Inspiration
Expiration

Fig 10.—The N_2 analyzer samples, analyzes, and records continuously the N_2 concentration of gas being inspired or expired. During inhalation of air *(left)* the N_2 analyzer records 79% to 80% N_2 in inspired and expired gas. The subject is then requested to take a deep breath of O_2 and breathe out slowly and evenly. During inspiration, the N_2 analyzer records 0% N_2. At the beginning of expiration, about 50 ml of pure O_2 (0% N_2) is expired *(phase I);* this is followed by about 200 to 300 ml of gas of rapidly rising N_2 concentration *(phase II),* which represents the washout of the remainder of the dead space gas by alveolar gas, and then by pure alveolar gas *(phase III).* The N_2 concentration of the last part of the expiration *(phase IV)* rises because of the progressive closure of the small airways at the bases of the lungs (see page 77). This is an idealized presentation of events that would follow inhalation of O_2 if functional residual capacity (including dead space gas) were 2,000 ml, volume of inspired O_2 2,150 ml, dead space 150 ml, and distribution of O_2 to the alveoli perfectly uniform.

O_2) being washed out by alveolar gas, which has a N_2 concentration of 40%. Phase IV is caused by the expiration of an increasing proportion of alveolar gas from the apices of the lung (see discussion on p. 77). The anatomic dead space is calculated by transforming the phase of rapidly rising N_2 concentration (phase II) into an ideal square front as diagrammed in Figure 7. (A sample record and calculation is given in Figure 69 and on p. 265.)

In adults, Radford has noted that anatomic dead space (in milliliters) equals the ideal weight of the patient (in pounds), as a convenient approximation. Anatomic dead space in general increases with increases in the size of the lungs. Consequently it is larger in larger persons, thus larger in men than in women and larger in patients with a greater functional residual capacity. In a given individual it is increased by an increase in lung volume or by drugs that relax airway smooth muscle, since this will dilate the airways. Anatomic dead space is greater during hyperventilation and in exercise, and is decreased by space-occupying lesions, by surgical removal of part of the conducting airway, and by tracheostomy.

Anatomic dead space is not routinely measured because it is of little value diagnostically, although of interest physiologically. In situations in which its size is of significance, such as in adjusting a respirator, the use of a value in milliliters equal to the body weight in pounds is adequate. The apparatus needed to measure anatomic dead space consists of a simultaneous record of a rapid gas analyzer (as in Figure 11) and expired gas volume (as in Figure 10).

'Physiologic' Dead Space

That portion of the inspired air that traverses the conducting airway and enters alveoli in volume/minute is called alveolar ventilation. In some patients, not all of this alveolar ventilation is equally effective in arterializing mixed venous blood; Figure 12,B shows ventilated areas of the lung that have no pulmonary capillary blood flow. The inspired air that enters these areas is wasted; the patient must expend energy to move this gas back and forth, but this accomplishes no respiratory function. Such gas is sometimes called "dead space" or "alveolar dead space." The volume of this "alveolar dead space" gas, however, is not the volume of all of these alveoli that have no blood flow, but only the volume of inspired gas that enters these alveoli on each breath. It (plus the anatomic dead space) is called the "physiologic dead space."

Figure 12,C, illustrates a similar condition varying only in degree; here, instead of no pulmonary capillary blood flow, there is reduced blood flow to alveoli pictured on the left. Ventilation is far in excess of that required to bring arterial blood P_{O_2} and P_{CO_2} to physiologic levels, and so a portion of the inspired gas entering these alveoli is wasted. This is also "alveolar dead space."

It is relatively simple to think of a volume of inspired gas that is ineffective in arterializing the venous blood—in one case because it never reached alveoli (Fig 12,A), and in another because it reached alveoli with no blood flow (Fig 12,B). It is much more difficult to visualize the effect on the arterial blood P_{O_2} and P_{CO_2} of alveoli that have ventilation and blood flow but in which the proportions of ventilation to blood flow vary widely (Fig 12,C). This nonuniformity will also produce a marked inefficiency of exchange between blood and gas, but the effect is hard to quantify. It has proved useful to represent this inefficiency consisting partly of an increased dead space (physiologic dead space) and partly an increase in right-to-left shunt (venous admixture). (See Riley schema in Appendix.)

The *physiologic dead space* can be calculated from measurements of

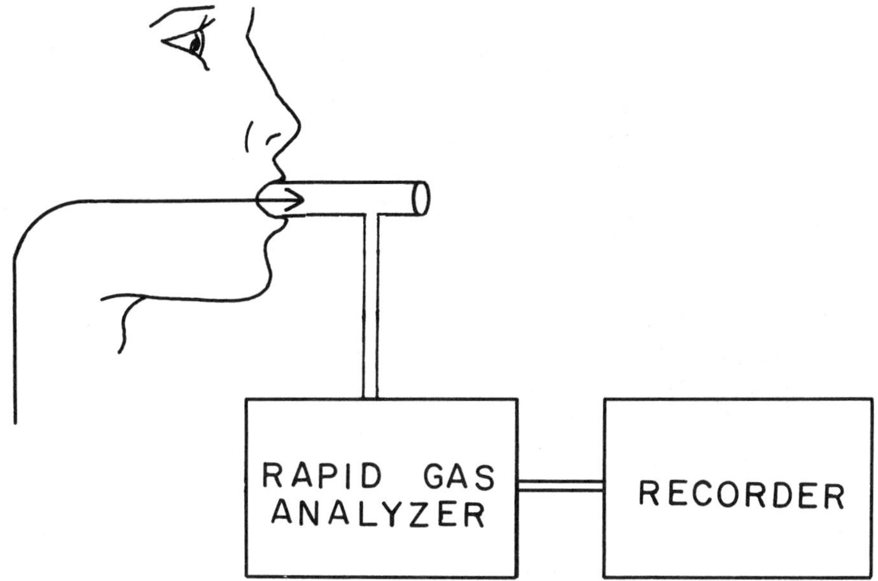

Fig 11.—Electrical methods for rapid measurement of gas concentration. A small sample of gas, entering or leaving the subject's mouth, is drawn continuously by a vacuum pump through rapid gas analyzers that measure gas concentration and send a signal to the recorder. CO or CO_2 may be analyzed by infrared absorption, O_2 by cell sensor, N_2 by emission spectroscopy, and a great variety of gases by mass spectrometry. The tubing conducting gas to the analyzers should have a small dead space and fast sampling rate. The apparatus should be able to sample, analyze, and record 90% of an abrupt change in gas concentrations in 0.05 to 0.08 sec. For a specific single-breath analysis, see Fig 10.

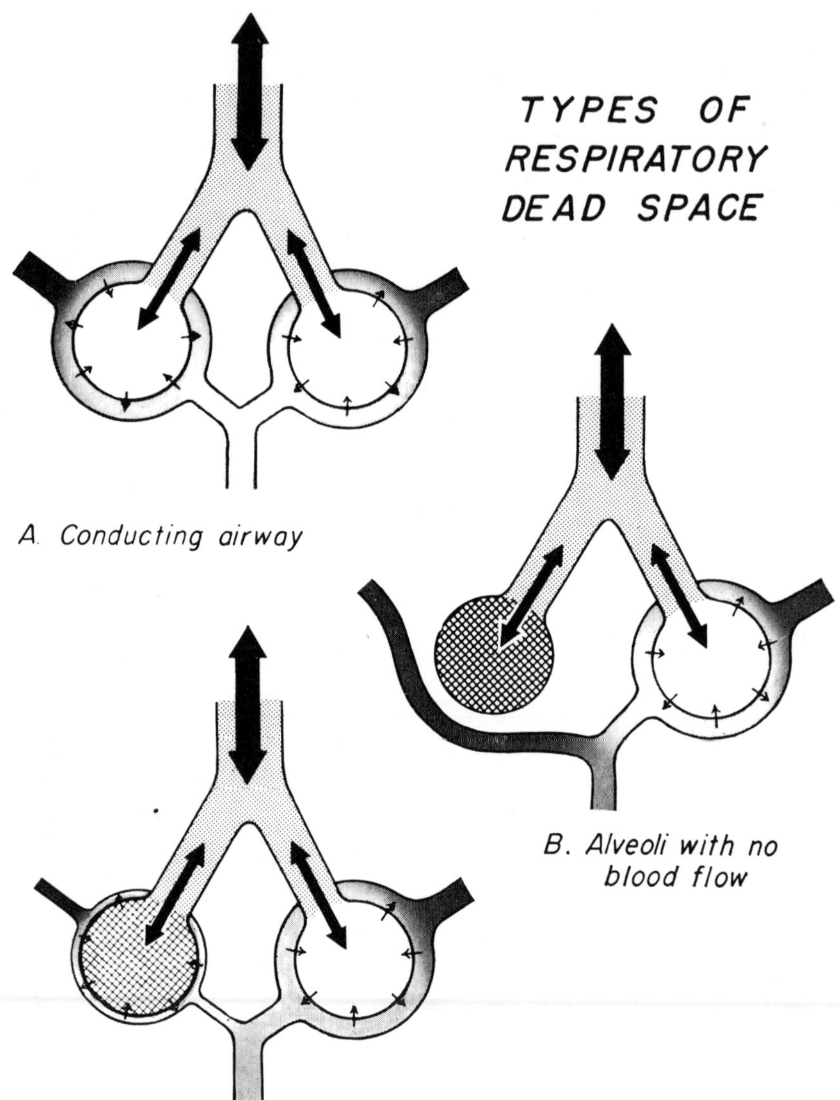

Fig 12.—Circular parts represent the alveoli, where rapid gas exchange occurs. Arrows in the conducting airways signify the tidal volume entering and leaving the whole lung and its distribution to different regions (see Fig 1). Width of the blood channel surrounding the alveoli indicates the volume of blood flow to each region: dark gray designates mixed venous blood entering and light gray indicates well oxygenated blood leaving the pulmonary capillaries. Anatomic dead space is stippled. Physiologic dead space includes this and some *(C)* or all *(B)* of the gas volumes ventilating crosshatched areas.

CO_2 elimination in the expired gas. Carbon dioxide is formed in the tissue and is carried in the venous blood to the pulmonary capillaries, where it enters the alveoli and is exhaled as part of the expired gas (Fig 13). Because inspired air contains practically no CO_2 (0.04%), all of the CO_2 in the expired gas must have come from the alveoli. Thus, the amount of CO_2 in an expired breath must equal the amount of CO_2 delivered from the alveoli. The amount of alveolar CO_2 expired can be calculated from alveolar volume times CO_2 concentration which should equal (tidal volume − dead space) (alveolar CO_2%/100) (see Fig 8). From these simple considerations we can obtain the relation (see Appendix, p. 263).

$$\text{Dead space} = \text{Tidal volume}\,\frac{(\text{alveolar } CO_2 - \text{expired } CO_2)}{\text{alveolar } CO_2}$$

This relationship, known as the Bohr equation, is based upon the conservation of matter. If you know one of either alveolar CO_2 or dead space volume, you can calculate the other. The difficulty is that there is no independent way to obtain a precise value of either dead space volume or alveolar CO_2 in the presence of nonuniformity of alveolar ventilation and pulmonary capillary blood flow. Today the widely accepted solution of the dilemma is to assume that arterial P_{CO_2} equals alveolar P_{CO_2} and to designate the value of dead space obtained with the Bohr equation as *physiologic dead space.* This is done because the arterial blood coming from all the alveoli approaches an integrated value of P_{CO_2} with respect to the different regions of the lung and to different times during the respiratory cycle; further CO_2 diffuses through body membranes so readily that its partial pressure in blood leaving any alveolus will always be equal to its partial pressure in the gas of that alveolus. The availability of carbonic anhydrase to plasma in the pulmonary capillaries will produce chemical equilibrium with the plasma bicarbonate and hydrogen ion.

While it is true that nonuniformity of alveolar ventilation with respect to alveolar capillary blood flow throughout the lung can produce a difference between the P_{CO_2} of mixed capillary blood and mixed alveolar gas in spite of diffusion equilibrium across any single individual alveolus (see p. 171), this difference is relatively small except in the presence of extreme nonuniformity of alveolar ventilation/alveolar blood flow or large venous-to-arterial shunts.

The difference between mixed venous (pulmonary arterial) P_{CO_2} and arterial P_{CO_2} is normally only 5 to 10 mm Hg; even if there were not equilibrium between alveolar gas and pulmonary capillary blood, the difference in absolute P_{CO_2} could not be more than 1 to 2 mm Hg.

The important point is that physiologic dead space equals anatomic

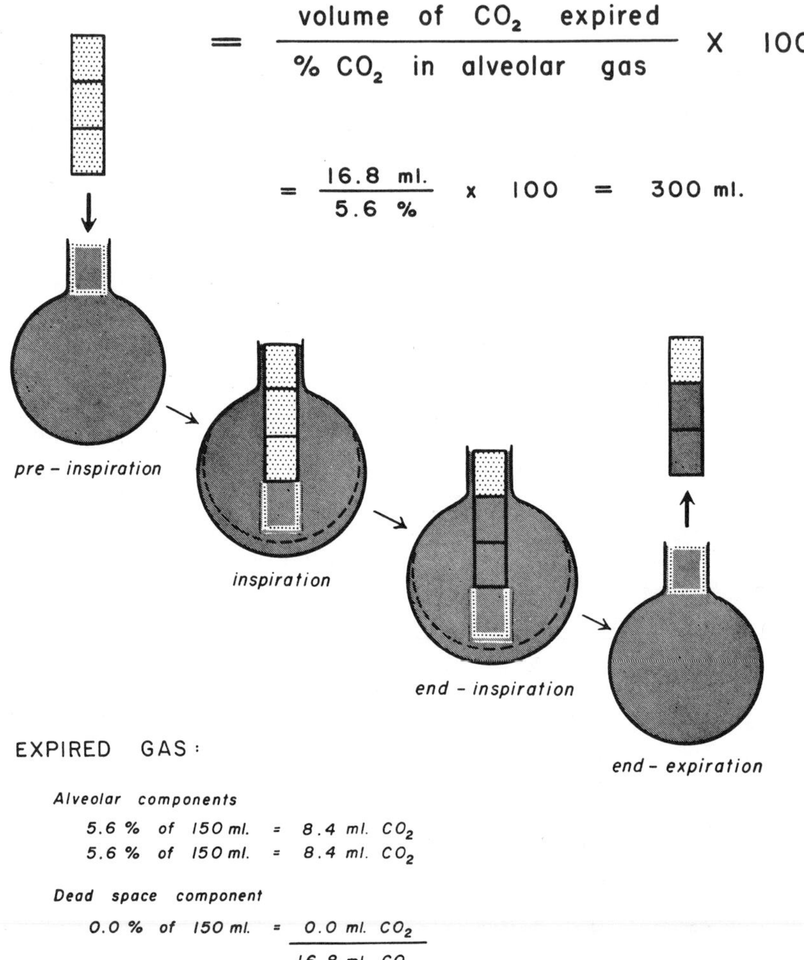

Fig 13.—Alveolar ventilation calculated on basis of expired CO_2. Each block represents 150 ml of gas. Dotted blocks represent inspired air (0.04% CO_2); shaded blocks represent alveolar gas (5.6% CO_2). During inspiration, 150 ml of dead space gas + 300 ml of inspired air enter the alveoli; dotted lines show preinspiratory lung volume. Almost instantly (end-inspiration) the inspired air mixes with alveolar gas and becomes part of it. During expiration, 450 ml of gas leaves the alveoli; 150 ml remains in the respiratory dead space, and 300 ml leaves as expired gas along with the 150 ml of dead space gas. Alveolar ventilation and volume of CO_2 expired for the breath are expressed as ml, corrected to BTPS (body temperature, ambient pressure, saturated with water vapor).

dead space plus an additional volume representing the effect of any inefficiency in pulmonary gas exchange that increases the difference between arterial and expired gas P_{CO_2} (Fig 12,B). Thus, the difference, physiologic dead space − anatomic dead space, is an index of nonuniform alveolar ventilation in respect to capillary blood flow. This relationship between alveolar ventilation and pulmonary capillary blood flow will be considered in more detail in chapter 7.

C. ALVEOLAR VENTILATION PER MINUTE

Calculated on the Basis of Tidal Volume, Anatomic Dead Space and Frequency of Breathing

This has been discussed on pages 28–31 and illustrated in Figures 7 and 8 (pp. 28 and 30). This calculated volume represents only the volume of fresh air reaching the alveoli per minute; it is wholly effective in arterializing venous blood only when the distribution of inspired gas is uniform in relation to pulmonary capillary blood flow. If distribution is not uniform, some of this alveolar ventilation is wasted or ineffective; even if the calculated volume is "normal," more inspired air must be delivered to the alveoli each minute to arterialize the blood.

Calculated on the Basis of CO_2 Elimination

The steady state output of CO_2 from the lungs must equal the rate at which CO_2 is washed out of the alveoli by alveolar ventilation, leading to the following equation:

$$\text{Amount of } CO_2 \text{ expired in ml per min} = \%\ CO_2 \text{ in alveolar gas}/100 \times \text{alveolar ventilation in ml per min}$$

This can be rearranged (and divided by the respiratory frequency per minute) to give the equation in Figure 13.

If we incorporate the assumption that alveolar P_{CO_2} equals arterial P_{CO_2}, this equation becomes the very useful relationship

$$\text{Alveolar ventilation (ml BTPS/min)} = 863\ \frac{\text{volume of } CO_2 \text{ expired (in ml STPD/min)*}}{\text{arterial } P_{CO_2} \text{ (in mm Hg)}}$$

*See p. 285 for a complete explanation of the factor 863, which converts CO_2 production measured as volume of dry gas at 0 °C and 760 mm Hg to that measured at 37 °C in water saturated gas and converts CO_2 concentration to partial pressure in alveolar gas, all at a barometric pressure of 760 mm Hg.

Arterial P_{CO_2} is remarkably constant in healthy humans at rest at about 40 mm Hg. (See chapter on regulation of ventilation.) This means the alveolar ventilation must be regulated by the body to match the CO_2 production rate. Any decrease in alveolar ventilation will cause arterial P_{CO_2} to rise. Conversely, an increase in alveolar ventilation will cause P_{CO_2} to fall. Therefore, in general clinical application an arterial P_{CO_2} over 40 mm Hg means alveolar hypoventilation (less ventilation than needed), and a fall in arterial P_{CO_2} below 40 mm Hg means alveolar hyperventilation. It is alveolar ventilation rather than minute ventilation that is important in gas exchange in the lung. Furthermore, alveolar ventilation is considered in relation to the body's needs (metabolic rate).

In an individual with uniform distribution of inspired gas and pulmonary capillary blood flow, alveolar ventilation calculated in these two ways—that is from anatomic dead space and physiologic dead space—should be equal. When there is nonuniform distribution, the calculation based on CO_2 elimination will yield lower values for alveolar ventilation because it measures the useful or effective alveolar ventilation and not the wasted or ineffective parts.

D. ALVEOLAR GAS COMPOSITION

The CO_2 and O_2 concentration in alveolar gas reflect the performance of the mechanical bellows process of the lung, which brings fresh inspired air into contact with the alveolar capillary blood. We have explained how to estimate alveolar ventilation from arterial P_{CO_2} (see equation on page 41). Alveolar P_{O_2}, when considered in combination with arterial P_{O_2}, would be a useful indicator of the overall exchange performance of the lung (see chapter on ventilation/blood flow) if we could measure it. Indeed, we will show how to calculate mean alveolar P_{O_2} by the use of the alveolar air equation.

It has been emphasized earlier in this chapter that marked uneven distribution of inspired gas occurs in pulmonary disease and different alveoli empty at different rates during expiration. This makes it difficult to call any "spot" sample of expired alveolar gas truly representative of all alveolar gas. We cannot, as in the case of CO_2, assume that arterial P_{O_2} equals the time average of expired alveolar P_{O_2}. In fact, the difference between them, which results from nonuniformity of alveolar ventilation/capillary blood flow and from possible failure of O_2 to equilibrate between alveolar gas and pulmonary capillary blood, is most useful as a measure of the severity of the abnormalities of these functions of the lung.

The alveolar air equation (see Appendix, p. 267) has been used extensively to solve complex problems in gas exchange. Although the equation itself is quite formidable, the principle underlying it is simple. The equation merely states that, at sea level, the total pressure of gases (O_2, CO_2, N_2, and H_2O) in the alveoli equals 760 mm Hg and that if the partial pressures of any three of these four are known, that of the fourth can be obtained by subtraction. Suppose, for example, it is desired to calculate the partial pressure of O_2 in alveolar gas:

$$\begin{array}{rl}
760 \text{ mm Hg} & = P_{O_2} + P_{CO_2} + P_{N_2} + P_{H_2O} \\
-\ \underline{47 \text{ mm Hg } P_{H_2O}} & \\
713 \text{ mm Hg} & = P_{O_2} + P_{CO_2} + P_{N_2} \\
-\underline{563 \text{ mm Hg } P_{N_2}} & \text{(assumed)} \\
150 \text{ mm Hg} & = P_{O_2} + P_{CO_2} \\
-\ \underline{40 \text{ mm Hg } P_{CO_2}} & \text{(measured as arterial } P_{CO_2}) \\
110 \text{ mm Hg} & = P_{O_2}
\end{array}$$

In the process of determining P_{O_2} by subtracting the P_{H_2O}, P_{CO_2}, and P_{N_2}, there are certain measurements and assumptions. It is generally agreed that the water vapor pressure at 37 °C is approximately 47 mm Hg, and this presents no problem. Alveolar P_{CO_2} is assumed equal to arterial P_{CO_2}. It is also assumed in the foregoing calculation that P_{N_2} = 563 mm Hg. This would be true if the respiratory quotient were 1.0, i.e., if the amount of CO_2 added to the alveoli were exactly equal to the amount of O_2 removed from the alveoli each minute; in this case the inspired N_2 would be neither diluted nor concentrated as it entered the alveoli, and alveolar P_{N_2} would equal moist inspired P_{N_2} (79.03% × 713 = 563 mm Hg). Actually, in most cases, more O_2 is removed per minute than CO_2 is added. The usual respiratory exchange ratio (R) is as follows:

$$R = \frac{200 \text{ ml } CO_2/\text{min}}{250 \text{ ml } O_2/\text{min}} = 0.8$$

This results in the N_2 molecules being slightly more concentrated, since the same number of N_2 molecules is now present in a smaller gas volume. If the alveolar N_2 rises to 81%, the alveolar P_{N_2} would rise to 577 and the alveolar P_{O_2} would fall to 96 mm Hg. It is therefore essential to calculate alveolar P_{N_2} accurately by determining the respiratory exchange ratio.

The changes in normal alveolar P_{CO_2} and P_{O_2} with changes in alveolar ventilation are shown in Figure 14.

E. HYPOVENTILATION OF THE LUNGS

Causes of Hypoventilation

Hypoventilation exists when an insufficient volume of fresh air enters the alveoli each minute relative to the metabolic activity of the body. As a practical matter hypoventilation is measured by an increase in arterial P_{CO_2} over 40 mm Hg.* Usually, hypoventilation in ambulatory patients with cardiopulmonary disease is due to mechanical factors limiting thoracic or pulmonary movements, but Table 3 shows clearly that hypoventilation can be caused in many ways.

Effects of Hypoventilation on Blood Gases

Since, by definition, hypoventilation supplies inadequate amounts of fresh air, it must lead to anoxemia, CO_2 retention, and respiratory acidosis (Fig 14). The sequence of events is as follows: Less O_2 now is added per minute to the alveoli by ventilation than is removed by the pulmonary capillary blood. Alveolar P_{O_2} falls, and arterial P_{O_2}, O_2 content, and percent saturation of hemoglobin decrease, resulting in anoxemia. Simultaneously, alveolar P_{CO_2} rises, because inadequate alveolar ventilation cannot remove the volume of CO_2 that is added to the alveoli by the pulmonary capillary blood. Since the P_{CO_2} of the blood at the end of the pulmonary capillaries (which has just left the alveoli) is in equilibrium with alveolar P_{CO_2}, end-pulmonary capillary and sys-

---

Fig 14.—Vertical hatched line represents values in a "normal" man with alveolar ventilation of 4.27 L/min, O_2 consumption of 250 ml/min, and R (gas exchange ratio) of 0.8. NOTE: (1) When alveolar ventilation exceeds this value, alveolar and arterial P_{O_2} rise, but there is little increase in arterial O_2 saturation because Hb is almost maximally saturated at the P_{O_2} achieved by "normal" alveolar ventilation. (2) When alveolar ventilation decreases to less than 3 L/min, arterial O_2 saturation falls sharply because of the steep slope of the O_2 dissociation curve at this P_{O_2}. (3) The line for blood CO_2 content, unlike that for arterial O_2 saturation, shows no abrupt inflection and is not flat until very high ventilations are achieved. Thus, an increase in ventilation that is ineffective in increasing the O_2 saturation is effective in decreasing the CO_2 content.

This chart applies approximately in a great variety of conditions. The lines apply exactly when (1) barometric pressure is 760 mm Hg, (2) O_2 consumption is 250 ml/min, (3) R is 0.8, and (4) gas tensions are the same in all alveoli and in the arterial blood. Figure 73 (p. 289) provides similar data for various values of R, alveolar ventilation, and O_2 consumption.

*It is assumed that the inspired P_{CO_2} is that of air, practically zero. Breathing in a poorly ventilated space or rebreathing from an apparatus that causes or permits the accumulation of CO_2 can raise the inspired P_{CO_2} and therefore elevate the alveolar and arterial P_{CO_2} above 40 mm Hg.

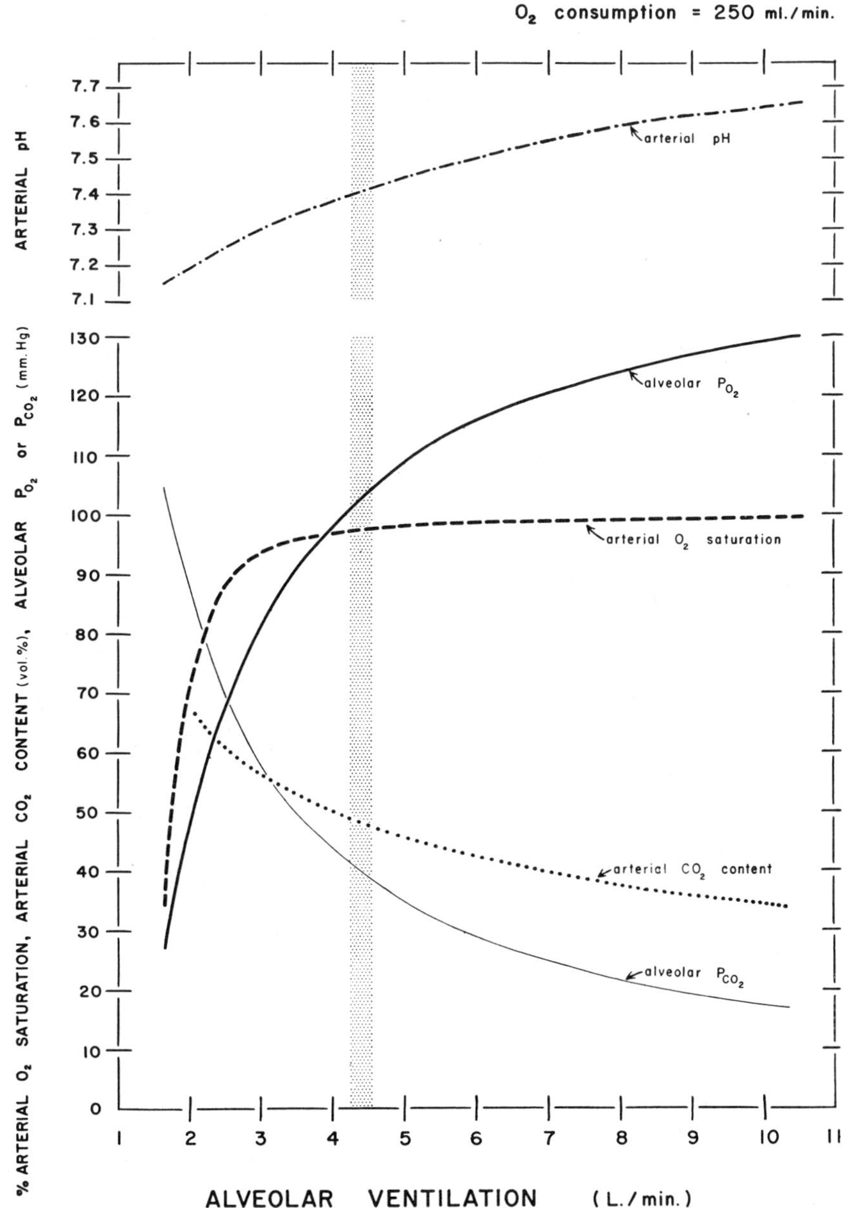
O2 consumption = 250 ml./min.
ARTERIAL pH
7.7
7.6
7.5
7.4
7.3
7.2
7.1
arterial pH
% ARTERIAL O2 SATURATION, ARTERIAL CO2 CONTENT (vol.%), ALVEOLAR PO2 or PCO2 (mm.Hg)
130
120
110
100
90
80
70
60
50
40
30
20
10
0
alveolar PO2
arterial O2 saturation
arterial CO2 content
alveolar PCO2
1
2
3
4
5
6
7
8
9
10
11
ALVEOLAR VENTILATION (L./min.)

TABLE 3.—POSSIBLE CAUSES OF HYPOVENTILATION

1. Depression of respiratory centers by general anesthesia, or drugs, cerebral trauma, increased intracranial pressure, prolonged anoxia or cerebral ischemia, or high concentration of CO_2.
2. Interference with neural communication between the respiratory muscles and the CNS respiratory centers produced by traumatic lesions of the spinal cord or peripheral nerve, by infections such as poliomyelitis or peripheral neuritis or by neuromuscular block produced by myasthenia gravis, botulinus or drugs, such as succinylcholine and by relaxation of the muscles of the tongue and pharynx, as during sleep.
3. Diseases of respiratory muscles.
4. Limitation of movement of thorax by arthritis, scleroderma, emphysema, thoracic deformity, or elevation of the diaphragm.
5. Limitation of movement of lungs by decrease in functioning lung tissue caused by disorders such as atelectasis, tumor or pneumonia, by decreased distensibility of lung tissue as in restrictive disease and congestion, or by pleural effusion or pneumothorax.
6. Limitation to movement of air through airways caused by obstructive lung diseases such as emphysema, bronchitis, or asthma, or by relaxation of the muscles of the tongue and pharynx, as during sleep.
7. Severe dysfunction of gas exchange caused by nonuniformity of alveolar ventilation/capillary blood flow, as in chronic obstructive lung disease.

temic arterial P_{CO_2} must also rise. A rise in arterial P_{CO_2} causes a fall in pH (respiratory acidosis; see chapter 9).

Hypoventilation always results in anoxemia and CO_2 retention when the patient is breathing air. This is shown graphically in Figure 14; the failure of arterial O_2 saturation to fall to the same extent as alveolar O_2 pressure is due to the shape of the O_2 dissociation curve (see p. 224).

The arterial blood can be well oxygenated despite severe hypoventilation, if a high concentration of O_2 is breathed; however, CO_2 cannot be eliminated properly without an adequate volume of alveolar ventilation.

F. HYPERVENTILATION OF THE LUNGS

The term hyperventilation refers to an increase in ventilation in excess of that required to maintain normal arterial blood P_{O_2} and P_{CO_2}. A listing of possible causes of hyperventilation is given in Table 4.

Effects of Hyperventilation on Blood Gases

Hyperventilation leads to a decrease in alveolar CO_2 tension and a rise in alveolar O_2 tension (see Fig 14, p. 45, and Table 4). The decrease in alveolar P_{CO_2} leads to a decrease in arterial blood CO_2 tension and content and to respiratory alkalosis, *but the increase in alveolar P_{O_2} produces only an insignificant increase in arterial O_2 saturation of normal individuals living at sea level.* Examination of the dissociation curves for CO_2 and O_2 (pp. 238 and 224) shows why the effect of hyperventilation differs with respect to blood CO_2 and O_2. The CO_2 content of the blood is influenced equally (though in opposite directions) by an increase or decrease in the arterial P_{CO_2}, and this holds true over the whole physiologic range of the CO_2 dissociation curve. However, the O_2 content and saturation of blood are *not* influenced in a *linear* manner by an increase or decrease in arterial P_{O_2}; arterial blood is almost completely saturated with O_2 at the arterial P_{O_2} present during quiet breathing of room air, and a further increase in arterial P_{O_2} caused by hyperventilation can add very little O_2 to the blood (see Fig 14, p. 45). On the other hand, when the arterial P_{O_2}

TABLE 4.—POSSIBLE CAUSES OF HYPERVENTILATION

1. Increased activity of the CNS respiratory center(s).
   a. *Infections,* such as meningitis and encephalitis, and *trauma, cerebral hemorrhage* and *tumors* are presumed to act by stimulation of the central mechanisms or by destruction of inhibitory regions.
   b. *Increased Metabolism.*—Hyperthyroidism, fever, and hot baths can increase ventilation out of proportion to the increase in metabolic rate, even causing metabolic alkalosis. Certain types of gram-negative bacteria can cause hyperventilation without fever.
   c. *Drugs and Hormones.*—Epinephrine (and, to a lesser extent, norepinephrine), some female sex hormones (particularly progesterone). Analeptic drugs stimulate respiration only when given in very large doses, as do salicylates. The site of action of these chemicals is not known precisely.
   d. *Volition or anxiety.*—This may be an acute reaction to the laboratory or may be a longer standing functional disorder such as hyperventilation syndrome or neurocirculatory asthenia.
2. Stimulation of peripheral afferents to the respiratory center.
   a. *Chemoreceptors* (carotid and aortic bodies) stimulated by metabolic acidosis (a decrease in arterial pH). A decrease in arterial P_{O_2} causes hyperventilation when neuromuscular mechanisms permit it, provided there are no serious mechanical limitations to increased ventilation. There are great individual differences in the ventilatory response to a decrease of the P_{O_2} of arterial blood.
   b. *Baroreceptors (Carotid and Aortic).* Low blood pressure causes hyperventilation either reflexly through the carotid and aortic pressure receptors mechanism or centrally by decreasing the cerebral blood flow and permitting medullary tissue P_{CO_2} to rise.
   c. *Sensory Nerve Endings.*—Stimulated by collapse of alveoli, as in pneumothorax, and atelectasis, by pulmonary hypertension and by irritation of nerve endings in the lower respiratory tract (as by ether vapor).

and saturation are low, hyperventilation both lowers arterial P_{CO_2} and *increases* arterial P_{O_2} and saturation.

When hyperventilation is chronic (as in residents at high altitude), compensatory mechanisms usually restore the blood pH to or toward normal and minimize the effects of hyperventilation on the body (p. 244).

G. DIAGNOSIS OF HYPO- AND HYPERVENTILATION

Because ventilation cannot be called inadequate or excessive unless related to the metabolic rate of the body, in the final analysis the adequacy of ventilation should be measured by its ability to maintain normal levels of arterial blood P_{O_2} and P_{CO_2}. The level of arterial P_{O_2} may be influenced markedly by nonuniform alveolar ventilation in relation to capillary blood flow in individual alveoli and possibly by impaired alveolar-capillary diffusion, while arterial P_{CO_2} is much less affected. Therefore, the level of arterial P_{CO_2} is a more trustworthy guide in the diagnosis of alveolar hypoventilation.

H. SUMMARY

*Hypo*ventilation with *air* leads to anoxemia, CO_2 retention, and respiratory acidosis. *Hypo*ventilation with *oxygen* usually leads only to CO_2 retention and to respiratory acidosis. *Hyper*ventilation with air "blows off" CO_2 and produces respiratory alkalosis, but adds little to the oxygenation of the blood (unless the alveoli were *hypo*ventilated at the outset).

II. UNIFORMITY OF ALVEOLAR VENTILATION

Up to this point we have regarded the lung as a uniform structure in which each alveolus has the same volume, the same distensibility, the same ventilation, the same blood flow, and the same facility for diffusion of gases across its alveolar-capillary membranes. If this were so, and all the fresh air inspired into the alveoli were distributed uniformly to alveoli of equal volume and with equal blood flow, then ventilation would be maximally effective in arterializing the mixed venous blood.

The real lung is not uniform. We know that differences exist between the ventilation and blood flow of different parts of the lungs, even in healthy subjects. In the remainder of this chapter we will discuss uneven distribution of inspired gas to alveolar volume, and in chapter 7 we will expand on the concept of uneven distribution of gas to blood flow and its effect on pulmonary function.

In the very simplest of lungs (Fig 15, *left*) the organ consists of a single chamber with pulmonary capillaries in its walls; in such a lung, ventilation is almost certain to be uniform throughout. As the lung becomes more complex, septa develop to a greater and greater extent. This increases greatly the surface for gas exchange, but also increases the opportunity for *uneven* ventilation. The human lung, with an estimated 300 million alveoli, is too complex to picture. In such a lung, even though healthy, alveolar ventilation is not absolutely uniform. In a very large percentage of patients with chronic pulmonary disease, alveolar ventilation may be decidedly uneven; in the same individual, poorly ventilated and hyperventilated areas may coexist side by side.

Figure 16 shows schematically the concept of even and of uneven

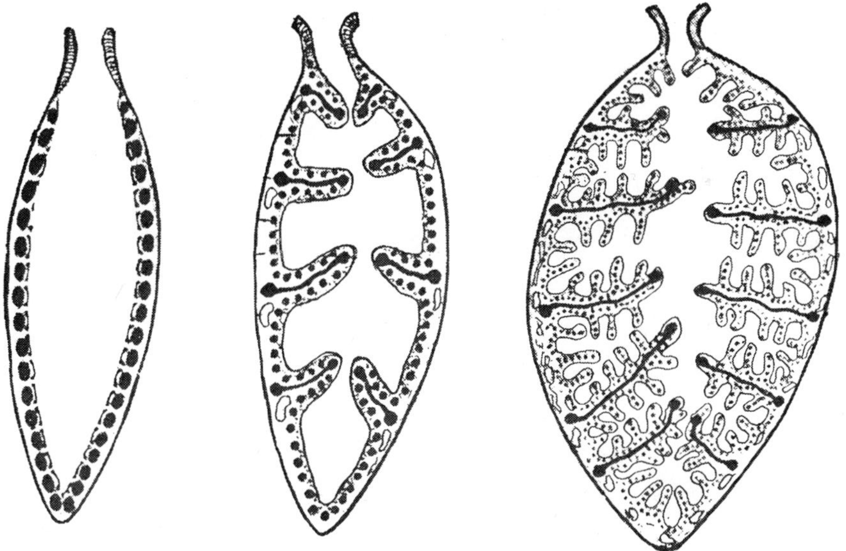

Fig 15.—Development of the multi-alveolar lung. *Left,* uni-alveolar lung of Proteus. *Center,* multi-alveolar lung of Siren with simple septa. *Right,* multi-alveolar lung of Rana with complex septa. Black dots in walls and septa represent pulmonary capillaries. (From Krogh A.: *The Comparative Physiology of Respiratory Mechanisms.* Philadelphia, University of Pennsylvania Press, 1941.)

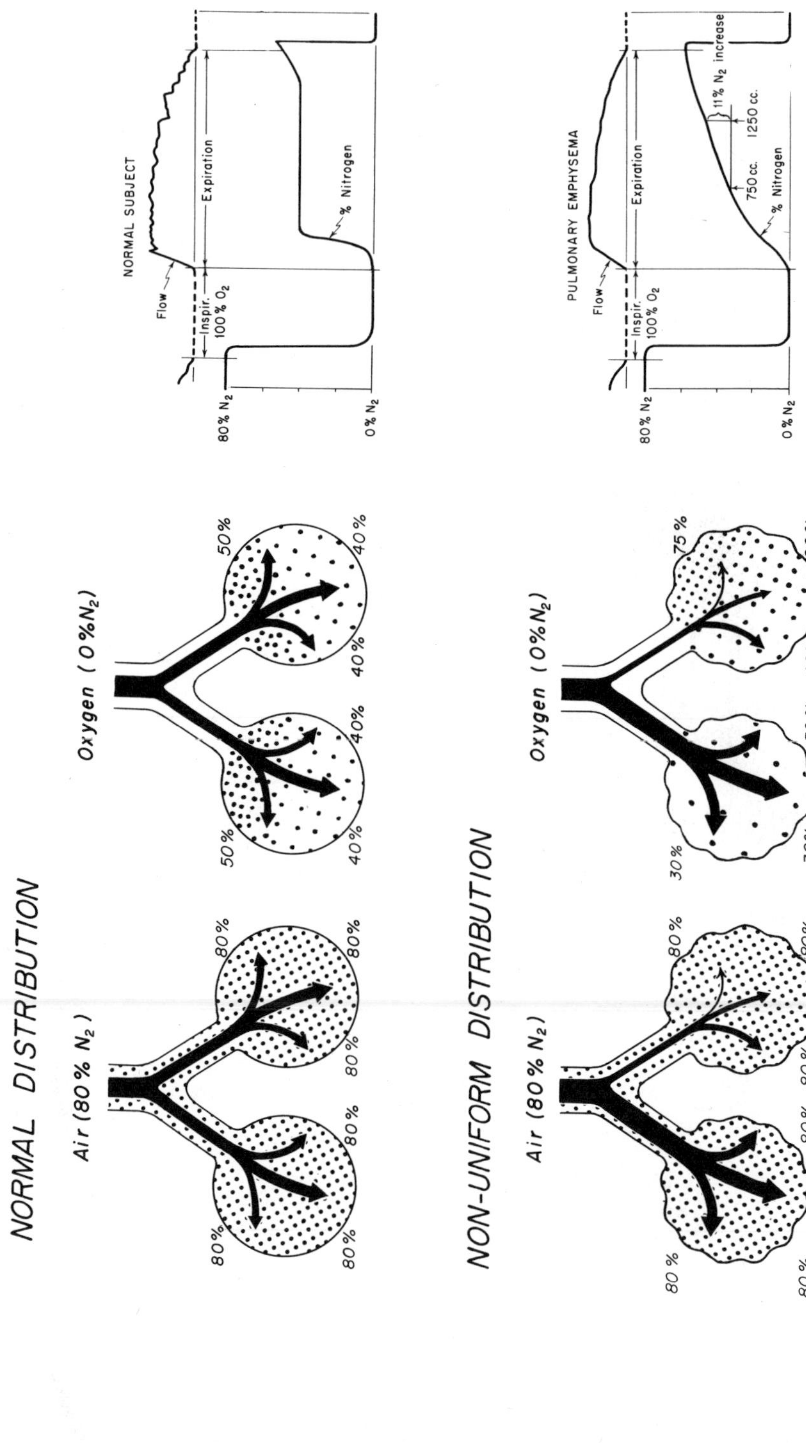

NORMAL DISTRIBUTION

Air (80% N_2)

80% 80% 80% 80% 80% 80%

Oxygen (0% N_2)

50% 40% 40% 40% 50% 40%

NORMAL SUBJECT

Flow

Inspir. 100% O_2

Expiration

% Nitrogen

80% N_2

0% N_2

NON-UNIFORM DISTRIBUTION

Air (80% N_2)

80% 80% 80% 80% 80% 80%

Oxygen (0% N_2)

30% 30% 30% 40% 75% 60%

PULMONARY EMPHYSEMA

Flow

Inspir. 100% O_2

Expiration

11% N_2 increase

750 cc. 1250 cc.

% Nitrogen

80% N_2

0% N_2

Fig 16.—In each case, the same volume of gas (air or O_2) is inspired, distribution being normal in one case *(above)* and nonuniform in the other *(below)*. N_2 molecules are represented by black dots. *Left,* schematic representation of alveolar N_2 during breathing of air; *center,* schematic representation of alveolar N_2 immediately after a single breath of O_2; *right,* actual records of N_2 concentration and gas flow during the next expiration.

The upper drawing represents a normal lung. Air contains 79.03% N_2 and mixed alveolar gas about 80% to 81% N_2 because the respiratory exchange ratio is less than 1; the blood absorbs more oxygen than it gives off CO_2, shrinking the gas volume and concentrating the nitrogen. Even in the normal person, the distribution of inspired gas in relation to alveolar volume is not completely uniform. In the upright position a greater volume of fresh inspired gas enters the lower alveoli than enters the apical alveoli during a large inspiration (see chapter on Mechanics). This accounts for the greater dilution of the nitrogen in the basal alveoli following a breath of air of O_2. But even breathing air, the nitrogen concentration will tend to be higher in the basal alveoli than in the apical alveoli because the greater blood perfusion rate promotes the absorption of O_2 more than it promotes the production of CO_2 magnifying the shrinking of the gas volume and concentrating the nitrogen further. However, when distribution of inspired air to the alveoli is grossly nonuniform, this would not be detected in the expired breath owing to the small changes in percent nitrogen. Breathing oxygen dilutes the N_2, the degree of dilution depending upon the fraction of inspired O_2 distributed to the various regions of the lungs. Thus, when there is nonuniform distribution, inhalation of O_2 magnifies its affect in the different areas.

ventilation. Let us assume that when an individual is breathing air, his lungs contain 2,000 ml of gas which has a N_2 concentration of approximately 80%. If he inspires 2,000 ml of O_2 into his *alveoli* and this O_2 is distributed evenly to each of the millions of alveoli in the lungs (in relation to its preinspiratory volume), each alveolus will now contain 40% N_2 (Fig 16, *top*). On the other hand, if the 2,000 ml of O_2 is distributed *unevenly,* some alveoli may get less than their share (hypoventilation) and others may get more than their share *(hyperventilation);* in this case the composition of alveolar gas will be decidedly *nonuniform* at end-inspiration (Fig 16, *bottom*).

It is impossible to put sampling needles into thousands of alveoli to determine whether gas composition is uniform or not, but it is possible to sample and to analyze the gas that leaves the alveoli on the expiration immediately after the inhalation of O_2. Figure 16 shows such records obtained with the N_2 analyzer. We are already familiar with this type of record (see Fig 10, p. 34) in which phase I represents pure dead space gas and phase II represents a mixture of alveolar and dead space gas. Phase III represents mixed expired alveolar gas. Even though this phase is a plateau in normal persons, this does not mean that N_2 concentration is the same in all alveoli after an inspiration of oxygen (see Fig 16, upper graph). In the upright individual the N_2 concentration of gas originally in the alveoli of the lung bases before the inspiration of O_2 is diluted more than N_2 in the alveoli of the apices (see chapter on mechanics). When an individual takes a breath of O_2 from residual volume, this oxygen initially starts filling the apex and, later, the base. However, the increase in volume of the alveoli in the apex is less related to its initial volume than for the alveoli in the bases because the alveoli of the apices start already partially distended (see Fig 27). In contrast, the volume of gas in the alveoli at the bases is initially small. The plateau in expired alveolar N_2 concentration therefore occurs because the proportional contribution of gas from the different alveoli to the expired breath remains relatively constant. However, as expiration progresses, alveoli with a greater N_2 concentration (in the apices of healthy patients) contribute an increasing fraction of the expired breath. This causes a slow rise in the mixed expired N_2 concentration.

The record of the expired N_2 concentration in nonuniform distribution (Fig 16, lower right) illustrates the error in considering a "spot sample of alveolar gas" to be truly representative of all alveolar gas. It is obvious that the first part of expired alveolar gas may differ markedly in gas composition from the last, and it requires little imagination to realize that the alveolar gas remaining in the unexpired residual gas may have yet a different composition.

In almost all diffuse lung disease the normally slight nonuniformity of distribution of inspired gas is grossly exaggerated, the inspired 100% O_2 is distributed unevenly to the various alveoli, and the end-inspiratory N_2 concentrations vary widely in different parts of the lung.

The slow rise of expired N_2 in phase III is frequently exaggerated in the terminal parts of a large expiration as it approaches residual volume, producing a sudden rise in mixed expired nitrogen concentration (phase IV, Fig 16; see chapter on mechanics). The lung volume at the start of this sudden rise is called the *closing capacity,* and the comparable volume above residual volume has been called *closing volume.*

The explanation for the onset of phase IV is that relaxation of lung tissue tension and external compression of airways in the bases of the lungs causes parts of the bronchi to begin to shut off—hence, the name. After this the greater proportion of gas comes from the apex, which has a higher nitrogen concentration.

A. TESTS OF DISTRIBUTION* OF INSPIRED GAS

These tests measure only the distribution of inspired gas to the alveoli just as though the lungs were an impermeable bag or bellows and the processes of diffusion and circulation did not exist. They require the use of gases such as N_2, H_2, or helium which are so poorly soluble that they do not pass in great quantity from the alveolar gas into the blood or pulmonary tissues, gases for which rapid analyzers are available.

Single-Breath Technique: Open Circuit

This has just been described to illustrate graphically the problem of distribution. The patient inspires a single breath of O_2 and then ex-

*The nomenclature used in discussing distribution is, like the lung, nonuniform! "Uneven ventilation" = "nonuniform ventilation" = "uneven" or "nonuniform distribution of inspired gas" = "nonhomogeneous ventilation or distribution" = "poor mixing." The problem of "nonuniformity" appears to be primarily one of uneven *distribution* to different air sacs, lobules or lobes rather than the slow *mixing within an alveolus* (either by mechanical mass flow or by interdiffusion of gases). This mixing occurs by diffusion, and the importance of the mechanism can be proven by studying the distribution of an inspiration of an aerosol of very large particulate size. When the next expired breath is collected, most of the aerosol is in it, except for a few particles that diffuse into the alveolar gas that is not expired. In contrast, an inspiration of a gas, say helium, mixes almost completely with alveolar gas and most of it remains in the lung during the next expiration. It has been shown by calculation that interdiffusion of gases within an alveolus is 80% complete in only 0.002 sec if the diffusion distance is 0.5 mm, or in 0.38 sec if the diffusion distance is 7 mm.

pires slowly and evenly into a spirometer or flow meter while the N_2 analyzer records continuously N_2 concentration. No measurements are made on the first 750 ml of expired gas because in some patients the last part of this may contain some dead space gas. However, the increase in N_2 concentration is measured over the next 500 ml of expired gas, which is certain to be alveolar gas during phase III. In healthy young adults, distribution is not perfectly uniform, but the N_2 concentration generally does not rise more than 1.5% throughout the expiration of this 500 ml of alveolar gas.† In older healthy individuals, the N_2 concentration may rise more rapidly from 750 to 1,250 of expired volume. However, in patients with severe emphysema, the N_2 concentration may rise as much as 16%. This exaggerated increase depends on uneven distribution of the gas *during inspiration* and also on *unequal rates of gas flow* from different regions of the lungs *during expiration.* If all regions emptied synchronously during expiration, the N_2 meter record would be horizontal even though the concentration of N_2 varied in different parts of the lung at end-inspiration.

Although the single-breath test for gas distribution is rapid and requires only a single breath of oxygen, it is uneven in healthy old people and is abnormal in almost any diffuse lung disease and therefore gives little diagnostic insight.

A single breath of air containing a small concentration of a chemically inert, relatively insoluble gas, such as helium, for which a rapid analyzer is available, provides the same information as the single-breath N_2 test. A record of the tracer concentration in the expired gas at the mouth compared to expired flow rate or volume is the mirror image of that for N_2 in Figures 10 and 16.

Multiple-Breath Techniques: Open Circuit

These tests are based on the rate of washout of pulmonary N_2‡ when O_2 is breathed (Fig 17). In the test the stepwise decrease in the alveolar P_{N_2} that occurs is followed continuously, breath by breath, by rapid

†If the expiration is very slow, the functional residual capacity very small, and the arterial blood O_2 saturation quite low, a slight change in N_2 concentration may occur between the 750 and 1,250 ml samples because the O_2 uptake greatly exceeds the simultaneous CO_2 elimination when 100% O_2 is inhaled.

‡As the concentration of pulmonary N_2 is reduced, some N_2 dissolved in the tissues and blood will enter the alveoli because the pressure of N_2 in blood and tissues is now higher than the alveolar P_{N_2}, and gases, like liquids, move from a region of higher partial pressure to a region of lower pressure. This N_2 can be corrected for, approximately, and need not concern us here.

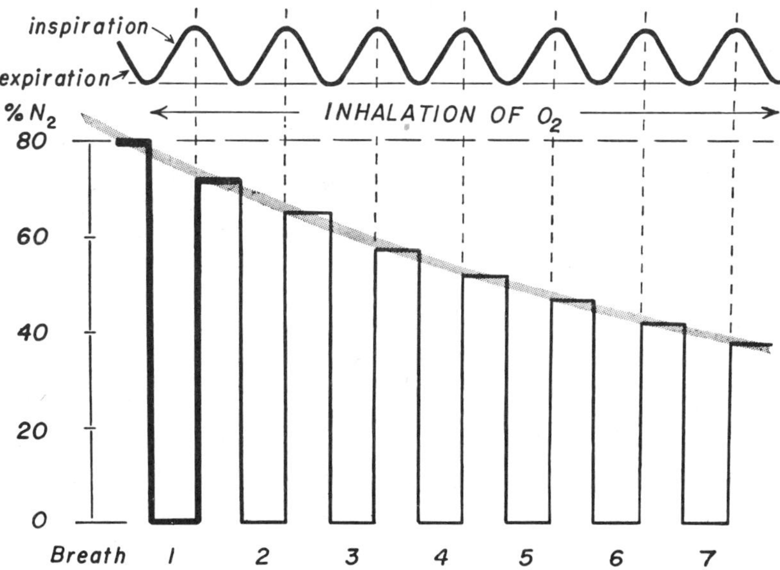

Fig 17.—Pulmonary nitrogen washout curve. A subject with uniform distribution of inspired gas breathes O_2 at constant tidal volume; N_2 concentration of respired gas is followed continuously with a N_2 analyzer. The N_2 record for the first breath *(broad line)* is similar to the N_2 analyzer record of the single-breath test in Figure 10, except that here the record is greatly compressed. Each plateau represents the N_2 concentration of expired *alveolar* gas. The resulting N_2 washout curve is a single exponential curve (see text).

electrical analyzers. The *actual* measurements of alveolar P_{N_2} breath by breath can then be compared with *theoretical* values that one would expect breath by breath if the inspired O_2 were distributed *evenly* to all the alveoli, i.e., if the lungs were a perfect, single mixing chamber. These theoretical values depend on the volume of gas in the alveoli being washed out (the functional residual capacity), tidal volume, dead space, and frequency of breathing.

An example of the calculation and measurements necessary for obtaining the theoretically perfect data follows. At the beginning of the test, the volume of alveolar gas is measured and is found to be 2,550 ml. The anatomic dead space is 150 ml. The first breath of O_2 is 450 ml. However, only 300 ml of O_2 plus 150 ml of dead space gas (the latter having the same composition as alveolar gas) enter the alveoli (Fig 13, p. 40). There is now 2,550 + 150 ml, or 2,700 ml, of alveolar gas with a concentration of 80% N_2 in the alveoli; this contains 2,160 ml of N_2. However, this volume of N_2 is now in a total gas volume of 3000 ml (300 ml of O_2 having been added), and so its new concentration is $^{2,160}/_{3,000} \times 100$, or 72% (see Fig 17, p. 55).

It may be simpler to consider that the initial alveolar N_2 concentration was diluted in the ratio, 2,700 ml/3,000 ml = 0.9. The theoretical N_2 concentration at the end of the second breath will be 0.9 × 72%, the concentration at the start of the second breath. In this manner the alveolar N_2 concentration will be successively 80%, 72%, 64.8%, 58.3%, and so on.

In this ideal case, in which the tidal volume is constant and the lungs behave as a single, perfect mixing chamber, a graph of alveolar (end-inspiratory) N_2 concentration against the number of breaths results in the type of curve shown in Figure 17. A curve that decreases by the same proportion over each successive interval is an exponential curve; such a curve, replotted on semi-log paper, yields a straight line.

A nitrogen clearance curve may be very steep (Fig 18, *top left*) if the lungs are washed out evenly and rapidly, or less steep (Fig 18, *top right*) if the lungs are washed out evenly but at a slower rate. In either case, a straight line results from plotting these values on semi-log paper (Fig 18, *bottom left*).

When there is uneven ventilation, there may be hundreds of different washout rates in different parts of the lungs, but as a rule the lung behaves as though there were a *poorly ventilated* portion and a *well-ventilated* portion, the first behaving like the lung in Figure 18, *top right,* and the other like the lung in Figure 18, *top left.* The curve obtained from the whole lung of this type is also shown (*bottom right,* dotted line). The extent of uneven ventilation is indicated by the *deviation*

Fig 18.—In each case, O_2 is breathed and the mean concentration of N_2 in the expired gas measured breath by breath. The graphs show mean expired (not alveolar) N_2 concentration plotted against the number of breaths (technique of Fowler, Cornish, and Kety). *Above,* data are presented on ordinary linear graph paper: *left,* rapid N_2 clearance, i.e., a well-ventilated lung; *right,* slow N_2 clearance, i.e., a poorly ventilated lung. *Below,* data are presented on semi-log paper, using the same N_2 clearance data as in the graphs above. *Left,* each line is a straight line, indicating that N_2 clearance proceeded in a regular fashion (exponential) from the well-ventilated and the poorly ventilated lung. *Right,* dotted line shows N_2 clearance curve that results from a patient with the *two systems* pictured above. The dotted line is not a straight line but can be analyzed in terms of two straight lines. Initially the curve is determined predominantly by the well-ventilated lung; after the 20th breath, this lung is cleared of its N_2 and the curve determined entirely by the N_2 clearance from the poorly ventilated lung. In this case, the uneven distribution must be on a regional basis.

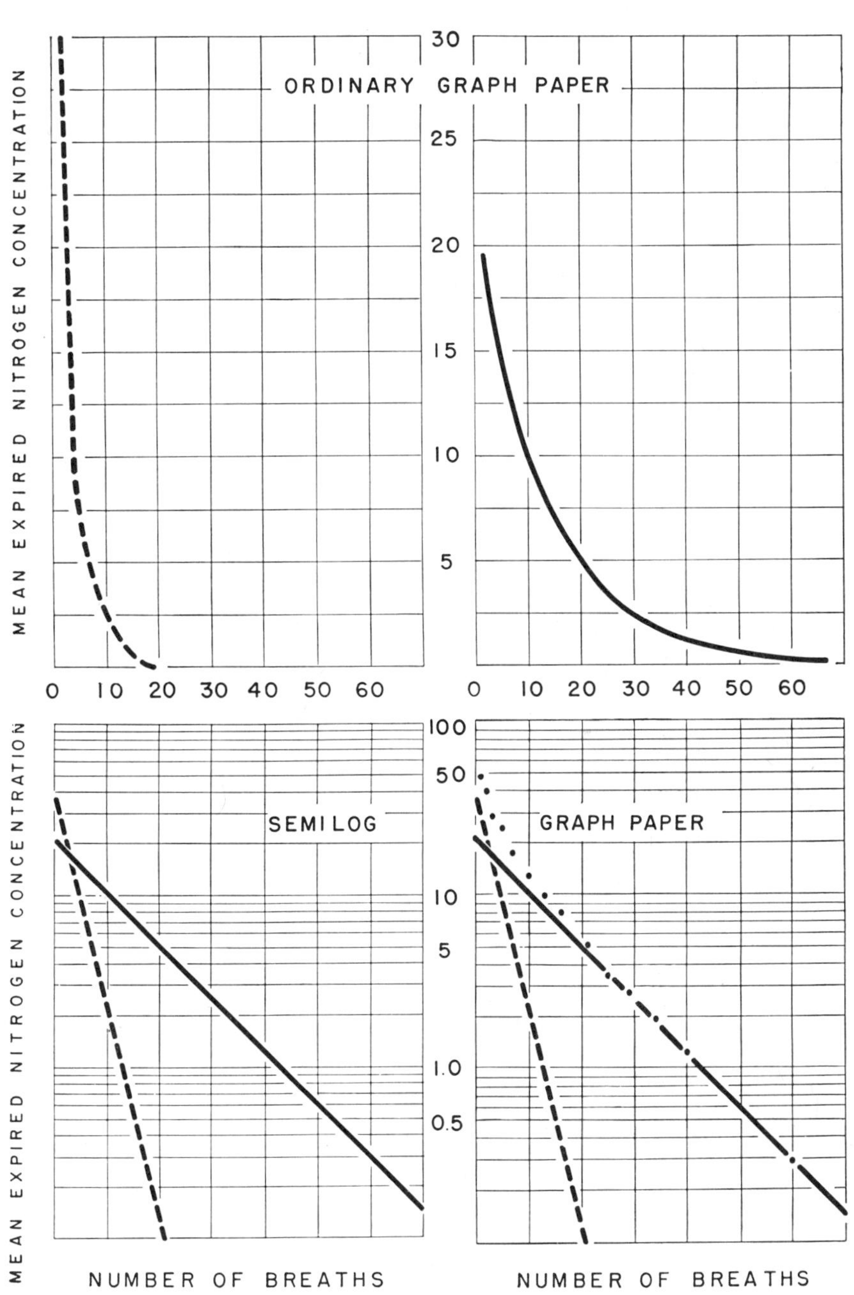
NITROGEN CLEARANCE CURVES
ORDINARY GRAPH PAPER
MEAN EXPIRED NITROGEN CONCENTRATION
30
25
20
15
10
5
0 10 20 30 40 50 60
0 10 20 30 40 50 60
SEMILOG
GRAPH PAPER
100
50
10
5
1.0
0.5
MEAN EXPIRED NITROGEN CONCENTRATION
NUMBER OF BREATHS
NUMBER OF BREATHS

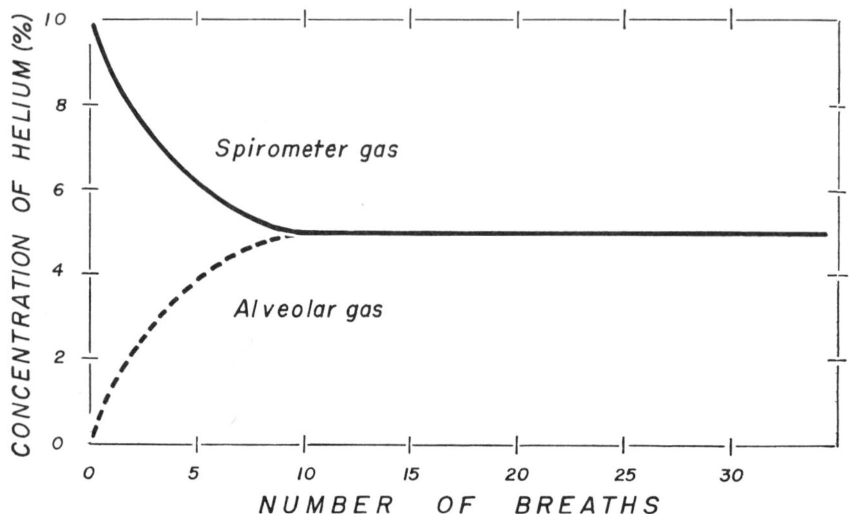

Fig 19.—Helium closed-circuit technique for measuring distribution of inspired gas. The method used is illustrated in Figure 4, (p. 17). Initially the bellows contains 10% helium and the lungs contain 0% helium. At equilibrium, concentrations of helium are the same in both bellows and lungs; the rapidity with which equilibrium is reached is influenced by the tidal volume. When this is allowed for, the curve affords an index of the uniformity of distribution or mixing efficiency. The solid line shows rate of *decrease* in concentration of helium, measured in the *bellows;* dotted line illustrates probable rate of *increase* in concentration of helium in the *alveolar gas.*

from a straight line of the *actual* values obtained in the patient. This test is seldom used because it is time-consuming and requires very precise measurements.

Multiple-Breath Technique: Closed Circuit

If a precisely measured quantity of a relatively insoluble foreign gas such as helium is added to a closed circuit (see Fig 4, p. 17), the *curve* of its dilution by alveolar gas, during rebreathing, gives an index of distribution (Fig 19). The rate may be an exponential one, indicating uniform distribution, or it may be *rapid initially* because of contributions from the *well-ventilated* areas and then *slower* because of less rapid exchange with *poorly ventilated* areas.

During rebreathing with a gas such as helium to an *equilibrium point* (equal concentrations of helium in lungs and bellows), the functional residual capacity can be measured as described in chapter 2. Nonuniformity has been judged by the number of breaths required to obtain 90% equilibration compared to the number calculated from tidal and lung volumes assuming uniform distribution *(index of mixing efficiency)*. Dead space volume assumed in the calculation is critical, the necessary gas mixing in the circuit is difficult to achieve, and the oxygen absorbed must be replaced precisely. The test has fallen into disuse because of these and other technical problems.

Distribution of inspired gas to different regions of the lung can be determined by having the patient inspire a radioactive gas (such as xenon 133) from a closed circuit and recording the output of radiation detectors placed in different positions over the chest (Fig 20), or observing the image on a scintillation camera. The radioactive gas must also be chemically inert, relatively insoluble in blood, and of short half-life so that it is not dangerous to the patient.

When the observed radioactivity reaches a maximum, the concentration of xenon in the alveoli is in equilibrium with that in the closed circuit. This provides a calibration for the output of the detectors in

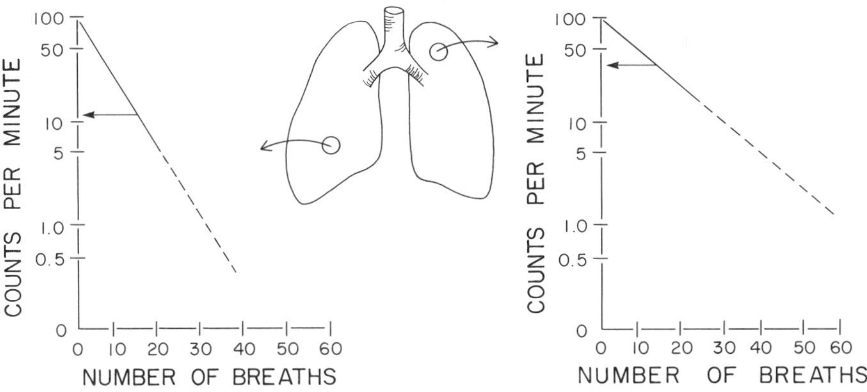

Fig 20.—Graphs of the decrease in alveolar xenon 133 concentration breathing air after having equilibrated with xenon 133 in a rebreathing circuit. The radioactive counts are expressed as percentage of the initial concentration. The circles indicate the location of the counters. The lefthand panel shows the counts over the base of the lung (approximately 21 cm below the apex). The righthand panel shows the counts over the top of the lung (approximately 4 cm below the apex). In both panels, the experimental disappearance curve is dotted after about 20 breaths to indicate that the values become less reliable as they have been corrected for the counts of xenon dissolved in the thorax wall.

terms of absolute xenon concentration. The successive output after each breath in relation to the output at equilibrium gives a clearance curve analagous to that for N_2 (see Fig 18) by having the patient breathe air and wash out the xenon. The "wash in" can be measured as well (see differential equation in Appendix). The inspiration of a single bolus of xenon can be used to measure the changes in volume of the different lung regions with changes in total lung volume (see chapter on mechanics) once the calibration is determined. Although radioactive gas methods require sophisticated instrumentation, they are available in most hospitals, and studies can be done even in the emergency ward.

Bronchospirometry

This is a method for obtaining quantitative measurements of the function of the two lungs separately. It involves catheterization of the left main bronchus by a tube fitted with a distal distensible cuff, so that all the gas ventilating the lung is conducted through this airway. When a double-lumen tube is used, the air to and from the right lung passes through a second channel, the opening of which lies in the trachea above the bifurcation. When a single-lumen tube is used, the gas to and from the right lung flows around the tube. In either case, the two lungs are separated as far as their gas flow is concerned, and it is possible to make measurements of the tidal volume of breathing, vital capacity, and O_2 consumption of each lung by means of two recording systems. Studies on normal subjects have shown that the right lung is responsible for about 55% of the ventilation and 55% of the O_2 consumption, and the left lung for 45% of each. Marked deviation from these ratios indicates predominantly unilateral pulmonary disease.

B. CAUSES OF UNEVEN VENTILATION

The causes of uneven ventilation are shown schematically in Figure 21*; the disturbances shown are not necessarily localized geographically to one lung but may be scattered throughout both lungs. *A* represents regional reduction of the number or quality of elastic fibers in the lung such as occurs in advanced pulmonary emphysema. *B* represents regional obstruction (partial) such as occurs in asthma, pulmonary

*Figure 21 actually is a deliberate simplification of the changes in the alveoli and airways that result in uneven ventilation. Study of chapter 4 will give the reader a better understanding of the factors causing nonuniform distribution of inspired gas.

CAUSES OF UNEVEN VENTILATION

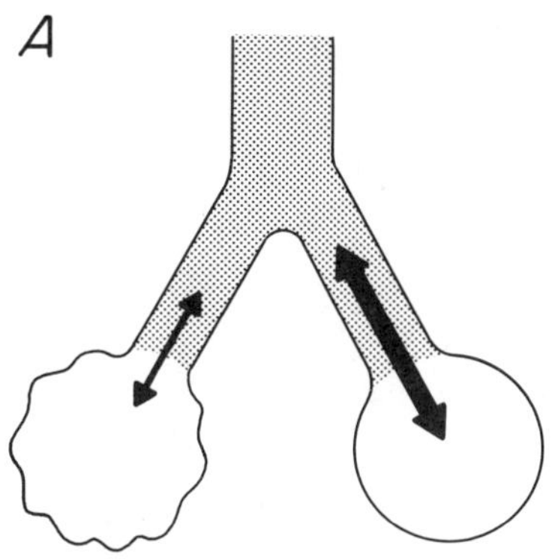

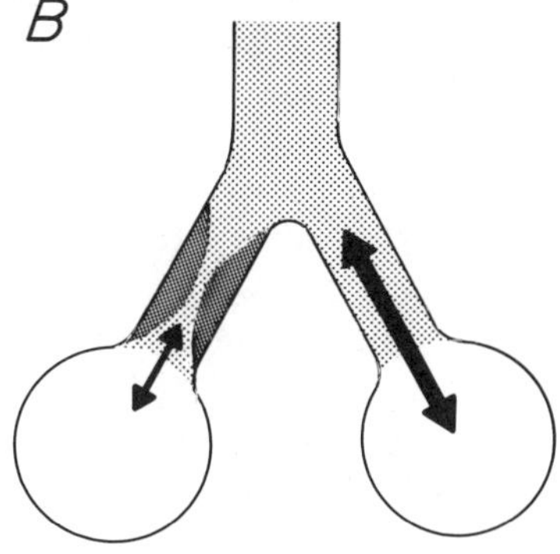

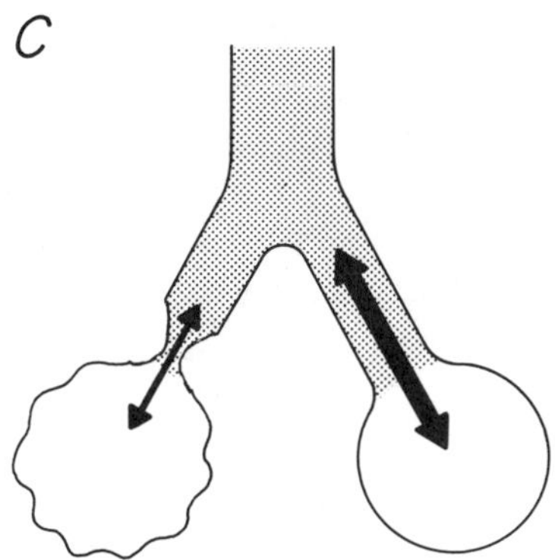

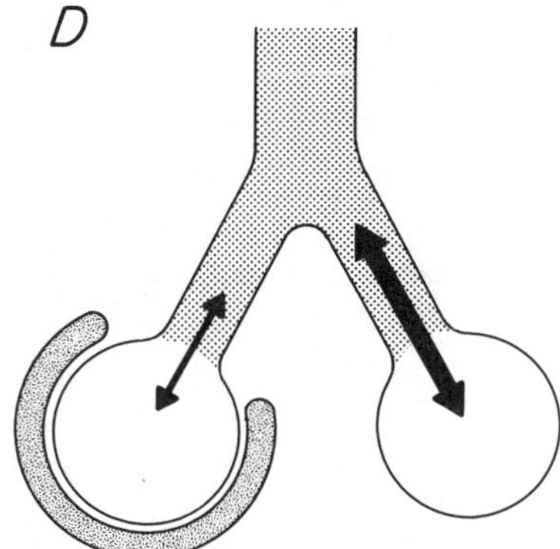

Fig 21.—Mechanisms responsible for nonuniform distribution of air ventilation. Circular areas represent the alveoli. Wavy lines in *A* and *C* represent alveoli that have lost their normal elastic recoil. Perialveolar band in *D* signifies alveoli that expand less than normally, although their elastic tissue is normal and there is no airway obstruction. Size of arrows indicates the volume of gas ventilating each region.

cysts, peribronchiolar or intrabronchial lesions. *C* represents combinations of A and B and is often seen in "obstructive emphysema"; the obstruction need not be bronchiolar constriction but may be of the dynamic compression type that occurs particularly on expiration (see p. 111). *D* represents regional changes in expansion of the type caused by fluid or exudate in the alveoli or interstitial spaces of the lung, pulmonary congestion, atelectasis, tumors, or restrictive disease. These changes may also be caused by nonuniform pulmonary expansion, such as occurs in every thoracic operation, or by nonuniform thoracic expansion. Paradoxical breathing may result from the last-mentioned disorder; for example, if the left phrenic nerve is cut so that the left hemidiaphragm cannot descend on inspiration, expansion of the right hemithorax on inspiration may actually pull up the left hemidiaphragm and draw air from the left lung into the right. Movement of gas from one region of the lung to another may also occur when the "time-constants" of different regions vary markedly.

Uneven ventilation is present to a slight degree in healthy young individuals and to a greater extent in older people, even if they are free from cardiopulmonary disease. Further, more uneven ventilation may be accentuated in a normal person by a change from the supine to the lateral recumbent position. For these reasons, the tests must be done under standard conditions in order to evaluate data properly.

Uneven distribution, although most pronounced in patients with emphysema, is a fairly frequent finding in patients with cardiopulmonary disease. Though not pathognomonic of any one disease, the presence of uneven ventilation, like the finding of râles, or radiologic shadows serves to call attention to an abnormality that may be identified more specifically by other physiologic tests or by radiologic, bacteriologic, or histologic studies. These tests of uneven distribution, then, do not replace other diagnostic procedures but provide a technique for the detection of pulmonary disease. One limitation of these tests is that they give no information regarding the distribution of pulmonary capillary blood flow to the various alveoli (see chapters 6 and 7). Patients with serious pulmonary vascular disorders may have no airway or alveolar disease; in these patients, data from tests of distribution of gas are normal.

C. EFFECTS OF UNEVEN VENTILATION

Hypoventilation of the *whole* lung invariably leads to anoxemia, CO_2 retention, and respiratory acidosis. *Uneven* ventilation in the presence of adequate, or even increased, total lung ventilation can also cause anoxemia and, to a lesser degree, CO_2 retention, unless pulmonary capillary blood flow is reduced regionally in proportion to the decrease in ventilation. However, it is not the uneven ventilation itself that causes this inefficiency in gas exchange, but the unevenness of alveolar ventilation in relation to pulmonary capillary blood flow (see chapter 7 on ventilation/blood flow ratios). The existence of uneven ventilation in respect to alveolar volume also prolongs the induction period of inhalation anesthesia because of the longer time required to establish a high concentration of the anesthetic gas in poorly ventilated areas.

D. SUMMARY

1. Inspired air must pass through a conducting airway ("anatomic dead space") to reach the alveoli where rapid gas exchange occurs; only air reaching *alveoli* raises alveolar P_{O_2} and lowers P_{CO_2} (the requirements for proper gas exchange), and therefore only alveolar ventilation is useful ventilation.

2. If the volume of inspired air reaching each alveolus is not uniform (with proper respect for the size of each alveolus) and unless alveolar capillary blood flow varies in proper proportion, some alveolar ventilation is wasted or ineffective.

3. In the diagnosis of alveolar hypoventilation or hyperventilation, the arterial P_{CO_2} is considered the most reliable index. If arterial, or end-expiratory, P_{CO_2} is increased above about 40 mm Hg, alveolar hypoventilation exists; if it is below 40 mm Hg, alveolar hyperventilation exists.

The total alveolar ventilation, that is, the fresh inspired air reaching the alveoli, may be calculated from the respiratory rate, tidal volume, and predicted anatomic dead space. However, this value is of less interest than the volume of fresh inspired gas that effectively ventilates the capillary blood, as indicated by the arterial blood P_{CO_2} (see p. 41). The calculated total alveolar ventilation may be useful if arterial blood P_{CO_2} is not known.

A decreased level of arterial P_{O_2} is not necessarily diagnostic of hypoventilation because uneven alveolar ventilation in relation to pulmonary capillary blood flow (see chapter 7) or impaired alveolar to capillary blood diffusion can reduce arterial P_{O_2} without increasing arterial P_{CO_2}. Considerable error may result from attempting to estimate alveolar ventilation from rate alone, tidal volume alone, minute volume alone, or from observation of the patient's respiratory *effort.*

4. Uneven distribution of inspired gas to alveolar volume is present to a slight extent in normal persons but is increased in almost all chronic parenchymal lung disease, which reduces its ability to discriminate among different pathological conditions. Nonuniform distribution of inspired gas indicates an inhomogeneity of lung mechanical performance, but the function of the lung in aerating capillary blood may not be as severely compromised if the capillary circulation adjusts to the alveolar ventilation in the different alveoli. Remember that *hyper*ventilation measured at the nose and mouth may be associated with *hypo*ventilation of many alveoli if gas is distributed unevenly throughout the lungs.

4

Mechanics of Breathing

Pulmonary gas exchange requires flow of gas to the alveoli and blood to the alveolar capillaries. In this chapter we shall discuss the forces and resistances that determine the flow of gas in and out of the lungs.

Air flows from a region of higher pressure to one of lower pressure. At end-expiration, when there is no air flow, alveolar gas pressure is equal to atmospheric pressure. If air is to flow into the alveoli, the alveolar pressure must be less than atmospheric during inspiration. Active contraction of the inspiratory muscles enlarges the thorax and further lowers intrathoracic pressure (normally subatmospheric, because the elastic lung tends to recoil inward, away from the thoracic cage). The decrease in intrathoracic pressure enlarges the alveoli, expands the alveolar gas, and lowers the total alveolar gas pressure to less than atmospheric so that air flows into the alveoli.

During inspiration, active muscular contraction provides (1) the force necessary to overcome elastic recoil of the lungs and thorax, (2) the force required to overcome frictional resistance during movement of the tissues of the lung and thorax, and (3) the force necessary to overcome frictional resistance to air flow through the hundreds of thousands of fine tubes and ducts of the tracheobronchial tree.

At end-inspiration, potential energy created by contraction of the inspiratory muscles is stored in the elastic tissues of the lungs and thorax. When the muscles of inspiration relax and no longer exert a force that distends the lungs and thorax, the elastic tissues of the lungs and thorax now recoil. If nonelastic tissue resistance and airway resistance are negligible, the elastic recoil causes the lungs and thorax to return very rapidly to the resting expiratory level even though expiration is completely passive. When the expiratory resistances opposing elastic recoil are abnormally great, active contraction of expiratory muscles may be needed, unless the time for expiration is long (see p. 92).

A. COMPLIANCE OF LUNGS AND THORAX

Elasticity is a property of matter that causes it to return to its resting shape after having been distorted by some external force. A perfectly elastic body, such as the spring in the upper part of Figure 22, will obey Hooke's law—i.e., when it is acted upon by 1 unit of force it will stretch 1 unit of length, when acted upon by 2 units of force it will stretch 2 units, and so on, until the elastic limit is reached or exceeded.

Some tissues of the lungs and thorax possess the property of elasticity. Like springs, these tissues must be stretched during inspiration by an external force (muscular effort); when the external force is removed, the tissues recoil to their resting position. Since elastic tissues obey Hooke's law just as springs do, springs are used in Figure 22 to depict the elastic properties of the lungs. The greater the muscular force applied, the more the springs are stretched and the greater the volume change on inspiration. This relation between force and stretch or between pressure and volume is dependent only on the change in distance or volume, measured under static conditions, and not on the speed with which the new position or volume is attained. The slope of the line that results from plotting the increase in volume against the external force (pressure) serves as a measure of the stiffness of the "springs" or the distensibility of the lungs and thorax; if the slope is more nearly vertical, the tissues are more distensible, and if more nearly horizontal, they are "stiffer."

Physiologists call this the "mechanical compliance" or, more simply, the "compliance" of the tissues; it is defined as the volume change per unit pressure change, and its units are L/cm H_2O.

Compliance is sometimes referred to as "elastic resistance."* In the popular usage of the word *resistance,* tissues with elastic properties do offer "resistance" to stretch. However, in scientific usage (electricity, aerodynamics), *resistance* involves a relationship between pressure and *flow* and is measured during motion, not under static conditions.

*"Elastance," which is the reciprocal of compliance, is an older term and no longer in common use. It is a measure of stiffness.

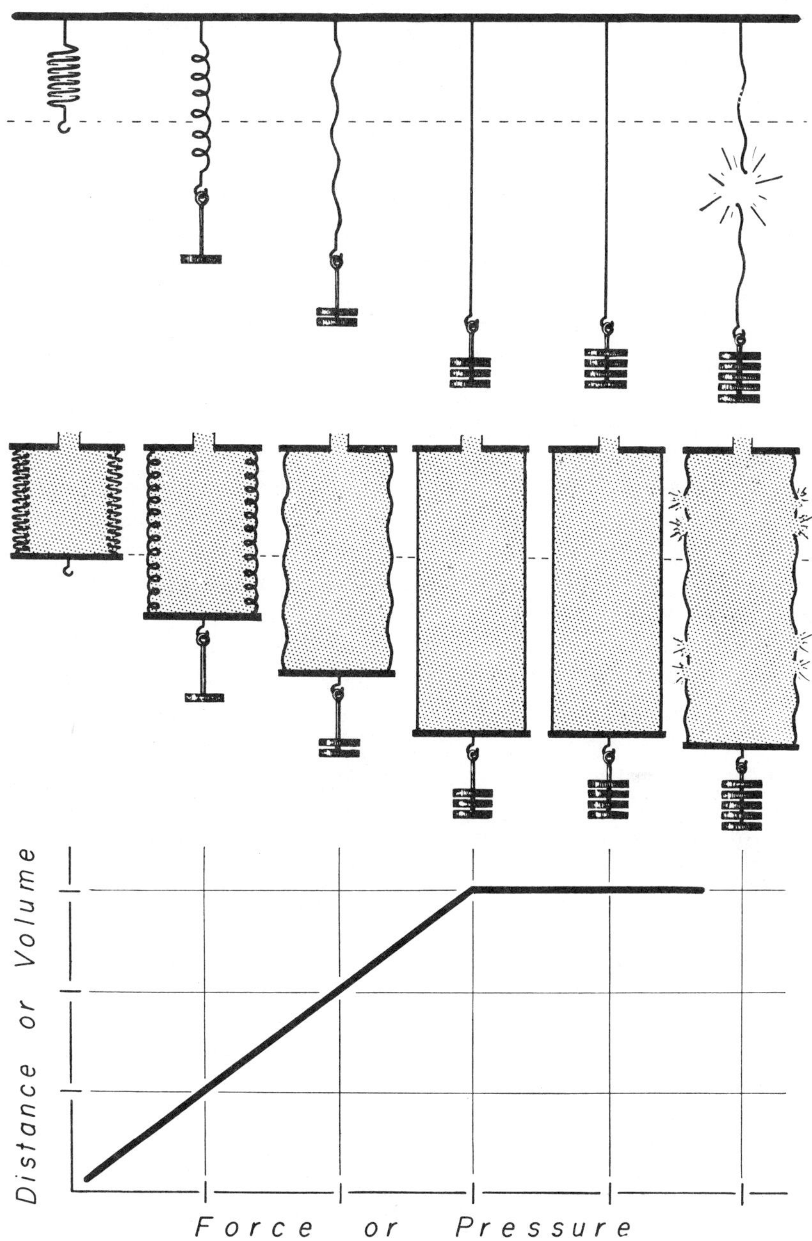

Fig 22.—For an elastic structure, the increase in length (or volume) varies directly with the increase in force (or pressure) until the elastic limit is reached. This linear relationship applies equally to normal lungs, over the physiologic range.

TABLE 5.—MEASUREMENT OF COMPLIANCE AND RESISTANCE

	DEFINITION	UNITS	MEASUREMENTS REQUIRED	CONDITIONS OF MEASUREMENT
Compliance	Volume change produced by a unit pressure change	L/cm H_2O	Pressure and volume	Static
Resistance	Pressure differential required for a unit flow change	cm H_2O/L/sec	Pressure and flow	Dynamic

Therefore *compliance* is used in considering *static* pressure-volume relationships and *resistance* in speaking of *dynamic* pressure-flow relationships (Table 5).

The system pictured in Figure 22 is a single elastic system; it has only one set of "springs." Actually, the elastic forces can be analyzed in terms of the elastic properties of the *lungs* ("lung springs") and the elastic properties of the thoracic cage ("thoracic springs") (Fig 23). The resting position of the lungs alone (out of the thorax, exposed to atmospheric pressure, and with no stretching force applied) is at the minimal air volume, which is less than residual volume. The resting position of the thoracic cage alone (lungs removed and no stretching or compressing force applied) is at a much greater volume, estimated by some to be about 55% of the vital capacity. The resting position of the lungs *and* thoracic cage, held *together* normally by the pleural surfaces, is somewhere between these two positions. This balanced or neutral position is called the *resting expiratory level,* and the contained gas volume at this level is the *functional residual capacity* (FRC). At this position, the "lung springs" are somewhat stretched and the thoracic springs somewhat compressed. Muscular energy is necessary to unbalance the lung-thoracic cage system toward either inspiration or further expiration. When the lungs and thoracic cage are acting together as a unit (as they normally do), they require more force for expansion to a given volume than does either component alone. Thus, if the compliance of the lung is 0.2 L/cm H_2O and that of the thoracic cage is also 0.2 L/cm H_2O, the compliance of the lungs and thoracic cage together (in series) is 0.1 L/cm H_2O.

$$\frac{1}{\text{Compliance (total)}} = \frac{1}{\text{Compliance (lungs)}} + \frac{1}{\text{Compliance (thoracic cage)}}$$

Measurement of Pulmonary Compliance

It is possible to determine the elastic pressure acting on the lungs alone by measuring the static "transpulmonary pressure." This is shown in

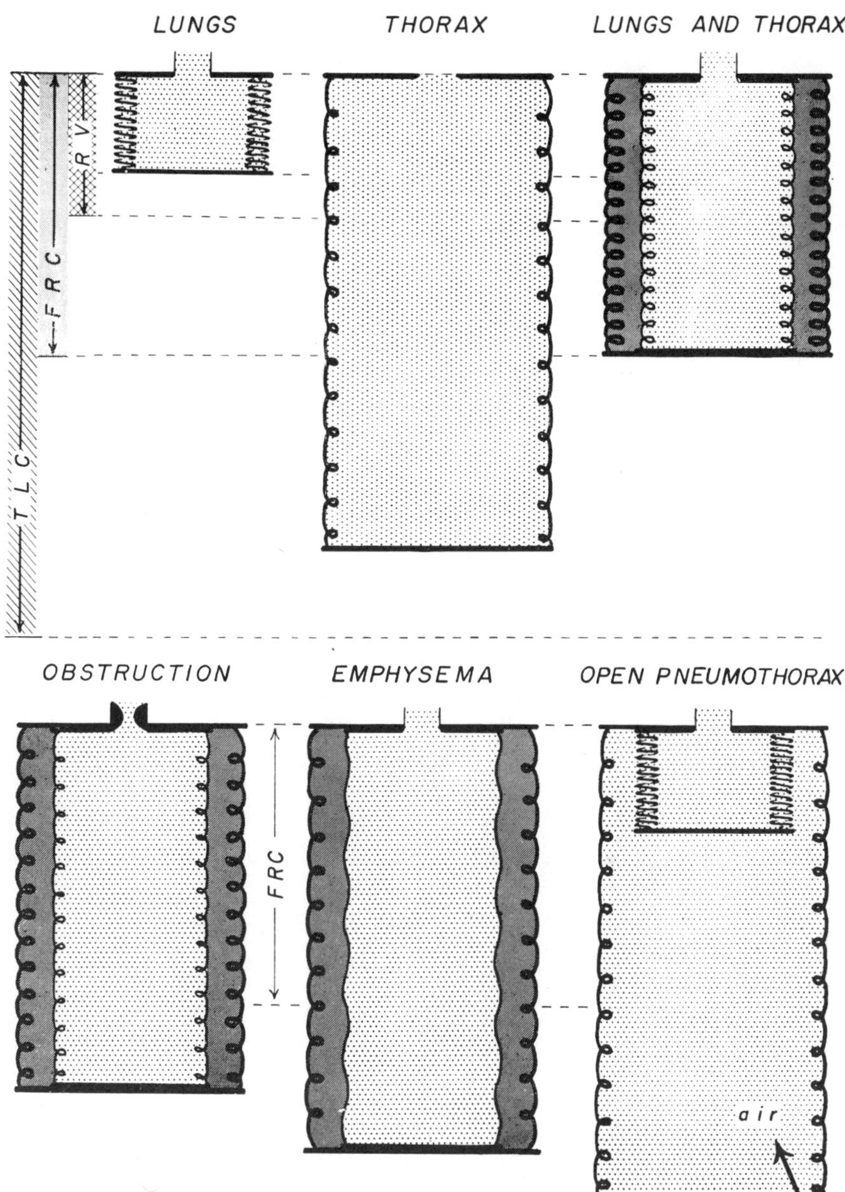

Fig 23.—*Top, left,* resting position of the lungs along; *middle,* resting position of the thoracic cage alone; *right,* resting position of the lungs and thoracic cage held together in normal manner by their pleural surfaces. *Bottom,* changes from normal resting position of the combined lungs and thoracic cage caused by obstruction, emphysema, or open pneumothorax. Dotted areas represent air-containing regions. Inner springs represent elastic tissues of the lungs; outer springs represent elastic tissues of the thoracic cage. Dark gray areas denote contact between visceral and parietal pleura.

Figure 24 *(2)*, as the pressure differential between the pleural space and the mouth. Transpulmonary pressure must be measured by getting between the lung and the chest wall (inside the chest but outside the lung). Because of the possibility of lung puncture, it is dangerous to measure intrapleural pressure directly in some patients with pulmonary disease, but a satisfactory approximation of changes in intrapleural pressure can be obtained by measuring pressure in the esophagus through a small tube or balloon in the esophagus with the patient sitting or semirecumbent. The esophagus is sufficiently passive so that the pressure changes follow accurately those outside the lungs but inside the chest wall. Because the esophagus has a slight tone of its own, the intra-esophageal balloon records pressure changes more faithfully than it measures absolute intrathoracic pressure.

Ideally, transpulmonary pressure should be measured under static conditions (no air flow) at a series of different inspiratory volumes. The patient with an esophageal balloon in the proper location is asked to inspire maximally from a spirometer, expire to a predetermined volume, then hold his breath while the new transpulmonary (mouth pressure minus esophageal) pressure is measured.* The procedure† is repeated several times at different volumes, and a pressure volume curve is constructed (multiple-breath technique, Fig 25,A). The pressure-volume curve is usually linear over the range normally used (although it is not when very large volumes above or below FRC are used). The compliance computed is, of course, an average value for the lungs. Compliance for individual lungs can be measured during bronchospirometry.

A pressure-volume curve can also be obtained from simultaneous records of (esophageal pressure–mouth pressure) and expired volume during a single slow expiration through a valve that periodically blocks expired flow momentarily (single-breath interrupted technique, Fig 25,B). When flow stops, the increment of alveolar pressure needed to produce gas flow through the airways disappears, the esophageal pressure decreases (becomes more negative) by the same amount, and al-

*Transpulmonary pressure can be measured satisfactorily with a differential strain gauge manometer.

†The lungs demonstrate considerable hysteresis; that is, the volume at a given transpulmonary pressure depends on the previous history of the lungs. For example, in Figure 25,A, the open circle point was obtained by inspiring to that volume from FRC. The volume is much less than that on the continuous curve at the same esophageal pressure, which was obtained by inspiring maximally (after several deep breaths) and then expiring to the same esophageal pressure as for the open circle point. Pressure-volume curves must be obtained by a similar procedure to be comparable, usually during expiration after a maximal inspiration, as in this example.

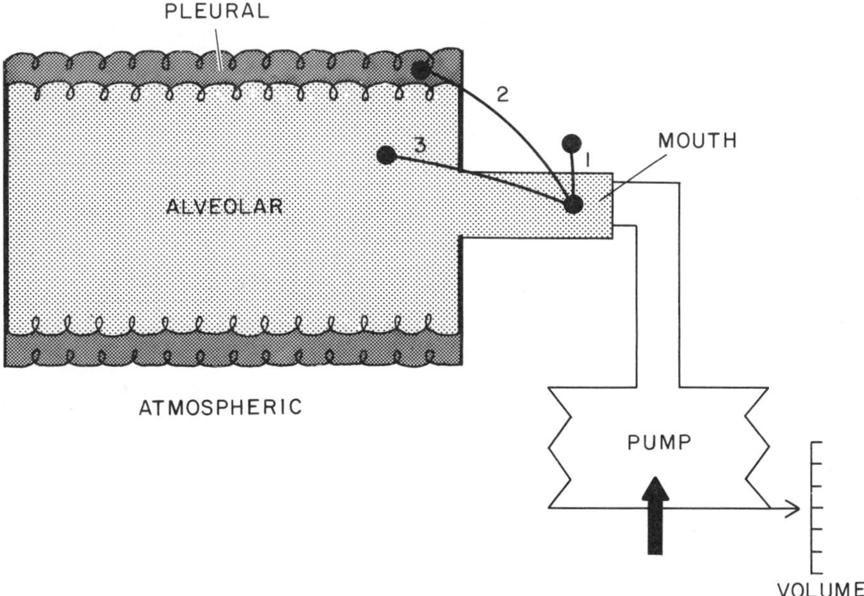

Fig 24.—Pressures concerned in the definition of thoracic mechanical properties. Schematic representation of the lungs and thorax is the same as in Figure 23. On inspiration, the pump (bellows) increases pressure in the airway above that in the lungs and air enters the lungs from the pump. The volume (at the increase of pressure) is indicated on the scale. On expiration pressure in the pump falls to atmospheric, and the unopposed elastic pressure of lungs and thorax produces expiration. The following pressure differences are measured continuously: *1,* transthoracic pressure (pressure difference between atmosphere and the mouth); *2,* transpulmonary pressure (pressure difference between the pleural cavity and mouth); *3,* airway pressure gradient (pressure difference between mouth and alveoli).

AIRWAY PRESSURE GRADIENT

PRESSURE DIFFERENCE	MEASURES	STATIC MEASUREMENT (if related to change in vol) PROVIDES DATA FOR CALCULATION OF:	DYNAMIC MEASUREMENT (if related to air flow) PROVIDES DATA FOR CALCULATION OF:
3	Airway pressure gradient		Airway resistance
2	Transpulmonary pressure	Pulmonary compliance	Pulmonary resistance* (tissue and airway)
1	Transthoracic pressure	Total compliance (pulmonary and thoracic)	Total respiratory resistance (pulmonary and thoracic)

*After subtracting pressure to overcome elastic recoil.

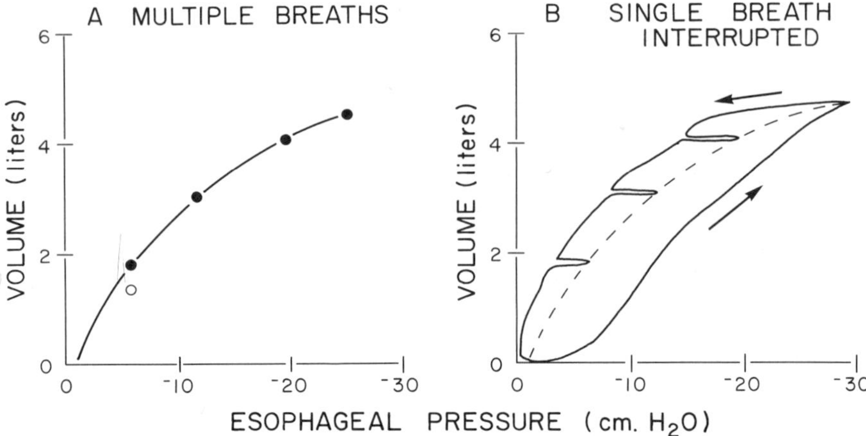

Fig 25.—Measurement of the lung pressure-volume curve and compliance. *Panel A, multiple breath technique.* The patient makes a maximal inspiration from residual volume and then expires to a given volume, holding his breath with open glottis at this point until the intraesophageal pressure stabilizes. This procedure is repeated for each experimental point and a curve connecting the points is constructed. It is necessary to follow the same procedure or lung hysteresis will alter the values. To obtain the point indicated by the open circle, the patient merely inspires from residual volume to the particular volume without first making a maximal inspiration. The intrapleural pressure is more negative than when the full correct procedure is used. *Panel B, the single-breath interrupted technique.* The patient inspires slowly from residual volume to vital capacity and then slowly expires. As he is breathing out the expiratory flow is interrupted (see Fig 31) long enough to permit the intrapleural pressure (minus mouth pressure) to stabilize. Each time this is done one point on the static pressure volume curve is obtained and the curve *(dotted line)* constructed between the points. Compliance is calculated as the change in volume per change in pressure over any particular region of the curve, generally around FRC. In both methods A and B, pressure on the abscissa is that across the lung, intrapleural (or esophageal) minus airway pressure. In method A, airway pressure equals atmospheric pressure, against which esophageal pressure is measured. In method B, airway pressure is not equal to atmospheric pressure so that esophageal pressure minus airway pressure should be plotted.

veolar pressure becomes equal to mouth pressure. The elastic pressure across the lung becomes equal to (esophageal pressure–mouth pressure) producing one point on the static pressure-volume curve. The dashed line in Figure 25,B, connecting similar points is thus a true static pressure-volume curve.

It is also possible to estimate compliance of healthy individuals by constructing pressure-volume curves during a series of tidal volumes of increasing depth, without breath holding. Figure 26 illustrates the principle involved; continuous recording of pressure and volume is required. Since compliance by definition should be measured under static conditions, values of volume and intraesophageal pressure must be selected only at points where there is no flow. Figure 26 shows points of "no-flow" at end-inspiration and end-expiration. Theoretically, at these points all of the transpulmonary pressure acts to balance the elastic recoil of the lung; none of it is needed to overcome frictional resistance since there is no net airflow out of the mouth. This value of compliance is called *dynamic compliance,* since it is not measured under truly static conditions. In healthy persons, pressure-volume slopes constructed in this way are usually quite similar to those curves obtained during static conditions.

Another method of obtaining dynamic compliance is to measure continuously respired gas volume (by rapidly responding spirometer or integrating pneumotachograph) and transpulmonary (esophageal) pressure during cyclic breathing, recording volume on the x-axis and change in esophageal pressure on the y-axis of a cathode ray oscilloscope. A loop is obtained (Fig 26,B). The change in esophageal pressure includes not only elastic pressure during inspiration and expiration, but also the pressure needed to produce flow in the resistance airways, lung tissue, and lung tissue hysteresis. These resistance components can be compensated by subtracting electrically a voltage proportional to the air flow rate. In practice this is easily done by varying the magnitude of the subtracted voltage until the loop becomes a line.

In many patients with pulmonary disease, and in some normal persons, pressure-volume curves constructed *during* breathing, especially at a rapid rate, yield values for *dynamic compliance* that are much lower than those obtained under static conditions. This is called frequency dependence of compliance.

The explanation for the frequency-dependence of dynamic lung compliance is based on the concept of "time-constants." Different lung regions fill and empty in different lengths of time, depending on how fast the air flows into them, against "resistance" to airflow and tissue movement, and how much air they can contain when full, limited by elastic recoil or compliance. Since the resistance and compliance both govern the time required to fill a given region, the characteristic time to fill that region, called its "time constant," is its resistance multiplied by its compliance.

$$\begin{matrix}\text{time constant} \\ \text{of region A}\end{matrix} = \begin{matrix}\text{resistance} \\ \text{of region A}\end{matrix} \times \begin{matrix}\text{compliance} \\ \text{of region A}\end{matrix}$$

$$\begin{matrix}\text{time constant} \\ \text{of region B}\end{matrix} = \begin{matrix}\text{resistance} \\ \text{of region B}\end{matrix} \times \begin{matrix}\text{compliance} \\ \text{of region B}\end{matrix}$$

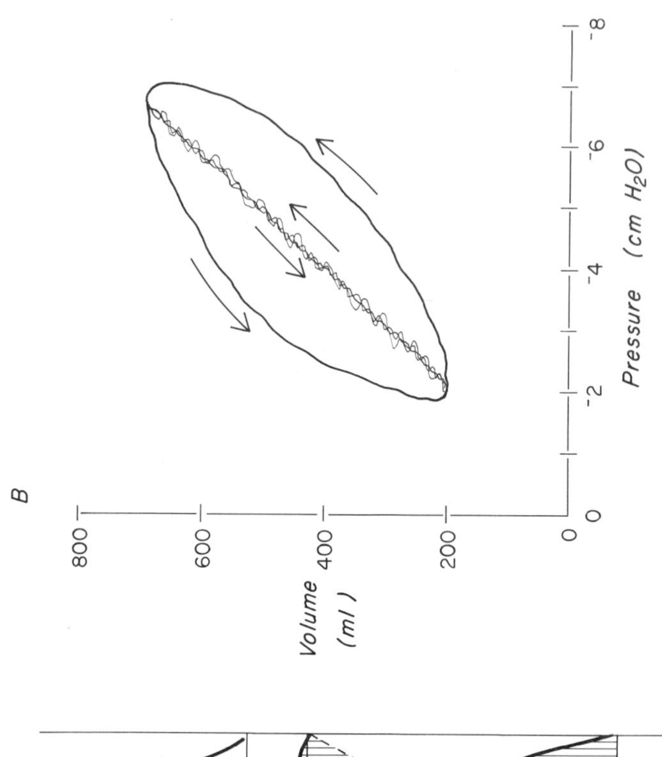
B
Volume
(ml)
800
600
400
200
0
0
-2
-4
-6
-8
Pressure (cm H_2O)

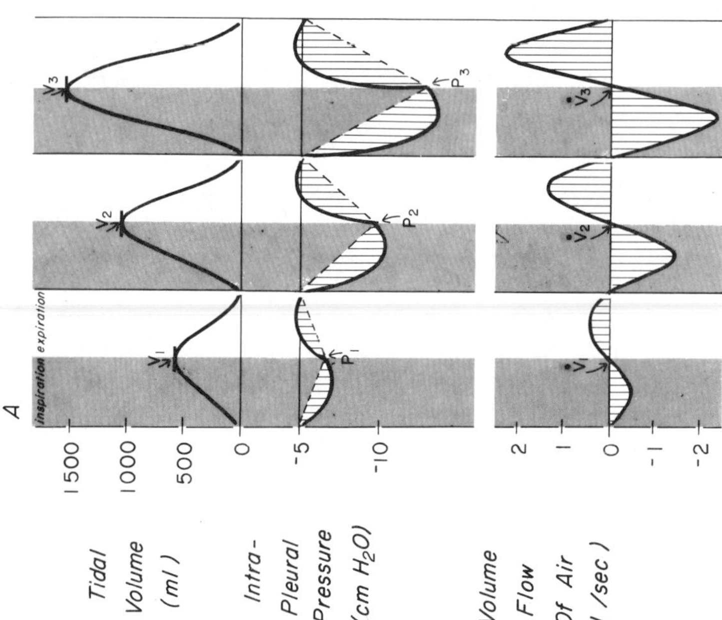
A
Tidal
Volume
(ml)
1500
1000
500
0
inspiration
expiration
V_1
V_2
V_3
Intra-
Pleural
Pressure
(cm H_2O)
-5
-10
P_1
P_2
P_3
Volume
Flow
Of Air
(l/sec)
2
1
0
-1
-2

Fig 26.—The measurement of *dynamic* compliance. *Panel A,* tidal volume, intrapleural (or esophageal) pressure, and volume flow of air are measured continuously and simultaneously, for three breaths, each deeper than the preceding one. At the end of inspiration, there is no air flow ($\dot{V}_1$, $\dot{V}_2$, and $\dot{V}_3$ = zero), and therefore the total transpulmonary pressure should be only that necessary to overcome elastic resistance. A pressure-volume curve can therefore be plotted from V_1 and P_1, V_2 and P_2, and V_3 and P_3. While these conditions are reasonably static in healthy lungs, in many diseased lungs with nonuniform distribution of inspired gas, even though total air flow at the mouth may be zero at the peak volume points (V_1, V_2, and V_3), gas may still be flowing from one region of the lung to another, so that the lung is not under static conditions. Measurement of compliance in this manner is *dynamic.* If there were no tissue and airway resistance, transpulmonary pressure would be required only to overcome elastic resistance; intrapleural pressure fluctuation during the respiratory cycle would then follow the straight lines (if the inspired and expired volumes were linear with respect to time). However, tissue and airway resistances do exist and additional pressure (that between the straight and the curved lines on the intrapleural pressure record) is required to overcome these (see Fig 33). *Panel B,* electrical subtraction method of measuring dynamic compliance. Intrapleural (or esophageal) pressure is displayed on the X axis and volume (integrated air flow) displayed on the Y axis of a cathode ray oscilloscope or X-Y recorder, producing the loop seen. Then an electrical voltage proportional to the instantaneous air flow is subtracted from the pressure signal and its magnitude adjusted to produce the straight line. This procedure subtracts a pressure equivalent to (air + tissue resistance) from the intrapleural pressure, leaving only the elastic pressure (the sign of this subtracted signal changes of course as air flow reverses direction). The slope of the line, volume/pressure, is dynamic compliance.

If one region has a shorter time constant than another, it fills more rapidly and is full earlier. A region with higher resistance or a larger compliance fills more slowly. With to-and-fro breathing, regions slow to fill may be incompletely filled at the moment when the individual starts to breathe out. This limits the volume entering that region to less than its full capacity. For this reason, volume change of the whole lung for a given inflation pressure is less than it would have been if breathing frequency had been slower and duration of each breath longer. Or, as breathing becomes more frequent, whole lung expansion becomes less. Apparent compliance of the whole lung ($\Delta V/\Delta P$) becomes less because ΔV becomes less for a given change in transpulmonary elastic pressure.

In lung diseases that affect different regions to a different extent, the tissue mechanical time constants are apt to differ. What this means is that in these patients static compliance cannot be estimated correctly by measuring dynamic compliance. However, a reduction of dynamic lung compliance measured at increased breathing frequency has been used to signal regional lung disease. A problem with the dynamic compliance test is that narrowing an air passage to half its diameter causes flow resistance to increase 16 times, virtually shutting off airflow to that region and eliminating its gas exchange at any practical breathing frequency except an abnormally slow rate. A decrease in diameter of this magnitude ought to be detected by any test for early lung disease. However, if 20% of the lungs fail to take part in a given test of lung function, this might not be interpreted as "abnormal" because "normal" values have a range of about $\pm 20\%$ around an average value predicted according to age, sex, height, and weight. Unfortunately, extensive or even incipient lung disease of 20% of the lungs is a serious portent of impending future disaster. This dilemma has not been solved.

Regional Expansion of the Lung

The alveoli in different regions of the lung in a sitting patient operate at different regions of their P-V curves at any given volume for the whole lung. Those at the base are less distended because of the lower transpulmonary pressure (more positive intrapleural pressure) at the base of the lung (or more simply, from the weight of the lung itself). Those at the apex are more distended, because of the greater transpulmonary pressure (more negative intrapleural pressure Fig 27, *left*). Those alveoli in the middle regions of the lung lie in between. Of course the alveoli in addition may have different P-V curves although the distension of externalized lungs with equal transpulmonary pressure throughout is remarkably uniform (Fig 27, *right*). The apical alveoli are more expanded in the normal breathing range (above FRC) (see discussion of closing volume, chapter 3). With a maximal inspiration beginning from residual volume, the effective change in alveolar volume is greater at the apex so the first part of an inspiration goes there; the later parts go to the more basilar alveoli. This gives rise to the "first gas in, last gas out" phenomenon, for when expiration occurs, the basal alveoli empty first.

If the patient is supine, the lower, or dorsal, alveoli are less distended than the upper, or ventral, alveoli, and the same relative

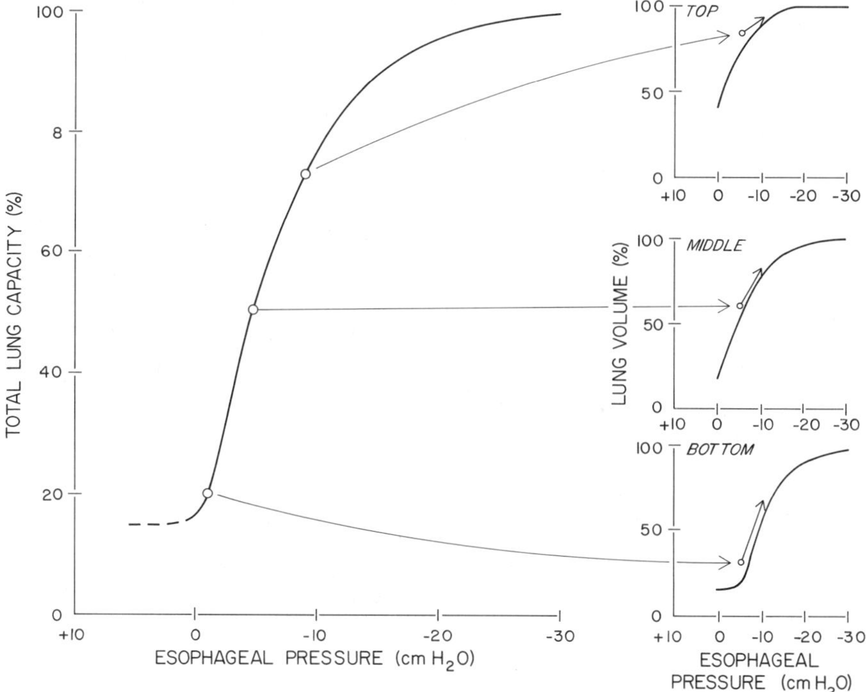

Fig 27.—Variations in the relative volume of different regions of the lung with midlung intrapleural pressure (esophageal pressure). All regions are considered to have the same pressure-volume curve, but transpulmonary pressure at the apex is about 4 cm of water more negative than in the middle region of the lung, while at the base it is 4 cm more positive. The three panels show volume for the top, middle, and bottom regions of lung plotted against esophageal pressure (transpulmonary pressure in the middle of the lung). The arrows indicate the volume excursions for a change of 5 cm of water in esophageal pressure over the normal tidal breathing range (-5 cm H_2O to -10 cm H_2O).

changes in volume occur, although the magnitude of the differences is reduced because of the shorter anterior-posterior depth of the thorax.

Measurement of Compliance of Lung-Thoracic Cage System

Figure 22 (p. 67) shows schematically how the elastic properties or the compliance of the lungs and thoracic cage may be measured by static pressure-volume measurements at different lung volumes. In actual practice, this measurement can be made in one of three ways:

1. A patient whose breathing has been suspended voluntarily or because of disease is intubated with a cuffed tracheal catheter or fitted with an air-tight mask (Fig 24) so that transthoracic pressure (*1* in Fig 24) can be measured. Measurement of the volume of air inspired at each of several positive pressure levels in the airway yields data for a pressure-volume curve.

2. The chest of an anesthetized patient is inflated through a cuffed endotracheal tube. The tube is occluded and the pressure measured under static conditions in the tube-lung system. The pressure measured is transthoracic (alveolar pressure-atmospheric pressure around the thorax). The volume change above the resting expiratory level caused by this inflating pressure is measured by opening the tube and measuring the volume of gas expired into a spirometer. The procedure is repeated at several volumes and a pressure-volume curve plotted.

3. A normal subject inspires a measured volume of gas from a spirometer, then closes his nose and mouth, opens his glottis, and relaxes his muscles of respiration. The elastic recoil of the lungs and thorax is now unopposed by active contraction of the inspiratory muscles; this produces an alveolar pressure (transthoracic) that can be measured by a mouth or nasal tube, because in a static system such as this, oral pressure equals alveolar pressure. Repetition of this procedure several times at different volumes produces a "relaxation pressure curve." Figures for compliance obtained by this method are larger and more variable than those for the second method mentioned because most subjects cannot completely relax their inspiratory muscles.

Although the pressure-volume relationship may yield a curved rather than a straight line, a value for compliance (volume change per unit pressure change) obtained over the usual range of tidal volumes may be used to compare the compliance of the lungs and thoracic cage in different individuals.

Measurement of Compliance of the Thoracic Cage

If data are obtained simultaneously for compliance of the lungs alone and of the lungs and thoracic cage together, one can calculate the compliance of the thoracic cage alone, using the equation on page 68.

Interpretation of Data For Compliance

Values for compliance, to have any diagnostic meaning, must be related to a predicted normal value for a person of the same lung volume. Equations for predicting normal values are given in Table 19 (p. 255).

'Static' Pulmonary Compliance

"Static" pulmonary compliance deals only with the elastic forces in the lung. *Dynamic compliance* includes these forces plus those of overcoming resistance in phase with lung volume, produced by slow regional time constants. Any difference between static and dynamic compliance implies differences in time constants of different parts of the lung.

Effect of Lung Volume

Pulmonary compliance varies with the initial volume of the alveoli that are to be distended by the applied transpulmonary pressure. If a change in transpulmonary pressure of 5 cm H_2O results in a volume change of 1 L, the compliance of the lungs is 1/5, or 0.2 L/cm H_2O. However, the volume change in one of the two lungs will be only 0.5 L (for the same change in transmural pressure), and compliance of one lung will thus be 0.5/5, or 0.1 L/cm H_2O. For one of the three right lobes, the volume change may be only 0.15 L and the compliance for one lobe only 0.15/5, or 0.03 L/cm H_2O. This does not mean that the tissues of one lobe or of one lung are stiffer than those of the two lungs measured together or that they differ in their elastic tissue components; it simply means that compliance is not really a meaningful term unless related to the amount of lung undergoing expansion. If one wishes to compare the elastic properties of the lungs of a newborn with those of a child or adult, one can correct for (in part) the difference in lung size by calculating the ratio:

$$\frac{\text{Volume change/original lung volume}}{\text{Pressure change}} \text{ or } \frac{\text{Compliance*}}{\text{FRC}}$$

*Compliance/FRC has been termed "specific" lung compliance or "distensibility."

Lung compliance "adapts" to a change in lung volume. If the lung is maintained at a reduced volume by placing elastic straps around the chest wall, compliance decreases and the intrapleural pressure at that lower volume becomes more negative, tending to restore it to its value at a more normal lung volume. Conversely, if a larger than normal lung volume is maintained, lung compliance is increased, again tending to make intrapleural pressure less negative and restoring it toward a more normal value. This tightening and relaxing process has been ascribed to changes in the surface tension of the alveolar walls.

The pulmonary compliance of newborn infants on this basis is 0.065 L/cm H_2O per liter of FRC, and that of adults is between 0.05 and 0.06.

If one wishes to relate the compliance of asthmatic, emphysematous, atelectatic, congested, pneumonic, or edematous lungs to that of normal lungs, one must know the FRC in each case, simply because the compliance of normal lungs changes directly with changes in FRC.

Tissues That Have 'Elastic Recoil'

Histologically identifiable elastic fibers, with characteristic staining properties, possess elastic properties. In addition, collagen, the reticulum of the lungs, pleura, bronchi and blood vessels, the surface tension of alveolar gas-liquid interfaces, the smooth muscle of bronchi and lungs, the pulmonary blood volume and bronchial mucus may be partly responsible for the elastic properties of the lungs. Similarly, numerous tissues may contribute to the elastic properties of the thoracic cage. Consequently, when one finds changes in compliance/FRC, one should not infer that these are due to changes in elastic fibers without studying also the other tissues or materials that contribute to the pressure-volume curve of the lung.

Of particular interest is a surface film presumed to line the alveoli that has remarkable surface tension–lowering properties. The first clue to this film and its properties was Von Neergaard's discovery that saline-filled lungs inflated considerably more for a unit change in transpulmonary pressure than did air-filled lungs. The conclusion was that air-filled lungs have greater elastic recoil than saline-filled lungs and that the difference is due to the surface tension of the air-water interface (this film acts as though it were elastic tissue in this respect). If this alveolar film were pure water or saline with a surface tension of 70 dynes/cm, its surface force would be great enough to cause alveolar instability and collapse. However, alveolar cells produce and secrete a phospholipid-protein material ("lung surfactant"), which can lower the surface tension of an air-water interface to extremely low levels (2 to 8 dynes/cm in the compressed state). This material helps to maintain alveolar stability. Pulmonary compliance can be modified by the quantity and type of material formed, and the concentration and condition of this material at the liquid-gas surface. The amount or characteristics of this surfactive material may be deficient in premature infants and in adults can be altered in many ways and in a relatively short time. In comparison, the elastic fibers of the lung are less labile.

Usefulness of Measurements of Compliance

1. When pulmonary compliance or maximal end-inspiratory esophageal pressure is abnormal, some pulmonary abnormality is present. The primary abnormality may, of course, be a change in FRC. When compliance/FRC is abnormal, one should suspect a change in the quantity or quality of the tissues of the lung, the presence of pulmonary edema, or an alteration in the surfactant lining the pulmonary alveoli.

2. Suitable measurements enable the physician to know whether a decrease in compliance is due to changes in the lungs, in the thoracic cage, or in both. This knowledge is useful therapeutically as well as diagnostically. For example, if the patient is unable to provide enough ventilation by his own muscular effort, methods providing much higher positive pressures may be used safely if it is the thoracic cage that is uncompliant. This is because alveoli rupture only when overdistended, and overdistention is caused only by large *trans*pulmonary pressures. Decreased compliance of the lungs is apt to be nonuniform, and a pressure that produces little ventilation of some regions may overdistend and even rupture alveoli in other regions. On the other hand, decrease in thoracic compliance usually affects the whole thorax and prevents grossly uneven alveolar distention at high inflation pressures.

3. Knowledge of the physical characteristics of the lungs and thorax enables the physician to select the proper type of mechanical resuscitator for a patient, and the anesthesiologist to provide the proper controlled ventilation for the lungs (in operations with the thorax open) or for the lungs and thorax (when the thorax is intact).

4. In cases requiring determination of pulmonary disability, measurements of compliance provide objective data on one type of physical basis for dyspnea and disability.

Pulmonary Compliance in Disease

Pulmonary Congestion

Normal resting lung compliance (uncorrected, for changes in lung volume) is decreased slightly when experimental pulmonary congestion is produced by sudden inflation of a pressure suit around the abdomen and legs or by rapid IV infusion of large volumes of fluid. Below resting lung volume, experimental increase in transpulmonary vascular pressure of 15 cm H_2O slightly increases the compliance of air-filled lungs, showing that full blood vessels help keep the air spaces open.

Pulmonary Edema

Compliance is reduced when edema fluid is present in the alveoli. The decrease is presumably out of proportion to the changes in FRC. Here, surface tension forces may be altered because of change in the character of the alveolar phospholipid film or because of changes in the geometric configuration of the air sacs. Froth may block additional bronchioles and prevent expansion of otherwise normal alveoli.

Restrictive Disease of the Lungs

Compliance is reduced in patients with pleural or interstitial fibrosis. This decrease is out of proportion to the reduction in FRC. It is known that collagen and "scar" tissue have length-tension (or pressure-volume) relationships different from those of elastic tissue. If, however, the affected areas receive no ventilation and become airless, FRC is reduced at the same time. Similar changes occur after repeated bouts of congestion accompanying mitral stenosis. Chest-strapping reduces pulmonary compliance but also reduces FRC. Fibrosis or sclerosis of the pulmonary vessels does not appear to alter pulmonary compliance.

Emphysema

When compliance is measured by static methods, it is usually increased in patients with emphysema. When measured during breathing, especially during rapid breathing ("dynamic" compliance), it is less than normal. The pressure-volume curve is usually shifted toward the left, which means that less transpulmonary pressure is required to maintain the lungs at FRC (or that normal transpulmonary pressure results in a large FRC). Maximal end-inspiratory esophageal pressure is less negative than normal. Figure 23 (*bottom,* center) shows that if there were complete loss of elastic recoil of the lungs but that of the thoracic cage remained normal, the thorax would enlarge toward its neutral position.

Other Lung Diseases

Compliance (uncorrected) is decreased in atelectasis and pneumonia.

Contraction of Bronchiolar Smooth Muscle

The compliance of saline-filled lungs of animals does not change when bronchoconstriction is produced. Presumably, the change of smooth muscle to a more contracted state does not change measurably the distensibility of the lung.

When airways are occluded in man by spasm, edema, congestion, or mucus, one would expect uncorrected compliance to decrease, and to decrease markedly when measured during rapid breathing. Tubocurarine (known to cause histamine release and bronchoconstriction) may decrease compliance (uncorrected); other muscle relaxants do not.

Thoracic Disorders

Poliomyelitis and kyphoscoliosis are often associated with changes in the lung characterized by decreased compliance (uncorrected); in some cases, compliance/FRC is decreased.

Pulmonary Artery Obstruction

Pulmonary artery ligation in the dog is followed, in several days, by a pronounced decrease in pulmonary compliance associated with congestive atelectasis; these changes are accompanied by decrease in the activity of the alveolar surfactant (noted as an increase in the surface tension of lung extracts). Compliance returns to normal in several weeks.

Anesthesia

General anesthesia in man is sometimes associated with a decrease in pulmonary compliance, possibly because of closure of alveolar units.

Vagotomy

In animals, bilateral vagotomy is followed by an increase in compliance but no change in compliance/FRC.

Hypothermia

In man, no change in compliance was noted after reduction of body temperature to 29°C.

Thoracic Cage Compliance in Disease

This may be decreased in patients with kyphoscoliosis (idiopathic, tuberculous, postpoliomyelitic), pectus excavatum, arthritic spondylitis following thoracoplasty, skeletal muscle diseases associated with spasticity or rigidity, and in abdominal disorders characterized by marked elevation of the diaphragm (the diaphragm and attached abdominal viscera represent one component of the thoracic cage). It may also be decreased in patients with marked obesity (Pickwickian types).

Effect of Decreased Compliance on the Patient

1. Decreased compliance forces the patient to do more muscular work to achieve adequate alveolar ventilation; this is particularly true when tidal volume is large (p. 100). Increased respiratory muscular effort is often associated with dyspnea and may eventually lead to fatigue and failure of the respiratory muscles. On the other hand, regularly repeated bouts of effort strengthen the breathing muscles just as physical training strengthens them elsewhere in the body.

Pulmonary compliance may be as low as 0.01 L/cm H_2O, or 5% of predicted normal value, in patients with severe diffuse alveolar fibrosis and diffuse carcinomatosis of the lungs. In such patients, a pressure differential of 50 cm H_2O would be required to inflate the lungs with 500 ml of air. Such pressures are greater than patients can produce over long periods and in excess of that routinely considered safe for a respirator.

2. Diseases altering pulmonary compliance rarely alter it uniformly throughout the lung. Uneven compliance (assuming that the intrathoracic pressure acting on the lung surface is uniform throughout) must lead to uneven expansion in different regions of the lung at end-inspiration; this contributes to uneven ventilation/blood flow ratios and nonuniform gas tensions.

The lung tissue distributes the force of elastic recoil by means of a network of fibers connecting the alveolar walls, and peribronchial spaces to the visceral pleura. In homogenous lungs the negative pleural pressure is transmitted by this pressure network to each of these internal surfaces. Picture a series of rubber bands tied end to end, with the far ends held between the fingers of each hand. Stretching out this linear array causes a recoil force on the fingers. All the rubber bands stretch the same amount, showing that this recoil force, or tension, is the same in each rubber band. Now suppose that instead of tying the ends of the rubber bands to each other we were to connect them to the walls of a bronchus or blood vessel. The force or pressure pulling on the wall would equal the force or pressure pulling on the pleural surface represented in this model by the fingers. Forces distribute equally throughout a homogenous elastic structure, whether linear, as described, or two dimensional, as a fishing net, or three dimensional, as a sponge or the lungs.

In nonhomogenous lungs, elastic forces pull unequally on different internal regions. Collapsed areas overstretch adjacent elastic fibers, which in turn exert a tension that tends to reopen the collapsed areas, particularly during a deep inspiration. On the other hand, a regional loss of elastic fibers reduces the tension on adjacent structures, letting them collapse, particularly during expiration. A chronic inflammatory process around a small bronchus may destroy the peribronchial tissue; this bronchus then collapses at the end of expiration because it lacks the external tension required to keep it open. Stiffening (fibrosis or edema) of lung tissue may cause a large negative pressure around the blood vessels during inspiration, causing transudation of fluid into the perivascular spaces. This perivascular fluid cuff shows up on chest x-ray films taken during the incipient stage of pulmonary edema.

3. Because of the increased energy requirement of deep breathing, especially when compliance is reduced, patients with low compliance usually breathe more rapidly and less deeply than do normal subjects (p. 100). As a rule, patients with decreased compliance (and no significant airway obstruction) have a normal or near-normal maximal voluntary ventilation (MVV) (p. 113), until vital capacity is reduced to 50% or less.

B. LUNG SURFACTANT

A decrease in the effective concentration of surfactant in the lungs can lower compliance. Surfactant can be sampled from an adult patient by performing segmental lung lavage, that is, washing the alveoli in a localized area of lung through a bronchoscope. The material washed out can be analyzed chemically or physically by measuring the tension-reducing effect of lung lavage material on the air-water interface in a Langmuir trough, when the surface film area is compressed. The failure of measured tension to lower to the normal range of 2 to 8 dynes/cm indicates the lack of sufficient material or the presence of inhibitory substances. The stability of bubbles in the lung lavage fluid is increased by surfactant, and represents another technique to measure its presence. At present, it is difficult to relate the recovery of surfactant to the events occurring at the alveolar level, and the test has limited diagnostic usefulness in the adult patient.

In order to detect a deficiency of lung surfactant in a fetus we can analyze the (lecithin*)/(sphingomyelin) in fluid obtained by amniocentesis. The primary surface-active component of lung surfactant is dipalmitoyl phosphatidyl choline, a form of phosphatidyl choline in which both fatty acids are palmitic. Analyzing lecithin, or better dipalmitoyl phosphatidyl choline, itself gives a measure of the amount of surfactant material secreted by the lung into the amniotic fluid. Sphingomyelin is a phospholipid that has no surface active properties and its concentration in the lung does not increase appreciably during gestation. Thus it provides a convenient reference for the total concentration of phospholipid in the amniotic fluid.

(Lecithin)/(sphingomyelin) increases during gestation, and its value provides an index of the maturity of the fetal lung. Phosphatidyl glycerol can be measured as well. It appears also to increase with gestation and is related to the appearance of surface active material, paralleling the concentration of dipalmitoyl phosphatidyl choline.

C. AIRWAY RESISTANCE

Just as a driving pressure is necessary in the circulation to pump blood through the arteriolar, capillary, and venular resistances (p. 137), so a driving pressure is necessary during inspiration to pull air through the upper airway, bronchial, and bronchiolar resistances into the alveoli and during expiration to push alveolar gas out through these tubes (Fig 28). The same equation applies as for blood flow:

$$\text{Resistance} = \frac{\text{driving pressure}}{\text{flow}}$$

The driving pressure along the airways is the airway pressure (*3* in Fig 24, p. 71), which is atmospheric pressure minus alveolar pressure during inspiration and alveolar pressure minus atmospheric pressure during expiration. The units are cm H_2O/L per second.

Airway resistance is created by friction between molecules of the flowing gas and between the gas molecules and the walls of the tubes.† When flow is laminar or streamlined (Fig 28), airway resistance varies

*Lecithin is the trivial name for phosphatidyl choline.

†In the case of a gas, the "friction" really means the momentum exchanged between molecules wandering back and forth across the stream, like cars entering a freeway.

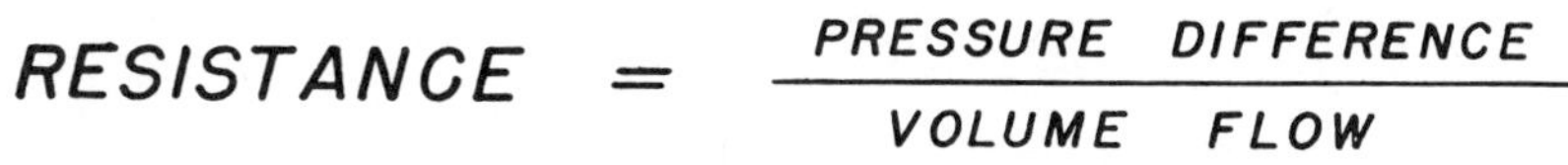

$$= \frac{\Delta P \ (cm.\ H_2O)}{\dot{V} \ (liters/sec.)}$$

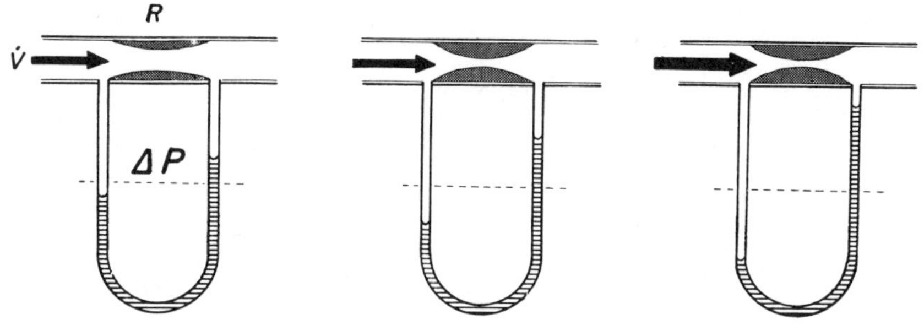

TYPES OF AIR FLOW

LAMINAR

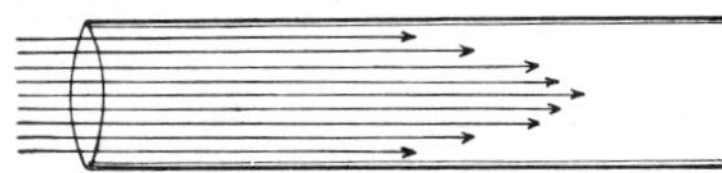

$$P = K_1 \dot{V}$$

TURBULENT

$$P = K_2 \dot{V}^2$$

TRACHEO-BRONCHIAL

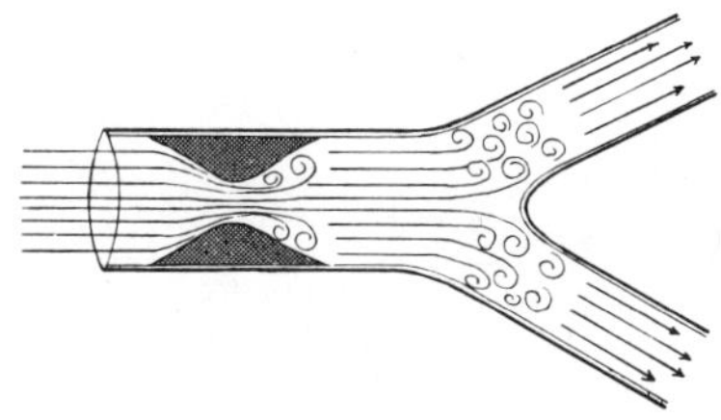

$$P = K_1 \dot{V} + K_2 \dot{V}^2$$

Fig 28.—*Top,* width of the arrow signifies volume flow of air ($\dot{V}$); shaded obstruction, degree of resistance *(R)* to flow. The U-tube manometer measures the pressure difference *(ΔP)* across the resistance. As resistance is increased, greater pressure is required to maintain the same flow. When flow is increased, another increment of pressure is needed. *Bottom,* pressure required when air flow is turbulent (or when there are eddies) is considerably greater than that when flow is laminar (see text).

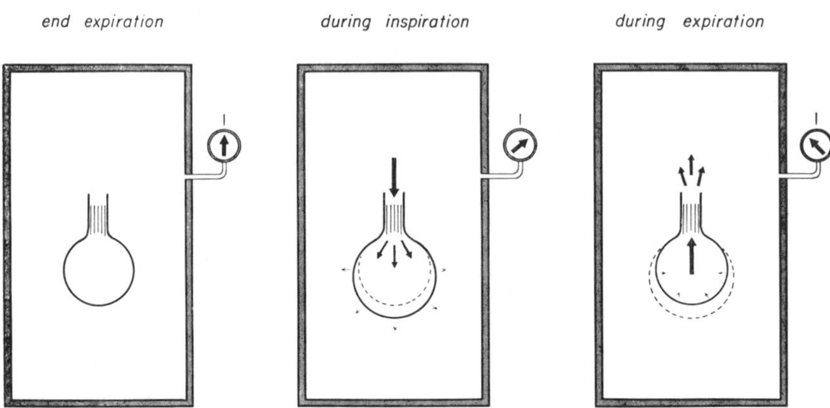

Fig 29.—Measurement of airway resistance: body plethysmograph technique. The rectangle represents the air-tight body plethysmograph. The patient is represented by alveoli and conducting airway, and his airway resistance by parallel lines in the conducting airway. The circle with pointer represents a sensitive gauge that continuously measures pressure in the box around the patient. During inspiration *(center)* the alveoli have enlarged from the original volume *(broken line)* to a new volume *(solid line)*; during expiration *(right)*, the alveoli have returned to their original volume. (See text.)

directly with the viscosity of the gas and the length of the tubes and *inversely* with the fourth power of the radius of the lumen of the tubes.

$$\text{Resistance to flow through a tube} = \frac{\text{viscosity} \cdot \text{length}}{(\text{radius})^4} \times \frac{8}{\pi}$$

Figure 28 shows the relationship among driving pressure, flow, and resistance. If the resistance, R, is small (short, wide tube) and the flow, $\dot{V}$, is small, only a small driving pressure is required *(top left)*. If R is increased (longer or narrower tube), more pressure is required to produce the same flow *(top center)*. If a greater flow is now required through the same resistance, more driving pressure is required *(top right)*.

Airway resistance also depends on the nature of air flow. Air flow may be laminar (or streamlined) or turbulent (Fig 28, *bottom*). As stated before, the pressure required to produce *laminar* flow is proportional to the volume flow ($\dot{V}$) times a constant (K_1), which is related to the *viscosity* of the gas; it is independent of the *density* of the gas. The pressure required for *turbulent* flow is proportional to the *square* of the volume flow ($\dot{V}^2$) times another constant (K_2), which is related to the *density* of the gas; it is independent of the *viscosity* of the gas.§

In smooth, straight tubes, turbulent flow occurs only at high velocities. However, the tracheobronchial tree has hundreds of thousands of branchings, and eddy formations may be set up at these; the pressure required for eddy flow is approximately the same as for turbulent flow. Turbulence (at low flow rates) or eddy formation is particularly apt to occur when there are irregularities in the tubes, such as might be caused by mucus, exudate, tumor or foreign bodies, or by partial closure of the glottis. Physicians sometimes administer 80% helium-20% O_2 to a patient with obstructed breathing in the hope that the airway resistance might be decreased by inhalation of a less dense gas. However, the *viscosity* of this mixture is slightly greater than that of air, and so the resistance to laminar flow is increased slightly, if there is any change. Inhalation of 80% helium-20% O_2 *will* decrease resistance when there is *turbulent* flow or eddy formation because the *density* of the gas mixture is low (0.33 times that of air).

Measurement of Airway Resistance

Airway resistance must be measured under dynamic conditions, i.e., during air flow. Three measurements must be made simultaneously and continuously in order to calculate airway resistance: (1) alveolar pressure, (2) atmospheric pressure, and (3) instantaneous air flow. Atmospheric pressure and instantaneous air flow (pneumotachograph) are easy to measure; alveolar pressure during flow can be measured with the body plethysmograph.

Figure 29 shows schematically the principle of the method. The patient (only the lung is pictured) is seated within the air-tight box; pressure is measured continuously in the box around the patient. One would expect that inspiration of 500 ml of air from the box into the patient's lungs would produce no pressure fluctuations in the box (if precautions are taken to prevent changes due to changes in temperature and humidity of the respired gas); actually the box pressure rises during inspiration. This is simply because gas flows only from a point of higher pressure to a point of lower pressure. At the beginning of inspiration, muscular action has enlarged the thorax and lowered alveolar pressure below atmospheric pressure. Throughout inspiration, alveolar gas (previously at atmospheric pressure) is now at subatmo-

§As a rule, resistance is measured at flow rates of about 0.5 L/sec as a convenient reference and to minimize the turbulent component of flow.

spheric pressure and so occupies more volume; this is the same as adding this increment of gas volume (resulting from the decompression) to the plethysmograph, so the pressure rises. The pressure change is registered by a very sensitive manometer. The reverse happens during expiration, when alveolar gas is compressed. From this measured pressure and appropriate calibrations, alveolar pressure can be calculated for any moment in the respiratory cycle. From these simultaneous measurements of alveolar pressure and flow (obtained with a pneumotachograph), airway resistance can be determined (see Appendix). The method is sensitive, rapid, objective, and specific for changes in airway resistance because the values do not include resistances attributable to the chest wall or lung tissues. It may be repeated as often as desired without tiring the patient.

Other methods (pp. 95, 107–113) provide data from which inferences regarding airway resistance may be drawn. For example, if the maximal expiratory flow rate, maximal voluntary ventilation (MVV), and forced expiratory volume are markedly decreased and the pulmonary resistance abnormally high and all return to normal after administration of a drug known to be a bronchodilator, one can infer that the results of these tests had been abnormal because of increased airway resistance rather than because of abnormal pulmonary tissue or thoracic cage resistance.

Normal Values for Airway Resistance

Normal values, using the body plethysmograph, during rapid, shallow breathing range from 0.6 to 2.4 cm H_2O/(L/sec) measured at flow rates of 0.5 L/sec in adults (see Table 20).

Interpretation of Data

Effect of a Previous Deep Inspiration

The subject is asked to pant during the measurement for technical reasons. However, panting is advantageous in that it opens the larynx and it permits measurements to be made near FRC, without a deep inspiration. A full inspiration can, at least temporarily, overcome the very increase in airway resistance that one wishes to measure. It is important to be sure that a deep sigh or full inspiration did not occur within a minute or two of the actual measurement.

Effect of Lung Volume

Airway resistance becomes less as lung volume is increased. Conductance is the reciprocal of resistance. It connotes the ease with which air flows through the tracheobronchial tree, whereas resistance implies the difficulty with which air flows. 1/R, or conductance, varies linearly with lung volume. For this reason it is important to know the lung volume at the moment that airway resistance is measured. Fortunately, instantaneous thoracic gas volume can be determined in the body plethysmograph at the moment that airway resistance is tested. For comparative studies, it is well to relate resistance (or better, conductance) to simultaneously measured lung volume. A forced vital capacity can produce an increase in tone of bronchial smooth muscle temporarily increasing airway resistance.

Effect of Inspiration and Expiration

During quiet breathing, airway resistance is slightly less during inspiration (presumably because the vocal cords are abducted and because the inspiratory traction of the pulmonary tissues widens the smaller airways and the more negative intrapleural pressure widens the larger airways) and slightly greater during expiration. However, the resistance does increase more toward the end of a maximal expiration in normal subjects.

Effect of Bronchodilators and Provocative Agents

The presence of abnormal bronchoconstriction can be demonstrated by measuring airway resistance before and after administration by aerosol of a bronchodilator, such as isoproterenol. Similarly abnormal sensitivity of the resistance airways can be brought out by administering, with care, histamine, cholinergic drugs (methachol is the most commonly used agent), or allergens.*

If one wishes to compare the airway resistance of different groups of patients, it is important that no bronchoconstrictor or bronchodilator agents be administered before the test. For example, inhalation of submicronic inert particles (carbon, aluminum, chalk, cigarette smoke) may lead to a twofold increase in airway resistance that may last 20 to 40 minutes.

Effects of Increased Airway Resistance on FRC and RV

Figure 30 shows that normally expiration is passive and complete in less than 3 seconds. If airway resistance were to increase abruptly during expiration (as it might at the beginning of an asthmatic attack),

*These tests are potentially dangerous and should only be carried out under close supervision with the ability to administer bronchodilators should excessive bronchoconstriction occur. The use of allergens is especially dangerous because of possible delayed effects.

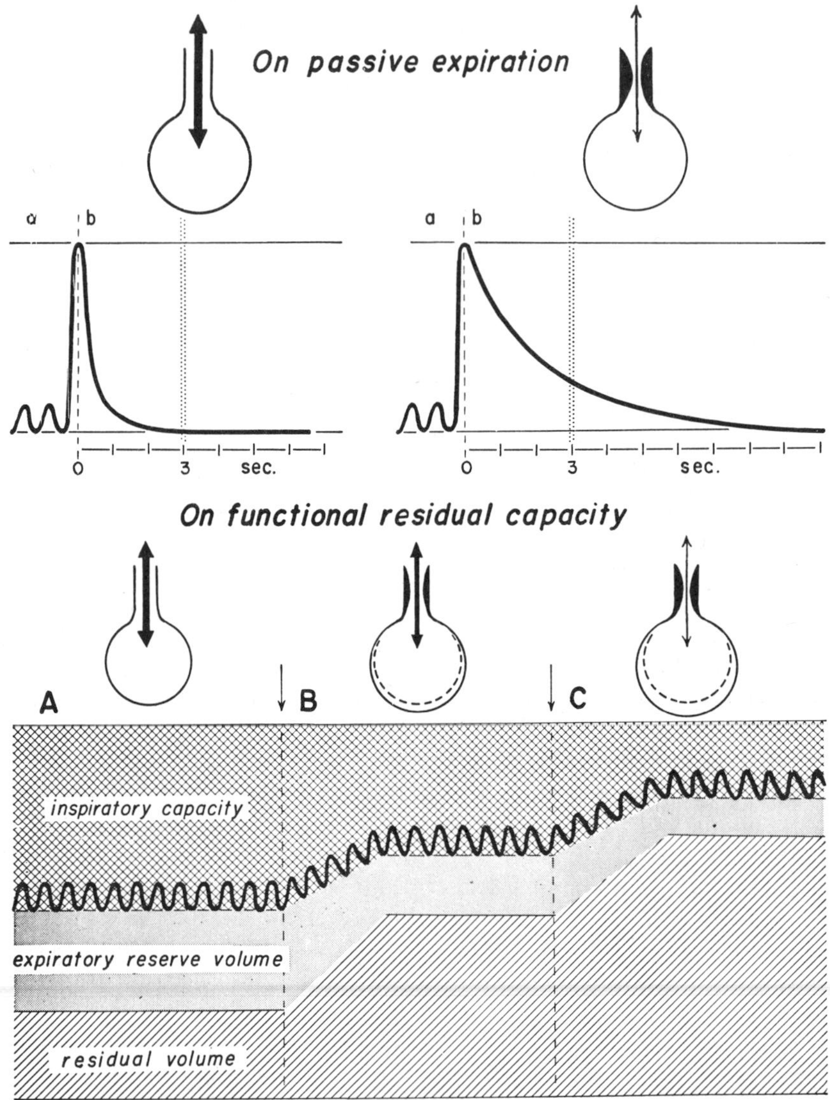

Fig 30.—*Top,* effect on air flow during expiration. *a* represents quiet breathing recorded on a slow kymograph. At *b* the kymograph is speeded and the patient takes a full inspiration and expires. *Left,* open airway, rapid expiration; *right,* partial expiratory obstruction, slow expiration (thickness of arrows signifies *rate* of flow; *volume* expired is the same in both cases). *Bottom,* effect on functional residual capacity. *Left to right,* increasing expiratory obstruction leads to increased functional residual capacity if time for expiration is limited. Dashed lines in lungs *B* and *C* represent the original functional residual capacity of *A,* when no expiratory obstruction was present.

the lung volume might not return to the resting expiratory level in this 3-second interval. Thus, if expiration is completely passive, expiration will not be complete if only 3 seconds is available for it. This means that FRC will be greater at the beginning of the next inspiration.

Detection of Abnormal Types of Resistance

The body plethysmograph method will detect elevated resistance only if it is present during panting. It will not detect abnormal resistance due entirely to a check valve (p. 111), which occurs only with a full and forced expiration, particularly in diseases affecting the smaller airways.

Interpretation of Measurements of Airway Resistance in the Presence of Small Airway Disease

The pressure drop along the tracheo-bronchial tree is fairly uniform, per unit length, until the last centimeter is reached. The so-called upper airways have 90% of the resistance and constitute 90% of the length; the "lower" airways, which have 10% of the resistance, have 10% of the length. Just before the alveolar ducts, the airways subdivide into very large numbers of passageways, with small diameters, but with a large total cross-sectional area, something like the bell of a trumpet. It is this last centimeter of length prior to the alveoli that has a truly "low resistance" of airflow. In this region, air velocities also are low, flow is laminar, not turbulent, and destruction of the walls by dusts, chemicals, or infectious agents can tear at the fabric of the lung. Such diseases may be relatively silent in that initially they do not interfere with breathing. They are difficult to detect by any method.

Usefulness of Measurement of Airway Resistance

The specific test of airway resistance enables the physician to determine whether a decreased MVV or maximal expiratory flow rate (see p. 104) is due to increased resistance in the airway or to numerous other factors. It provides an objective test that is suitable for judging pulmonary disability because the patient cannot voluntarily influence the result of the test. It is also useful in evaluating therapy on an individual basis.

Airway Resistance in Patients

Asthma

Airway resistance is always increased during the asthmatic attack and may be increased twofold to threefold in the symptom-free interval between attacks. The resistance, as in normal persons, is greater during expiration, but inspiratory resistance is also greater than normal. The increased resistance in asthma is sometimes, but not always, acutely reversible by the inhalation of a few breaths of bronchodilator aerosol and is usually reversed by vigorous therapy. The asthmatic diathesis can be determined during a symptom-free interval by a bronchial provocation test.

Emphysema

Airway resistance is usually increased and only slightly reversible, even by vigorous bronchodilator therapy. Much of the increased airway resistance in emphysema appears to be due to collapse of airways during expiration. The finer airways do not have rigid walls and are generally kept open by traction of the elastic tissues of the lung; this traction is diminished in emphysema if elastic tissue is diminished or altered and so the fine tubes collapse during expiration (check valves). Larger airways have their own structural tissue, but this appears to be modified or damaged in emphysema, and even the larger air ducts may collapse during expiration. In addition, during a forced expiration, positive intrapleural pressure is developed because muscular contraction decreases the volume of the thoracic cage faster than air leaves the lungs. This positive pressure exceeds the pressure in the lumen of bronchioles on the tracheal side of the partial obstruction and tends to collapse the walls further. (The pressure required to collapse airways and limit flow is far lower in patients with emphysema than in normal individuals.) Finally, alveoli that have lost varying amounts of their elastic tissue tend to empty in a disorderly manner, and the orifice of the air duct may be closed or may be occluded prematurely by adjacent inflated air sacs.

Other Obstructive Diseases

Airway resistance is increased in a wide variety of disorders in which fibrous tissue, tumors, effusions, etc. constrict, compress, impinge on, or obstruct airways.

Added Resistances

The physician occasionally imposes additional airway resistance (external or internal) on the patient by the use of narrow tracheotomy tubes, long and narrow endotracheal tubes, bronchospirometers, breathing tubes, and valves. Patients with weakened respiratory muscles often suffer severe distress with the addition of even small external resistances.

D. TISSUE RESISTANCE: PULMONARY RESISTANCE AND TOTAL RESPIRATORY RESISTANCE

In addition to the frictional resistance caused by the flow of gas molecules through the airways, there is another frictional resistance in the pulmonary and thoracic tissues themselves. This is the result of displacement of the tissues during inspiration and expiration; the tissues involved include the lungs, rib cage, diaphragm, and abdominal contents. Pulmonary resistance is defined as airway plus pulmonary *tissue* resistance. Total respiratory resistance is pulmonary plus thoracic *tissue* resistance. Like airway resistance, tissue resistance can be measured only during motion; the force needed to overcome it is related to the rapidity or quickness of motion. At the beginning of inspiration, when air flow has not yet begun and the tissues are not moving, resistive force is zero. It becomes maximal at the time of the maximal rate of air flow (even though maximal inspiratory *volume* has not yet been reached). It is zero again at end-inspiration when flow and movement stop; at this point the elastic force is maximal (Fig 26) because the maximal volume has been reached.

At the end of inspiration, the elastic tissues are under stretch and tend to recoil. This elastic or recoil force is available to overcome frictional resistance in tissues and airway resistance. Just as there is friction in the moving tissues during inspiration, so there is friction of motion during expiration, and again the frictional force is greatest at the moment of maximal movement or volume flow. The greater the amount of elastic force dissipated in overcoming frictional resistance in the *tissues,* the less is the elastic force available for overcoming *airway* resistance. When the force available for causing air flow is reduced, expiration is slowed.

Measurement of Pulmonary Resistance

Pulmonary Resistance

The transpulmonary pressure during flow (Fig 24) overcomes elastic recoil, airway resistance, and "pulmonary tissue resistance." If one subtracts from the total transpulmonary pressure (measured with an esophageal balloon) that which is required to overcome elastic recoil,* the remaining transpulmonary pressure is that required to overcome

*This requires knowledge of the pressure-volume curve of the lungs and the assumption that it is a straight line.

airway and pulmonary tissue resistance. Pulmonary tissue resistance cannot be measured independently, but can be calculated by subtraction if airway resistance is known.

Another method for the measurement of total pulmonary resistance is the electrical subtraction method (Fig 26) analagous to the method used for determining lung compliance. In this technique a voltage proportional to the rate of change of lung volume, equal to the rate of airflow, is subtracted from the total transpulmonary pressure (mouth pressure minus esophageal pressure). This voltage is varied to produce an "S"-shaped line on the cathode ray oscilloscope. The line is a segment of the pressure-flow curve of the lung and the voltage subtracted is proportional to the transpulmonary pressure necessary to overcome lung elastic recoil. By knowing the slope of the pressure-flow line, the pulmonary resistance is calculated.

The interruption of airflow momentarily by an electrical shutter can also be used to estimate the transpulmonary pressure related to airflow (Fig 25,B, single-expiration method of measuring lung compliance). The sudden decrease in transpulmonary pressure (mouth minus esophageal pressure) upon cessation of airflow is caused by the disappearance of the pressure gradient required to overcome airway resistance and to overcome the viscous resistance of the lung itself. Therefore, the magnitude of change in transpulmonary pressure during interruption of airflow is directly proportional to pulmonary resistance.

Measurement of Total Respiratory Resistance

This resistance is measured by the interrupter technique, illustrated in Figure 31, which requires recording only pressure at the mouth. When expired airflow is interrupted by the shutter (downstream from the pressure recording point), mouth pressure rises. If we can make the important assumption that the lungs and chest wall continue to exert the same pressure during the interruption as they did during airflow before the interruption,† then the increase in mouth pressure during interruption again equals the pressure that had been required to produce airflow through the airway resistance and to overcome the viscous resistance of tissues just prior to interruption. In patients who have an unusually high airway resistance, pressure equilibra-

†During the brief occlusion (generally 0.1 sec), mouth pressure continues to rise as the thoracic muscles increase their expiratory effort under neuromuscular control. A pressure increment during interruption is not seen in the transpulmonary pressure difference (esophageal pressure minus mouth pressure) because once airflow has ceased this equals the elastic forces and does not change significantly at constant lung volume.

INTERRUPTER TECHNIQUE

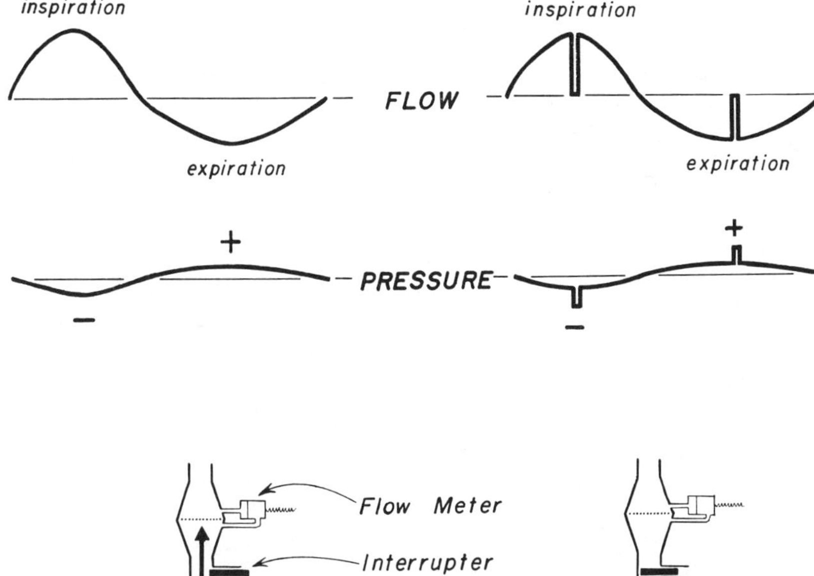

FREE FLOW

INTERRUPTED

$$\text{RESISTANCE} = \frac{\text{PRESSURE}}{\text{FLOW}}$$

Fig 31.—Method for measuring "airway" resistance. Simultaneous measurements of trans-airway pressure (pressure difference between alveoli and mouth) and of flow are required to measure airway resistance. Here the subject breathes through a flow meter; air flow can be interrupted very briefly at any time without the subject's knowledge and pressure measured on the tracheal side of the obstruction. At random times during the respiratory cycle, the flow is interrupted momentarily at the mouthpiece by a shutter and static pressure measured (tracheal pressure). In a static system, the mouth or tracheal pressure is equal to alveolar pressure, if the glottis is open. This measurement of "airway" resistance probably includes tissue resistance as well (see text).

tion between the mouth and alveoli does not occur instantaneously and the interrupter technique may give erroneous results.

The total respiratory resistance can also be determined by measuring simultaneously and continuously the air pressure and flow at the mouth while very rapid airflow cycles (above 3 cycles/sec) are produced by a piston pump or loud speaker (Fig 32). This is called the forced oscillation method. The elastic forces opposing volume changes of lung and thorax decrease as frequency of oscillations increases, while the inertial forces, which include inertia of the lungs, thorax, and the airway gas itself, increase as driving frequency increases. The total opposing force, which can be measured as (peak-to-peak pressure difference)/(peak-to-peak flow), is a combination of the resistance and the so-called *reactance,* which in turn has elastic and inertial components. Reactance is minimal at the rapid pump frequencies of 3 to 8 cycles/sec, at which point only viscous resistance remains (see Appendix). This value of resistance varies nearly proportionately to airway resistance in patients; it includes some element of lung tissue and thoracic cage resistance as well as of airway resistance.

Interpretation of Pulmonary and Respiratory Resistance

Values for pulmonary resistance and total respiratory resistance reflect primarily the airway component. Consequently, these measure-

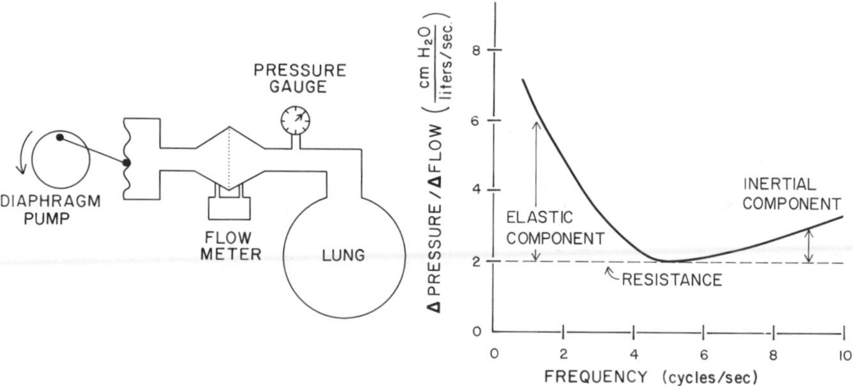

Fig 32.—Pulmonary oscillatory method of measuring total respiratory resistance. The diaphragm pump produces rapid cyclic breathing, the flow rate is measured by the pneumotachograph and the pressure at the mouth by the pressure manometer gauge. Elastic resistance to expansion of the lungs + thorax decreases with increasing frequency; the inertia, partly of the lungs and thoracic tissues, but mostly of the air itself, increases as frequency increases. The minimum point occurs at the resonant frequency of the lungs + thorax combination at which point resistance is that of air flow and tissue movement alone.

ments are increased in patients with airway obstruction. The component due to lung tissue resistance, which includes lung hysteresis, is about 20% of the pulmonary resistance in healthy young men. It may be increased in patients with pulmonary sarcoidosis, pulmonary fibrosis, diffuse carcinomatosis, asthma, or kyphoscoliosis. It is rarely increased to the extent of being an important or limiting resistance.

Total respiratory resistance exceeds airway resistance by about 25% in normal persons and consequently is not much greater than pulmonary resistance. Theoretically, thoracic cage resistance could be calculated from total respiratory resistance minus pulmonary resistance. No measurements of this resistance have been made in patients with thoracic disorders.

E. COHESION

In certain abnormal conditions, such as atelectasis and collapse of the lung during thoracic surgery, the surfaces of the smaller air ducts are held together by surface tension forces (cohesion). In such cases, another factor opposes inspiration, because no air movement occurs until an "opening pressure" has been built up in the airways. This "opening pressure" for bronchi is small (1 or 2 cm H_2O), but that for alveoli is large (10 to 12 cm H_2O). Attempts to overcome atelectasis by a high endotracheal pressure are hazardous if some of the airways are open, since the high pressure results in distension of their alveoli and may lead to alveolar rupture. In thoracic surgery, once a lung has been permitted to collapse to "minimal volume," the surfaces of the airways are likely to stick together by cohesion. Probably because of this phenomenon, positive pressure applied to the nose, mouth, or endotracheal tube will inflate only the lung in the closed hemithorax, even though the compliance of a lung and its hemithorax is less than for the lung alone (on the open side). Once this opening pressure is exceeded, the lung on the open side will receive more ventilation than the other, if both are inflated by the same pressure.

F. INERTIA

The inertia of the lung-thoracic cage system is so small during normal breathing that it can be neglected at atmospheric pressure. It may contribute more in hyperbaric environments or during very rapid breathing cycles (greater than 3 cycles/sec).

G. THE WORK OF BREATHING

Work, in the physical sense, is force × distance, or pressure × volume. The cumulative product of *pressure* and the *volume* of air moved at each instant is equal to *work* ($W = \int PdV$). If one knows the mechanical work done and the O_2 consumed by the respiratory muscles in doing this work, the efficiency of ventilation can be calculated as follows:

$$\text{Efficiency} = \frac{\text{useful work}}{\text{total energy expended}} \times 100$$

Work of Moving Only the Lungs

This is calculated from records of transpulmonary pressure and volume during breathing. The principle is illustrated in Figure 33, which shows a block attached to a wall by a spring. In the upper set of diagrams, the block is resting on a "frictionless" surface such as ice. In this case, as the block is moved by an external force, the distance moved is proportional to the force *(solid arrow)* even during movement, since the only force required is that to stretch the spring. In the lower set of diagrams, the block is resting on a rough surface and two forces are required to move it. One is the force required to stretch the spring; this *(solid portion of the arrow)* depends on the distance moved and is the same as in the upper diagrams. The other *(broken arrow)* is the force required to overcome friction. This force increases when the speed of movement increases and becomes zero when the block comes to rest. The graphs show the force-length changes corresponding to each movement of the block. When friction is present, the line deviates from the straight line; the shaded area between the straight line and the curve represents the additional *work* to overcome friction during movement.

Similarly, during inflation or deflation of the lungs, the amount of pressure required at any given instant depends not only on the pressure to overcome elastic recoil but also on the pressure to maintain movement of air through the airways and movement of the tissues of the lungs. The greater the rate of volume change (volume flow/min) the greater is the pressure used in overcoming friction. In Figure 33 *(top, left)* is shown a pressure-volume curve during breathing. Since work $= \int PdV$, the shaded area between the diagonal and the ordinate represents the work in overcoming the elastic resistance, whereas the shaded area between the diagonal and the curved line represents the additional work of moving nonelastic tissues and overcoming airway resistance.

Work of Moving the Lungs and Thoracic Cage

This is done normally by the muscles of respiration. It is difficult to estimate by direct means. However, if a patient is no longer breathing spontaneously as a result of neuromuscular disease, deep anesthesia, or the injection of drugs that produce neuromuscular block, his ventilation can be maintained by a pump respirator (Fig 24, p. 71).* This permits measurements of the work required for normal pulmonary ventilation because, under these conditions, the lungs, thorax, and gas are moved by the pump respirator.

It is easy to measure the work of the pump respirator, and the respirator must be doing the amount of work that would have been done by the respiratory muscles under these conditions. The work done by the respirator is calculated from simultaneous measurements of (1) the force acting on the thorax to cause inspiration (the pressure difference between the mouth and the atmosphere; *1* in Fig 24), and (2) the volume of air breathed. Normal values are 0.5 KgM/min during rest. The work of breathing increases disproportionately as the minute volume increases and reaches a maximum of about 250 KgM/min when a subject breathes maximally (about 200 L/min).

O_2 Consumption of Respiratory Muscles

The O_2 consumed by the respiratory muscles in a healthy person is normally such a small fraction of the total body metabolism that it is difficult to measure. It does become measurable as the O_2 cost of additional ventilation during performance of the test for maximal voluntary ventilation or when the patient is made to breathe through a known, added resistance. From such measurements and other data, it has been calculated that the mechanical efficiency of the respiratory muscles is low (5% to 10%), so that 10 or 20 times the O_2 is required to perform the mechanical work as is needed for a similar amount of heat energy. It is difficult to estimate the O_2 cost of additional ventilation if cardiac work is increased simultaneously.

It is certain that the respiratory muscles of many patients with cardiopulmonary disease do more work and require more O_2 than those of resting subjects. It would be interesting and important to determine the mechanical work of breathing, the O_2 consumption of the respiratory muscles and the efficiency of breathing in normal subjects and in

*Attempts have also been made to measure the work of breathing in subjects who have been instructed to relax voluntarily all the muscles of respiration while they are on the respirator; it is not certain, however, that such voluntary relaxation is complete.

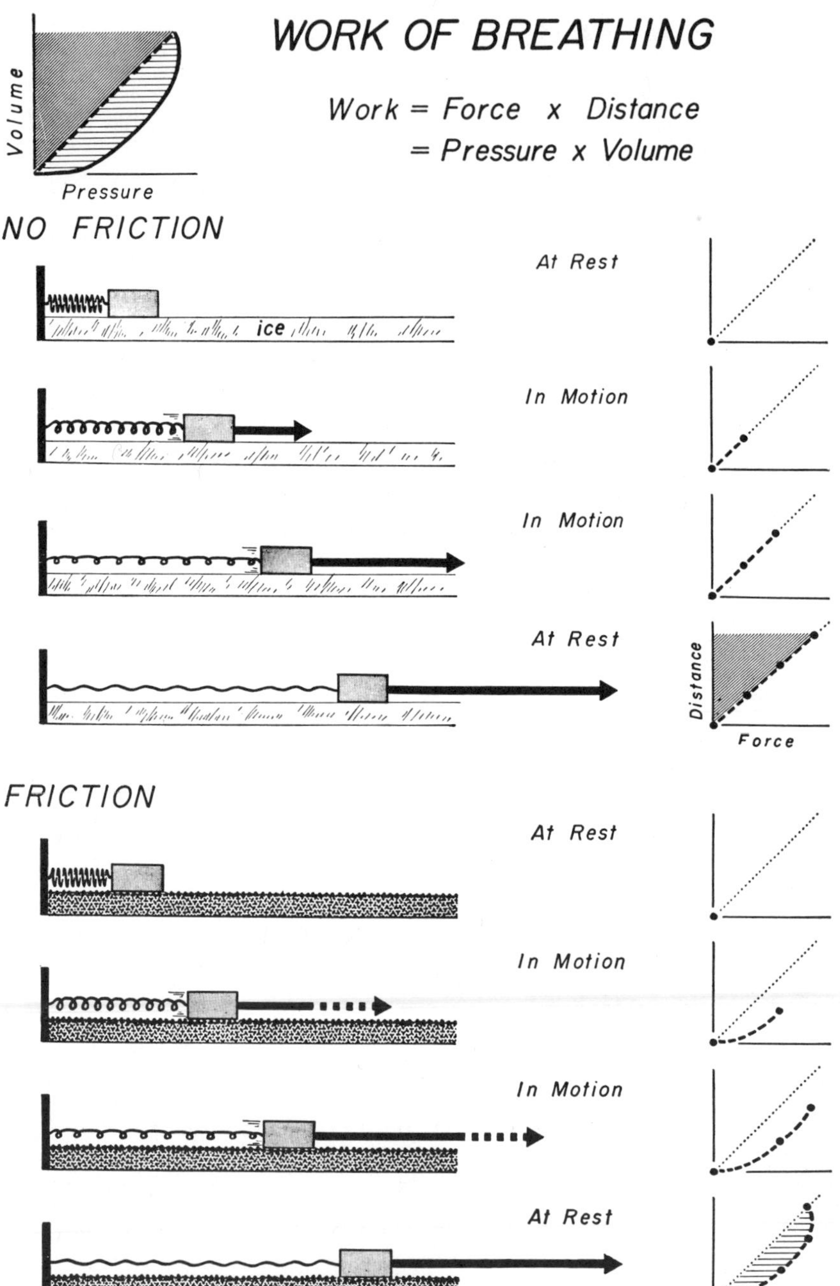

Fig 33.—*Solid arrow* represents the force required to move the block a certain distance when there is no friction and only the elastic resistance of the spring must be over-

patients with respiratory impairment. Some studies have indicated that the "O_2 cost" of additional ventilation (above the resting level) is greater than normal in patients with emphysema and in obese patients.

Minimal Work of Breathing

It is possible, with our knowledge of the mechanics of breathing, to offer rational explanations of breathing patterns in patients with pulmonary disease. The optimal rate and depth of breathing should be that which produces the required alveolar ventilation with the minimal amount of work on the part of the respiratory muscles. If the alveolar ventilation required is 4.0 L/min, this can be achieved by rapid, shallow breathing or slow, deep breathing. Some combinations that will give an alveolar ventilation of 4.0 L/min (assuming a respiratory dead space of 150 ml) are as follows:

FREQUENCY, BREATHS/MIN	TIDAL VOLUME, ML	MINUTE VOLUME, L/MIN	ALVEOLAR VENTILATION, L/MIN
10	550	5.5	4.0
15	417	6.3	4.0
20	350	7.0	4.0
30	283	8.5	4.0
40	250	10.0	4.0

If we examine these factors for the best compromise between rate and depth, we see that as the rate increases, the depth decreases, and therefore the elastic forces decrease. However, the minute volume increases (because dead space ventilation/min increases), so that air flow must increase and the resistive forces must be greater.

The best compromise in normal subjects, so that the required alveolar ventilation is obtained by the least sum of these forces, occurs at about 15 respirations per minute, because the work expended in respiration in normal individuals is so small, other factors may be relatively more important in determining respiratory rate and depth. In patients with very stiff lungs (decreased compliance), the best combination occurs at more rapid rates, to minimize the elastic factor. On

come. *Broken arrow* shows the additional force required to overcome friction; this is needed only during movement of the block (see text). The graphs of force vs. distance are straight lines when there is elastic resistance alone, but are curved when there is frictional resistance as well; the shaded area in the graphs above the diagonal line represents the *work* required to overcome elastic resistance; that below the diagonal line represents work to overcome frictional resistance.

the other hand, asthmatic patients, who have increased airway resistance as the dominant mechanical problem, do not select rapid respiratory rates because they would require a greater minute volume and therefore higher rates of air flow.

For example, patient G.L. had a respiratory rate of 30 to 40 per minute. Lung compliance (esophageal balloon) was 0.013, which is about 1/17 normal. The airway resistance was within the normal range. Autopsy showed pulmonary carcinomatosis, which was the cause of his stiff lungs, but there was no airway obstruction. This patient was breathing frequently because of the greatly increased effort involved in breathing deeply. This phenomenon also occurs in some patients who have pulmonary restrictive disease, pulmonary scleroderma, and other lesions restricting or constricting the lungs and chest.

H. MAXIMAL INSPIRATORY AND EXPIRATORY FORCES

These forces are measured under static conditions by having the subject expire or inspire maximally against a mercury or other manometer. The maximal pressure is usually measured by a manometer connected to a tube in the mouth. Precautions must be taken so the patient does not use his buccal muscles to develop pressure. A small leak in the mouth tube (e.g., an 18-gauge needle) can minimize this effect. A normal person can develop 60 to 100 mm Hg or more positive or negative pressure, depending on the degree of effort. This is a test predominantly of muscle strength, with a small contribution of lung elastic recoil.

It is particularly useful in studying patients in whom the MVV is decreased but pulmonary compliance and resistance are normal; reduction in maximal inspiratory or expiratory force may point to muscular weakness as the critical factor causing the decrease in MVV.

I. TESTS OF OVERALL MECHANICAL FUNCTION OF LUNGS AND THORAX

So far, we have discussed compliance and resistance and specific tests to measure specific properties of the lungs and thorax. For initial purposes, it is customary to use relatively simple procedures to test the mechanical function of the lungs. These tests are not completely objective because they require cooperation of the patient; furthermore, they are not analytical because they measure several properties of the lungs and thorax simultaneously. Nevertheless, they represent the proper initial approach. They are often diagnostically useful per se; when they are not, the result obtained usually suggests the proper direction for additional, more precise study of the patient.

Spirograms

Spirographic tracings of normal breathing, forced inspiration and expiration (Fig 34), plus maximal voluntary ventilation made on a rapidly moving kymograph (Fig 35) permit analysis of many characteristics of the breathing pattern and provide a permanent record for comparison with later tracings. Some of these characteristics follow:

Times for Normal Inspiration and Expiration.—Normally, expiration requires about 1.2 times as long as inspiration. In patients with expiratory obstruction or with disease in which the elastic recoil (which normally aids expiration) is diminished, expiratory time is prolonged.

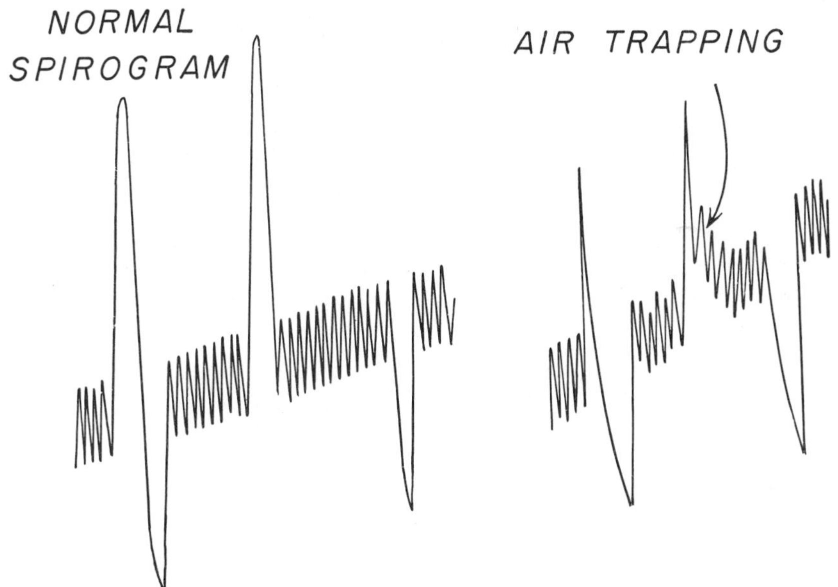

Fig 34.—Spirograms of normal individual and patient with emphysema. In each case, a patient performs the following maneuvers *(left to right):* (1) vital capacity test, (2) maximal inspiration followed by normal breathing, and (3) maximal expiration followed by normal breathing. *Left,* spirogram of normal individual. *Right,* spirogram of patient with emphysema; note *(a)* slow return to resting expiratory level ("air trapping") following maximal inspiration, and *(b)* prolongation of expiration (the latter shown more clearly in Figure 30, where a rapid kymograph is used).

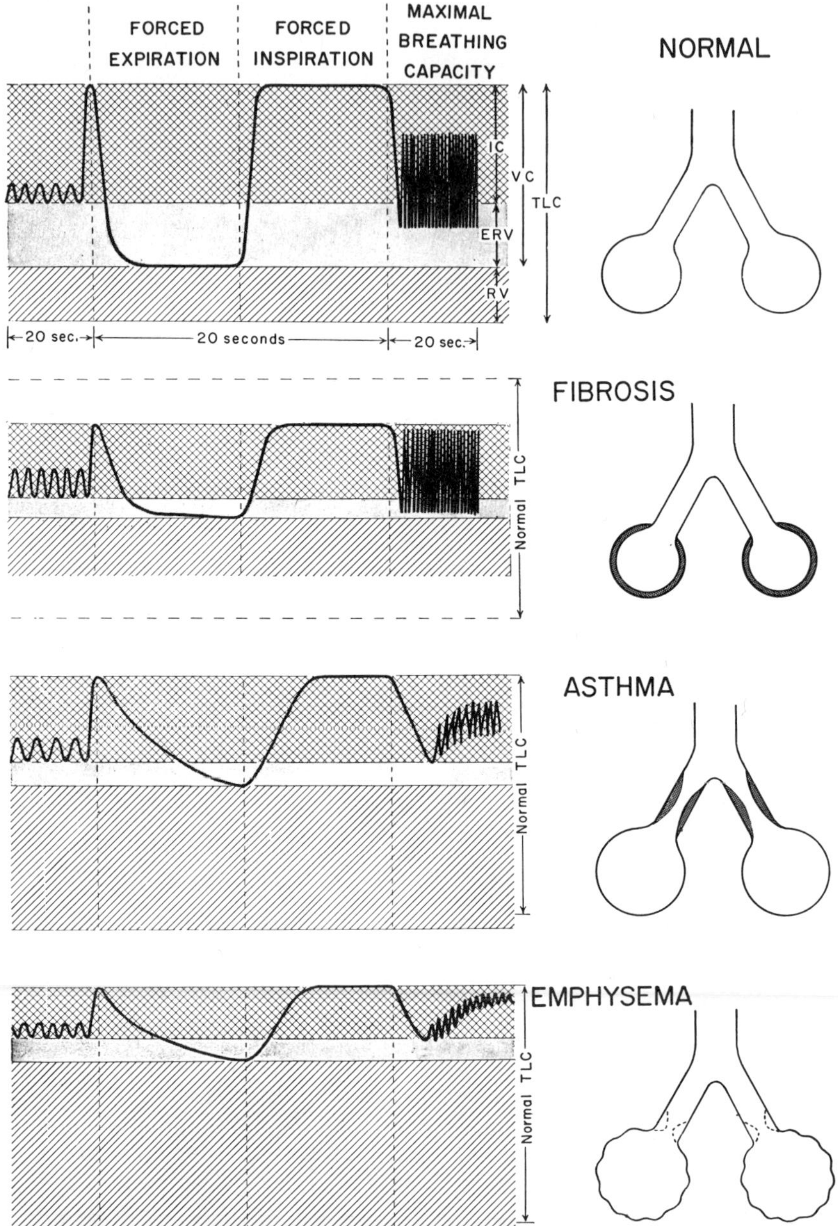

Fig 35.—In each illustration, the patient *(left to right) (a)* breathes quietly (slow kymograph), *(b)* takes a maximal inspiration, then expires as completely, forcefully, and rapidly as he can (rapid kymograph), *(c)* from the position of complete expiration, makes a max-

Time for Return to Resting Expiratory Level.—If a normal individual inspires maximally and then permits his chest to return passively to the resting expiratory level, all of the inspired air is expelled before the next inspiration occurs (Figs 30 and 34). In patients with predominantly expiratory obstruction, this maneuver may be followed by a slow steplike return to the normal base line, during which several breaths may occur before the resting expiratory level is reached. This phenomenon, called "air trapping," may be noted to an even greater degree in emphysema, partly because of associated obstruction and partly because after rapid overdistention of the lung, the lung returns more slowly to its original volume. This abnormally slow return to the resting expiratory level may also occur after a maximal expiration. If patients with air trapping are taught to breathe out slowly, they can often breathe out more completely. This is one of the rational objectives of breathing exercises.

One- and Two-Stage Vital Capacity.—The "two-stage vital capacity" refers to the procedure in which the inspiratory capacity and expiratory reserve are determined separately and then added (see p. 9). In asthma and emphysema, the two-stage value may exceed the one-stage by as much as 1 L. This is because of the air trapping that occurs when maximal expiration follows a maximal inspiration. If the two-stage value is smaller than the one-stage, it is likely that the subject is not cooperating fully.

Maximal Inspiratory and Expiratory Flow Rates.—Alterations in the pattern of breathing become more apparent when maximal, forced inspiratory and expiratory efforts are made. Figure 35 shows records from normal persons and from patients with pulmonary disease. Quantitative measurements of air flow can be made directly from the spirometer record if a rapid paper speed is used; such values are identical to those using the more expensive electrical flow meter or pneumotachograph, if air flows do not exceed 500 L/min.

At least a dozen different methods have been used to read numbers from the forced expiratory volume record (Fig 36). Some, like

---

imal, forced inspiration (rapid kymograph), and *(d)* performs the maximal breathing capacity test (slow kymograph). Timed vital capacity can be measured from *(b)* and maximal and mean expiratory and inspiratory flow rates can be calculated from *(b)* and *(c)*.

The spirogram is shown in proper relation to total lung capacity, vital capacity, functional residual capacity, residual volume, expiratory reserve volume, and inspiratory capacity of each patient. The "lungs" on the right are similar to those pictured in Figure 21. "Fibrosis" refers to restrictive types of fibrotic disease.

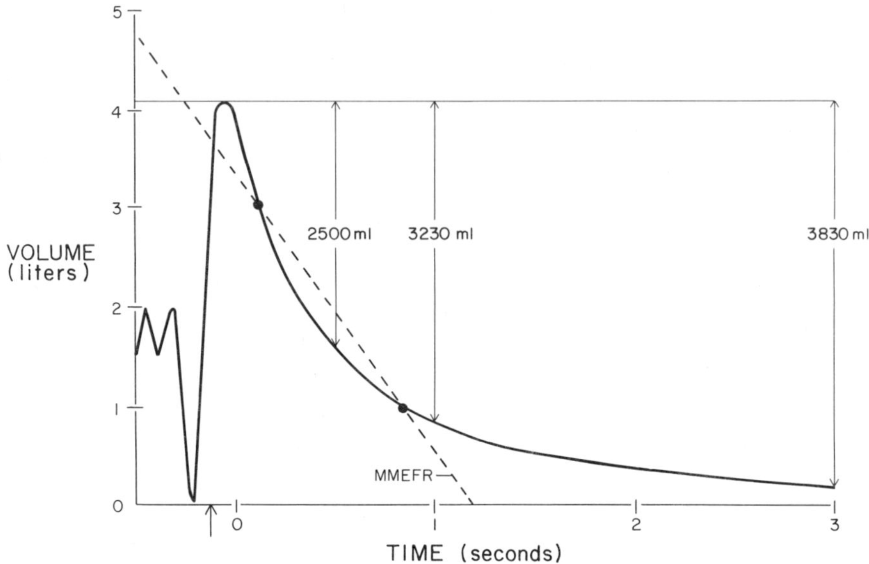

Fig 36.—A rapid spirographic tracing with calculation of air flow indices. The paper speed was increased 20-fold at the arrow. The vital capacity was 4,060 ml. Forced expired volume (FEV); 0.5 seconds was 2,500/4,060 = 62%; 1.0 seconds was 3,230/4,060 = 80%; and 3.0 seconds was 3,829/4,060 = 94%. The maximum expiratory flow rate (MEFR), the average expiratory flow rate between 200 and 1,200 ml was 1.9/0.25 = 7.6 L/sec.

"peak flow," emphasize the maximal rate of outflow that usually occurs early during forced expiration. For maximal expiratory flow rate (MEFR) the subject is asked to inspire maximally and then blow out as hard and as fast as he can. The first 200 ml of expired gas is disregarded and the flow rate is measured between 200 and 1,200 ml of expired gas. Other measurements such as the "maximal midexpiratory flow rate" (MMEFR) stress airflow during the middle part of the volume expelled. This measurement of change in volume and change in time begins when 25% of the vital capacity has been expelled and ends after 75% is expelled. Still others—for example, the flow at a volume that is 25% of vital capacity (MEF 25%)—lean heavily on the flow measured near the tail end of the forced vital capacity record.

Flow-Volume Curves

Conventional spirometry records the forced respiratory maneuvers as the expired or inspired volume versus time. Since the instantaneous change in volume versus time is gas flow, it is possible to compute and plot the spirogram as flow versus time or flow versus volume.* The more commonly used approach is the *flow-volume curve* presentation. The advantage of flow-volume curve is that instantaneous flow can be determined at any point in the vital capacity rather than relying on mean values for flow calculated from two or more points on the volume versus time record. The flow-volume curve can be displayed very conveniently on a cathode ray screen (or any x-y recorder) (Fig 37), with the flow plotted on the vertical axis and volume plotted on the horizontal axis.

During a forced expiration, the pressure drop along the bronchi (Fig 38) results in an intraluminal pressure close to atmospheric (mouth pressure is atmospheric), whereas pleural pressure is greater than atmospheric (pleural pressure = alveolar pressure minus lung elastic pressure).† The pressure difference across the bronchial wall tends to collapse the wall during forced expiration (called *dynamic compression*). On the other hand, a forced inspiration does not produce this collapsing tendency, because the pressure in the pleural space is subatmospheric, therefore tending to open rather than close the bronchi. The rate of inspiratory airflow, therefore, is a function of the airway (plus tissue) resistances and the inspiratory effort of the subject. The determinants of expiratory airflow are interrelated in a more complex fashion because of dynamic compression of airways during expiration, and increased effort does not result in increased rates of expiratory flow (provided the subject exerts sufficient effort to raise pleural pressure sufficiently). The bronchi near the bottom of the lungs always collapse somewhat earlier or more easily during expiration than those near the top because gravity causes static pleural pressure to be less negative near the bottom then near the top. This is thought to account for the phase IV (closing volume) seen in the single breath N_2 tracing (see Fig 10).

The rate of air flow during forced expiration in a healthy young man is initially very rapid (400 L/min), though there is considerable slowing at end-expiration. If he exhales maximally and then breathes in as hard and fast as he can, the air flow is again rapid (300 L/min), but this rate can be maintained during inspiration until the lungs are full (Fig 35). A marked reduction in flow rates indicates that a mechanical problem exists that may be present during either expiration or in-

*Flow is measured by electrical differentiation of the volume signal of the spirometer or by a pneumotachograph.

†Pleural pressure exceeds atmospheric pressure during forced expiration due to the action of the respiratory muscles. During a passive expiration, as in quiet breathing, pleural pressure approximates atmospheric pressure.

spiration, or both. Flow rates may be reduced to as low as 20 L/min. Such severe reduction in expiratory flow rate is particularly serious because it decreases the patient's ability to cough and so to remove secretions from his airway

The test does not give information as to the specific mechanical factor involved and does require cooperation of the patient; in these

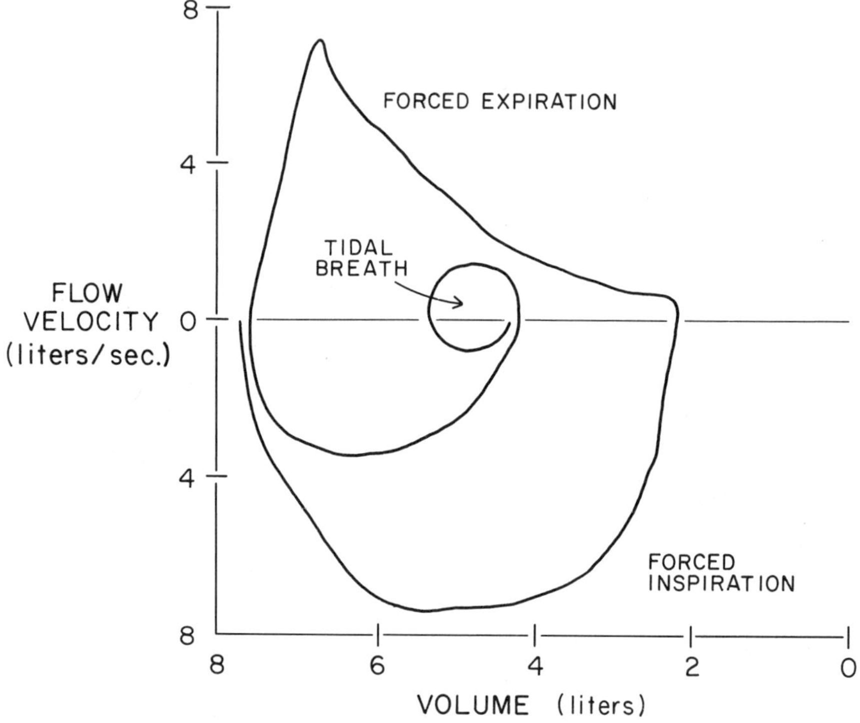

Fig 37.—Flow-volume loop of a normal subject. This plot indicates total lung volume on the abscissa and flow measured at the mouth (with a flowmeter) on the ordinate, expiratory flow upwards and inspiratory flow downwards. Total lung volume was calculated from the FRC (measured separately) and the inspired or expired lung volume. Tidal breathing is indicated by the small loop with its origin at FRC (4.2 L). The subject slowly inspired to TLC, then forcibly exhaled to RV followed by a forcible inspiration to TLC. These maneuvers generated forced expiratory and forced inspiratory flow-volume loops. Note that peak expiratory flow occurs early in expiration and is followed by rapidly decreasing flow indicating dynamic compression of the airways. Peak inspiratory flow slightly exceeds peak expiratory flow and is maintained for a longer period since the airways remain patent during inspiration. The respiratory maneuvers depicted are analogous to those depicted by the more conventional spirometric representation of volume versus time (see Fig 36).

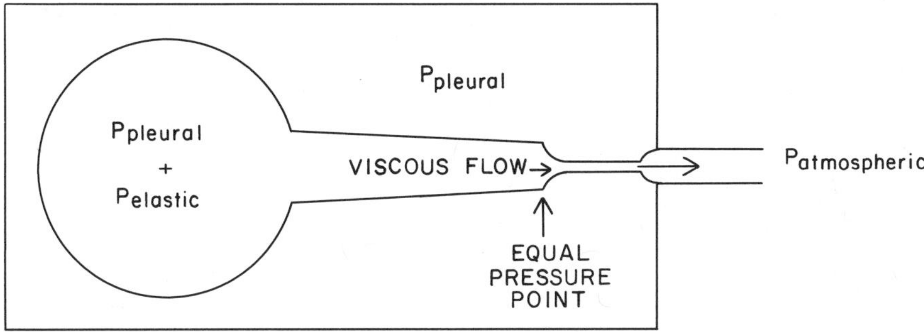

Fig 38.—Collapse of the airways during expiration: The total pressure in the alveoli equals pleural pressure + the elastic pressure of the lungs. Flow in the airway requires a pressure drop owing to the viscous resistance of the gas. If the air flow is rapid enough, or the airway resistance great enough, this pressure drop will become equal to and then greater than the elastic pressure, the airway transmural pressure becomes zero or less and the airways will tend to collapse. The point along the airway where this occurs is called the *equal pressure point.* With a forced expiration the equal pressure point moves closer to the alveoli because as the flow rate increases so also the viscous pressure drop increases, but the elastic pressure remains the same. Cartilage in the large airways helps to oppose the tendency to collapse during forced expiration.

respects, it suffers from the same defects as the maximal voluntary ventilation test (maximal breathing capacity, see below). However, the test is much simpler, it is less fatiguing, is easily repeatable, and clearly separates inspiratory and expiratory difficulties.

If one measures "intrathoracic pressure" during the test (esophageal balloon technique), one can determine whether the subject is making his maximal effort; if not, lack of comprehension, lack of cooperation or neuromuscular, muscular, or metabolic disturbances may be responsible.

Forced Expiratory Volume ("Timed Vital Capacity").‡—This is a very simple test that measures the volume that is expired by maximal effort in a specified time. The time may be the first second ($FEV_{1.0''}$), or the first 3 seconds ($FEV_{3.0''}$), or the interval between 0.25 and 0.75 seconds ($FEV_{0.25-0.75''}$), for example. In the United States, $FEV_{1.0''}$ and $FEV_{3.0''}$ are commonly used (1- and 3-second "timed vital capacity"). The patient makes a forced expiration into a spirometer and total expired volume in one second, or other desired time period, obtained from a record or by computer processing. The volume in 1 second can

‡See Table 6 for terminology.

TABLE 6.—TERMINOLOGY FOR MEASUREMENTS OF VENTILATORY CAPACITY

MEASUREMENT EXPRESSED IN TERMS OF:	NAME OF TEST (SYNONYMS IN PARENTHESES)	ABBREVIATION	REMARKS
A Single breath			
1 Volume	Forced vital capacity (Fast vital capacity)	FVC	Always refers to *expiratory* effort unless qualified by "inspiratory"
2 Volume in a unit time	Forced expiratory volume ("timed vital capacity")	FEV_t	Must be qualified by a time interval. $FEV_{1.0''}$ = vol. expired in 1 sec; $FEV_{0.25-0.75''}$ = vol. expired between 0.25 and 0.75 sec
	Percentage expired ("% timed vital capacity")	$\%FEV_t/VC$	Refers to volume of forced expiration (in time specified) related to vital capacity
		$\%FEV_t/FVC$	Refers to volume of forced expiration (in time specified) related to *forced* vital capacity
3. Volume/time	Maximal expiratory flow rate	MEFR	Refers to L/min for specified portion of a forced expiration; MEFR 200–1,200 is flow rate for the liter of expired gas after 200 ml has been expired
	Maximal inspiratory flow rate	MIFR	Refers to L/min for specified portion of a forced inspiration
	Maximal mid-expiratory flow	MMF	Refers to L/min measured for the middle half of FVC
4. Flow at a particular volume	Maximal expiratory flow volume	MEFV	PEF refers to peak expiratory flow; MEF 50% is instantaneous flow at 50% of FVC; MEF 25% is flow at 25% of VC
B. Repeated breaths			
1. Volume/time	Maximal breathing capacity	MBC	Usually attained by voluntary effort, occasionally exercise produces greater values
	Maximal voluntary ventilation	MVV	Maximal volume obtained by voluntary effort

be expressed either as percent of that particular forced vital capacity (i.e., $\%FEV_{1.0''}/FVC$) or as percent of the vital capacity performed without relation to speed (i.e., $\%FEV_{1.0''}/VC$). It has sometimes been expressed in terms of percent of *predicted* vital capacity.

A normal individual can expire 83% of his vital capacity in 1 second, 94% in 2 seconds, and 97% in 3 seconds, and it makes little difference whether forced vital capacity, vital capacity, or predicted vital capacity is used. This is not true in patients with pulmonary disease; a patient with interstitial pulmonary fibrosis may expire 83% or more of *his* vital capacity in 1 second (because he has a markedly reduced vital capacity) but only 50% of his *predicted* (normal) vital capacity. The

$FEV_{1.0''}/FVC$ (in terms of actual vital capacity) is reduced in patients with obstructive pulmonary disease but not in those who have restricted expansion without obstruction.

Maximal Voluntary Ventilation (MVV); Maximal Breathing Capacity (MBC).—Maximal breathing capacity (MBC) is the maximal volume of gas that can be breathed per minute. Maximal voluntary ventilation (MVV) is the maximal volume that can be breathed per minute by voluntary effort (Fig 35).

As a rule, maximal ventilation can be attained only by voluntary effort, although in some patients with severe pulmonary disease, exercise ventilation or ventilation induced by inhalation of high concentrations of CO_2 may exceed the MVV, probably because voluntarily forced expiration occludes airways partially or completely.

In the MVV test, the patient is instructed to breathe as deeply and as rapidly as he can through a low resistance system for 15 seconds. The patient should be permitted to choose his own frequency and tidal volume; the frequency is usually between 40 and 70/min, and the tidal volume is about 50% of vital capacity. Maximal figures are rarely attained by insisting upon repeated performance of the entire vital capacity, because the extremes of inspiration and expiration are performed with undue expenditure of time and energy. During performance of the test, it is important to use large-diameter breathing valves, large-diameter breathing tubing, and low inertia spirometers to attain reproducibility of results.

Significance of MVV Values.—The ability of a patient to breathe at sustained high velocity depends on many factors: the muscular force available, the compliance of the lungs and thoracic cage and the resistance of the airway and pulmonary thoracic tissues. Figure 35 shows that MVV is reduced out of proportion to decrease in vital capacity in patients with obstruction of the airways or with emphysema. This illustration also shows that air trapping and a large increase in functional residual capacity may occur during the test; in extreme cases, this results in an MVV that is less than the exercise or even the resting minute volume.

On the other hand, MVV may be fairly well maintained in some patients with restrictive types of pulmonary restrictive disease, even though there is marked reduction in vital capacity (Fig 35), because the major defect in these patients is a limitation to expansion of the thorax. Similar values have been obtained in healthy individuals whose chests have been strapped tightly. The addition of as much as 90 lb on the chest and abdomen results in only a slight decrease in MVV in healthy subjects; the effect of such a weight over long periods of time is not known.

J. SUMMARY

Tests of respiratory mechanics are commonly used for screening for the presence of lung disease. Simple forced expiratory spirometry can frequently provide diagnostic data for the underlying mechanisms of altered mechanical function. In special circumstances, additional tests of lung resistance and compliance are required to provide objective evidence for pulmonary diagnosis.

5

Regulation of Respiration*

Previous chapters have considered overall ventilation of the lung, dead space (wasted) vs. alveolar (effective) ventilation, the distribution of ventilation to different areas of the lung, the diagnosis and effects of hypoventilation and hyperventilation, and the mechanical changes that occur in the thorax during the ventilatory cycle. In this chapter, we will consider mechanisms that the body has available to sense inadequate alveolar ventilation, to correct it, and the reasons for the measures used to test them.

A. OVERVIEW OF THE RESPIRATORY CONTROL SYSTEM

The respiratory control system is designed to sense the adequacy of ventilation and to adjust the level of ventilation to the bodily need for O_2 and the requirement to eliminate CO_2 (Fig 39). The primarily controlled variables are the arterial P_{CO_2} (and pH) and arterial P_{O_2}. Other sensory inputs may modulate the effects of these primary variables (see below). The respiratory control system consists of (1) the peripheral chemoreceptors and other receptors with their afferent nerves, and (2) central CO_2-sensitive neurons (central chemoreceptors), both sense and deliver information to (3) the respiratory centers (medullary and pontine) where the sensory information is coordinated and neural output is initiated to (4) the respiratory motor neurons, the efferent nerves and respiratory muscles. Two parallel neural pathways project to the

*We wish to acknowledge the assistance of Professor Sukhamay Lahiri with this chapter.

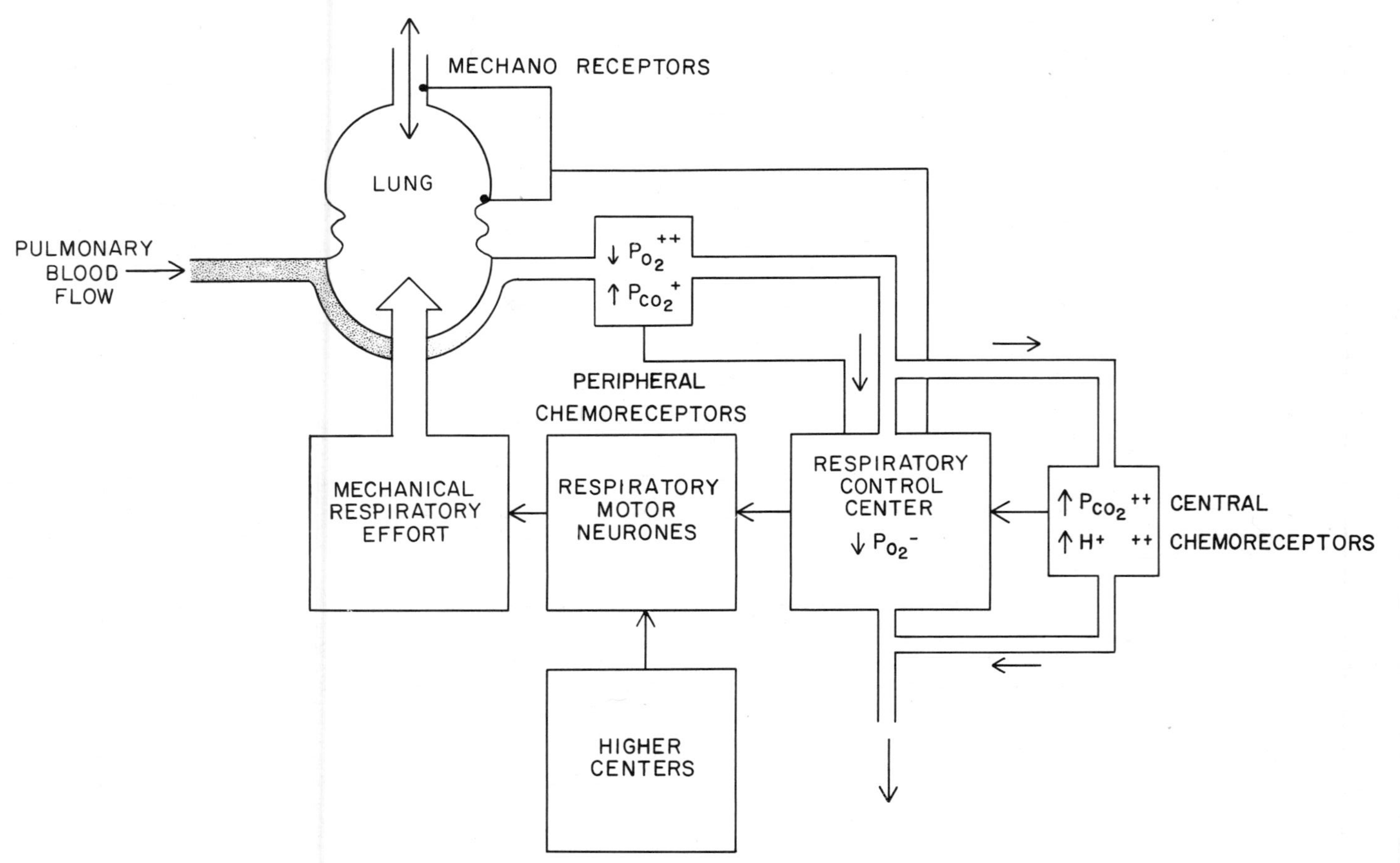
MECHANO RECEPTORS
LUNG
PULMONARY BLOOD FLOW
$\downarrow P_{O_2}$ ++
$\uparrow P_{CO_2}$ +
PERIPHERAL CHEMORECEPTORS
MECHANICAL RESPIRATORY EFFORT
RESPIRATORY MOTOR NEURONES
HIGHER CENTERS
RESPIRATORY CONTROL CENTER
$\downarrow P_{O_2}$ −
$\uparrow P_{CO_2}$ ++
$\uparrow H^+$ ++
CENTRAL CHEMORECEPTORS

Fig 39.—A simplified schematic model of the ventilatory control system. The thin line arrows represent nerve impulse traffic. Mixed venous blood enters from the left, flows through the alveolar capillaries, passes through the left heart and then through the chemoreceptors and the carotid and aortic bodies, which primarily sense a decrease in blood Po_2 but also sense changes in blood Pco_2. The arterial blood also supplies the brain-stem respiratory centers, which are very sensitive to increases in arterial Pco_2 and depressed by a decrease in Po_2. $\downarrow Po_2^{++}$ means that a decreased arterial Po_2 produces a large *increase* in ventilation; $\downarrow Po_2^{-}$ means that a decrease in arterial Po_2 results in a moderate *depression* of ventilation. $\uparrow Pco_2^{+}$ means that an increase in arterial Pco_2 results in hyperventilation; $\uparrow Pco_2^{++}$ means the hyperventilation is very large. $\uparrow H^{++}$ means that an increased $[H^+]$ causes a large hyperventilation. A change in pH should be assumed where there is a change in Pco_2. A decreased pH accompanies an increased Pco_2, and the effects of the two modalities cannot be distinguished with certainty.

spinal motor neurons to control respiratory muscles one by voluntary and one by involuntary systems. Altered activity of respiratory muscles is ultimately responsible for changes in ventilation in response to altered arterial blood gas composition. In addition, the higher cerebral centers permit voluntary control over respiration.

B. REGULATION OF VENTILATION

Since hypoventilation during air breathing leads to hypoxemia, CO_2 retention, and respiratory acidosis, one would suppose that compensatory mechanisms would be activated by a decrease in O_2, an increase in CO_2, or a decrease in pH. In normal persons, all three of these do increase pulmonary ventilation, although the relative sensitivities of these mechanisms differ considerably. The useful compensatory mechanisms are those that increase primarily the tidal volume and therefore increase alveolar ventilation (Table 7). Typical ventilatory responses to altered inspired P_{O_2} or P_{CO_2} or blood pH are shown in Figure 40.

Effect of an Increase in Arterial P_{CO_2}

The normal respiratory center is exquisitely sensitive to a rise in arterial P_{CO_2} and responds promptly with an increase in tidal volume and alveolar ventilation; with a further increase an arterial P_{CO_2}, frequency of breathing is also increased (see Table 7). Hypoventilation leads to a rise in arterial P_{CO_2}; the latter, by stimulation of medullary neurones,

TABLE 7.—Pulmonary Ventilation in Response to CO_2 Excess*

Concentration of CO_2 in Inspired Air (%)	Tidal Volume (mL)	Frequency (breaths/min)	Minute Volume (L/min)	Alveolar Ventilation (L/min)
Effects of CO_2 Inhalation on Ventilation (More than 20 normal subjects studied at each concentration of CO_2)				
0.03	440	16	7	4.6
1.0	500	16	8	5.6
2.0	560	16	9	6.6
4.0	823	17	14	11.3
5.0	1,300	20	26	22.5
7.6	2,100	28	52	47.9
10.4	2,500	35	76	69.0

*All data are mean values; alveolar ventilation was calculated using predicted anatomical dead space, taking into account increases in tidal volume.

increases ventilation and restores arterial P_{CO_2} to nearly normal levels. However, this mechanism is readily depressed by anesthesia, drugs, severe anoxemia, or cerebral injury or by high, narcotic concentrations of CO_2 itself. Under these conditions, ventilation does not increase sufficiently and the arterial P_{CO_2} remains elevated. Arterial P_{CO_2} may rise when there is mechanical limitation to ventilation, so that even a sensitive respiratory center cannot cause sufficient hyperventilation to restore normal arterial P_{CO_2}. The mechanism for the CO_2 effect is probably a change of $[H^+]$ in specialized chemoreceptors of the central respiratory neurones located in the medulla. The carotid chemoreceptors normally contribute in a minor way to the CO_2 response, although their relative contribution to the CO_2 response increases during hypoxia.

Effect of a Decrease in Arterial P_{O_2}

Hypoxemia stimulates ventilation through reflexes initiated in the chemoreceptors primarily of the carotid bodies by a decrease in arterial P_{O_2}. These bodies are perfused directly by arteries arising from the external carotid, and "sample" the arterial blood as it flows through them very rapidly.* If these structures are removed or inactivated, little or no hyperpnea occurs in response to a lowered arterial P_{O_2}. The "low O_2 stimulus" is not decreased O_2 *content* or *saturation* of the arterial blood, but decrease in the *partial pressure* or *tension* of O_2 (P_{O_2}). In anemia, CO poisoning or sulf- or methemoglobinemia, the defect is solely a reduction in active hemoglobin: the O_2 content of arterial blood may be reduced greatly with no appreciable change in arterial P_{O_2}. In these conditions there is no hypoxic stimulus to the chemoreceptors and no increased ventilation.

Although these O_2 receptors are sensitive to slight changes in arterial P_{O_2}, the effect on ventilation is relatively small near the normal range of arterial P_{O_2}. When normal men are subjected for short periods of time to increasing degrees of uncomplicated O_2 lack by the inhalation of hypoxic gas mixtures, there is no significant increase in respiration until arterial P_{O_2} is about 60 mm Hg (inspired O_2 about 16%). The chemoreceptor mechanism functions even during deep anesthesia or moderately severe depression of the CNS. It is of interest that the hyperpnea of hypoxemia becomes well defined in most individuals at approximately the arterial P_{O_2} that marks the beginning of the steep slope of the O_2 dissociation curve (see Fig 65, p. 224).

*Aortic bodies that are perfused by small vessels arising from the ascending aorta contribute to the response to hypoxemia in a minor way.

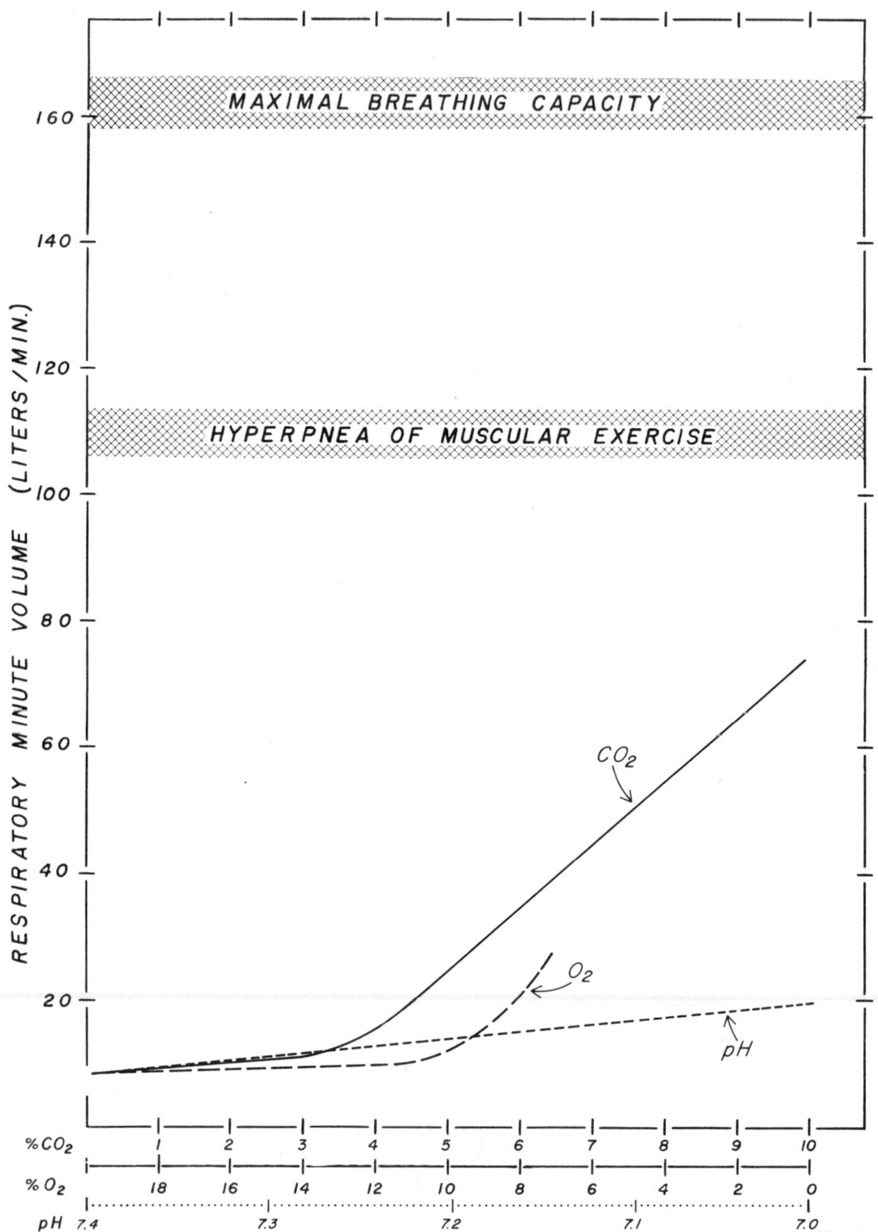

Fig 40.—The hyperpnea produced in normal man by breathing low O_2 or high CO_2 mixtures and in patients with acidosis, is contrasted with maximal possible hyperpnea (maximal breathing capacity) and with minute volume obtained during severe muscular

Effect of Acidosis

A decrease in pH can lead to an increase in tidal volume and alveolar ventilation. The Kussmaul type of breathing in diabetic or renal acidosis is an example of this. Both central and reflex chemoreceptor mechanisms are involved.

Other Factors Influencing Pulmonary Ventilation

Irritant and Other Protective Reflexes

Irritant receptors occur throughout the respiratory tract. They lie between airway epithelial cells and respond to particulate or gaseous irritants. The impulses travel in myelinated fibers in the vagus. A respiratory reflex causes apnea, closure of the glottis, and bronchial constriction when irritant materials enter the upper airway. Coughing produces forceful expiratory effort when foreign, irritating materials enter the lower respiratory tract. A swallowing reflex results in closure of the glottis and inhibition of inspiration when food is passing from the mouth to the esophagus. A submersion reflex causes apnea and bradycardia when water enters the upper respiratory tract; this is especially well developed in diving animals.

Pulmonary Stretch (Hering-Breuer) Reflexes

The best-known of these is the "inflation" or "inhibito-inspiratory" reflex, which checks respiration when the lungs have been inflated to a certain volume or degree of stretch. The receptors are probably within airway smooth muscle. The large myelinated afferent nerve fibers run in the vagus nerves. The very slow, deep breathing that follows experimental section of both cervical vagus nerves is due to loss of this check mechanism so that each inspiration becomes longer. A less well-known member of this group is the "deflation" or "excito-inspiratory" reflex, which causes earlier and more rapid inspiration and acceleration of respiratory frequency; it is initiated by deflation or collapse of portions of the lungs.

A third stretch reflex produces a maximal inspiration following a greater-than-normal inspiration and presumably provides a mechanism

---

exercise. The increased minute ventilation produced by one regulating factor may be opposed by the changes resulting in other regulating factors. When a gas mixture containing a reduced oxygen concentration is inspired, minute ventilation increases because of stimulation of the peripheral chemoreceptors. At the same time arterial P_{CO_2} is decreased and arterial pH increased, which tend to oppose the increase in minute ventilation.

for reinforcing deep inspiration when this is required. Chest wall mechanoreceptors can also influence respiration. These include tendon receptors and muscle spindles with their gamma motor neurones.

Thoracic Chemoreflexes (Von Bezold-Jarisch Reflexes)

These include the coronary and pulmonary chemoreflexes. The pulmonary reflex is also called the juxta capillary (or J reflex) because the receptor is believed to be in the wall of the capillaries. Stimulation results in reflex bradycardia, and hypotension, and apnea followed by rapid, shallow breathing. This response is produced by the injection or inhalation of minute amounts of a wide variety of chemical substances so that they reach either the pulmonary or the coronary circulation; afferent impulses travel in slowly conducting nonmyelinated fibers in the vagus nerves. This reflex may be activated by capillary vascular congestion or interstitial alveolar edema. The effects in experimental animals are dramatic and sometimes catastrophic, but may vary in different species and their physiologic or pathologic significance in man is still obscure.

Circulatory Factors

Increase or decrease of pressure in the carotid sinus and aortic arch leads to increase or decrease in the number of impulses from these vascular receptors (pressure, baroreceptors, or stretch receptors) to the respiratory center. Since these baroreceptor impulses are inhibitory, increase in arterial blood pressure reflexly diminishes pulmonary ventilation and decrease in blood pressure augments it.

Serious hypotension also appears to result reflexly in constriction of the arterioles supplying the carotid and aortic bodies so that ischemia of these structures may occur and cause intense respiratory stimulation. (The metabolic activity of the chemoreceptor tissue, though slight, exceeds the supply of O_2 when blood flow is very sharply curtailed and then local PO_2 and pH decrease and PCO_2 rises to stimulant levels.)

A decrease in cerebral blood flow may also permit the accumulation of stimulant materials such as CO_2 in the cells of the respiratory center and augment respiratory activity; an increase in cerebral blood flow may produce the reverse effect.

Reflexes From Joints

Back and forth motion of a limb produces afferent impulses that reflexly increase the rate and occasionally the depth of breathing.

Pain Receptors

Pain may cause either respiratory stimulation or inhibition, depending on the character, origin (visceral or somatic), and intensity.

Temperature

Increase in body temperature increases pulmonary ventilation, sometimes so tremendously that severe alkalosis and tetany follow. This effect results in part from warming the brain by the blood.

Supramedullary Regulation

Supramedullary areas exert important effects on the medullary respiratory center; these include cortical areas that mediate voluntary control of respiration and midbrain centers that mediate changes in respiration with altered affective states.

C. TESTS OF VENTILATORY CONTROL

Ventilatory control is tested by providing a stimulus to perturb the respiratory control system and measuring the subsequent ventilatory response. The stimuli usually applied are short-term increases in inspired CO_2, which tests predominantly the central respiratory chemoreceptors, or transient alveolar hypoxia (decreased inspired O_2), which tests predominantly the peripheral chemoreceptors. Voluntary hyperventilation is useful to evaluate the integrity of the neuromuscular apparatus. Evaluation of ventilatory responses during exercise and during sleep can be useful to determine the integrity of the respiratory control mechanism under these conditions. During these tests, the subject should be isolated as far as possible from external stimuli to minimize possible effects of conscious ventilatory control.

While the nature of the stimuli utilized to test respiratory control are reasonably well defined, determination of the response of the respiratory center is more difficult to quantitate. Direct measurement of the output of the respiratory center neurones would be ideal, although this approach is not yet possible. Indirect methods that have been used to evaluate the output of the respiratory center are (1) integrated electrical activity of the phrenic nerve, (2) integrated electrical activity (EMG) of the diaphragm, (3) inspiratory force generated by the respiratory muscles, (4) work performed during inspiration, and (5) lung ventilation. Lung ventilation is the simplest parameter to measure, although it can be greatly influenced by factors other than respiratory center output as discussed below. Diaphragmatic EMG, inspiratory force, and inspiratory work are more difficult to measure but may more directly indicate respiratory center output.

The diaphragmatic EMG is measured using electrodes in a catheter placed in the esophagus and positioned near the diaphragm. This technique provides the most direct evaluation of the response of the respiratory muscles to their stimulation by neural output from the respiratory center. However, its use is limited by its technical difficulty.

The force generated by the respiratory muscles is estimated by measuring the negative pressure at the mouth with the onset of inspiration against a closed shutter (called the *occlusion pressure*). Since there is no airflow, the mouth pressure reflects the static mechanical forces in the respiratory system generated by the respiratory muscles in response to the respiratory center output. The pressure change is measured 0.05 to 0.15 seconds after closure of the shutter in order to minimize conscious or reflex changes in muscle tone that occur during longer occlusion.

The work of inspiration requires intrapleural pressure and simultaneous volume measurements as described in chapter 4 (Mechanics). Pressure is measured with an esophageal balloon, which makes this procedure more cumbersome than measurement of occlusion pressure.

Response to Increased CO_2

Ventilatory Response to CO_2: Steady-State Method

In this method, the subject breathes a gas mixture containing increased concentrations of CO_2 and the change in ventilation (or one of the other parameters of respiratory center output) at steady state is measured. It normally requires 10 to 15 minutes to reach a steady state of ventilation. Five percent CO_2 in O_2 is commonly employed as a test gas, although greater reliability can be achieved by using several additional CO_2 concentrations, such as 3% and 7.5%. Ventilation is measured during the test by flowmeter, breath by breath, by collecting the expired gas, or calculated from the respiratory frequency and tidal volume. Normal persons show an approximately fourfold increase in ventilation during the breathing of 5% CO_2, but the response is quite variable depending on innate sensitivity of the respiratory center, reversible factors such as drug ingestion, or wakefulness, and day-to-day variation. A less variable index of response can be calculated if an arterial blood sample is obtained at the steady-state level of ventilation. A normal response is an increase in ventilation of 1.5 to 2.5 L/min per

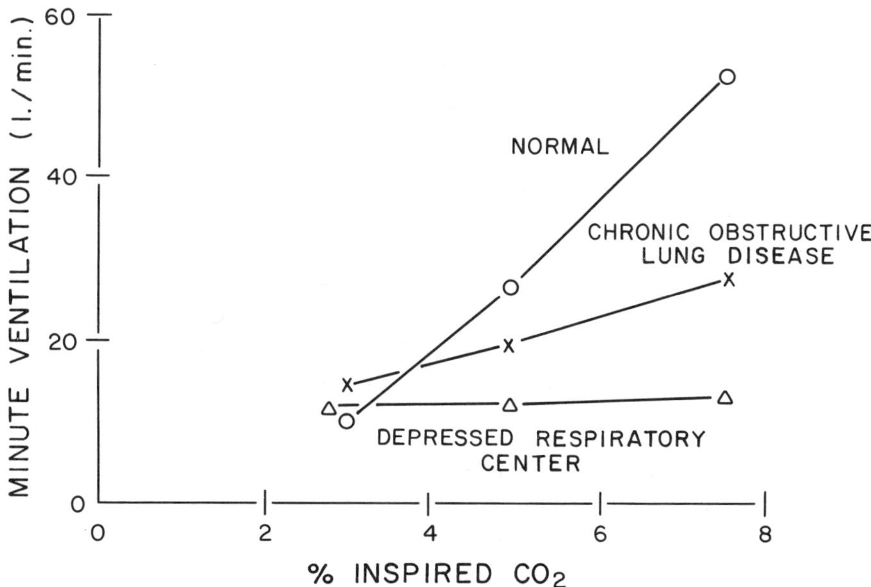

Fig 41.—Steady-state CO_2 response test. The subjects breathed gas mixtures containing 3%, 5%, and 7.5% CO_2 in air until a steady level of minute ventilation was attained (approximately five to six minutes). Subjects breathed room air for about ten minutes between each test gas. The normal subject *(circle)* shows an approximately linear increase in minute ventilation over this range of inspired CO_2. The subject with moderately severe emphysema *(x)* shows a blunted ventilatory response to CO_2. The subject with nonresponsive respiratory center *(triangle),* in this case due to previous inflammatory disease of the brain, shows essentially no ventilatory response to exogenous CO_2.

mm Hg rise in arterial P_{CO_2}. An example of the steady-state CO_2 response test performed in a normal subject and in one with emphysema is shown in Figure 41.

Ventilatory Response to CO_2: Rebreathing Method

The rebreathing method for evaluating response to CO_2 presents a constantly increasing stimulus to the respiratory center. This is accomplished through a progressive increase in alveolar and arterial P_{CO_2} as the subject rebreathes from a small bag. The expired CO_2 is continuously monitored and minute ventilation is calculated from the tidal volume and respiratory frequency. Expired, alveolar, and arterial CO_2 can be considered as equivalent under these rebreathing conditions (see chapter 9). Results are expressed as a change in ventilation per unit change in arterial P_{CO_2}. The volume of gas in the rebreathing bag should slightly exceed the vital capacity in anticipation of hyperventilation with increasing CO_2. The gas in the bag should be enriched in oxygen in order to forestall the development of hypoxia (with its attendant respiratory stimulation) during the rebreathing period. The gas in the bag should contain approximately 46 mm Hg P_{CO_2} at the start of the test to facilitate rapid equilibration between the bag, alveolar gas, and mixed venous blood (see rebreathing P_{CO_2} test in chapter 9).

Response to Decreased O_2

Tests for evaluating the response to O_2 lack are not as well standardized as those for evaluating increased CO_2. Steady-state and rebreathing techniques can be employed as described for the high CO_2 tests. It is important during these tests to maintain a relatively constant alveolar CO_2 in order to prevent fluctuations in the CO_2 stimulation of respiratory chemoreceptors. This can be accomplished during steady-state measurements by the addition of CO_2 to the respired gas. The use of low oxygen tests is limited by the effects of the consequent hypoxemia on cardiovascular and CNS function. The patient should be observed during the procedure and resume breathing air or 100% O_2 as soon as possible. Severe hypoxemia can produce unconsciousness and brain damage.

A test that minimizes possible fluctuations in alveolar CO_2 and avoids much of the systemic effects of hypoxemia is to administer one to three breaths of 100% nitrogen. The bolus of blood with a low P_{O_2} reaches the peripheral chemoreceptors before there has been any decrease in arterial P_{CO_2} secondary to the resulting increase in minute ventilation. Thus, in healthy individuals, the transient hypoxemia results in a prompt stimulation even though the arterial P_{O_2} does not decrease to the low levels required to excite the carotid body in a steady-state test. It is advisable to repeat the test several times and then accept the one with the greatest response because variations in the timing of the arrival of the blood with a low P_{O_2} affect the increment in minute ventilation.

Voluntary Hyperventilation

Voluntary hyperventilation can assess the intactness of the cerebral voluntary centers, the cooperation of the patient, and the ability of respiratory muscles and lungs to increase ventilation. In contrast to the maximal voluntary ventilation test (see chapter 4), end-tidal or arterial P_{CO_2} is also frequently measured, and the goal is a comfortable level of ventilation that can be sustained for about one minute. The test is useful to evaluate the ability of a patient with CO_2 retention to voluntarily return arterial CO_2 to a normal level or to evaluate the ability of a patient with depressed CO_2 response to increase minute ventilation.

D. INTERPRETATION OF ALTERED CO_2 OR O_2 RESPONSE

Response to Increased CO_2

Since the respiratory control system is a homeostatic regulated mechanism, interruption at any point in the system may influence the ventilatory response to CO_2. There are three general conditions that account for most of the abnormalities in CO_2 response when measured in the pulmonary function laboratory. The first is an alteration of the central respiratory chemoreceptors (medullary and pontine) resulting in decreased response to changes in arterial P_{CO_2}. An evaluation of respiratory center sensitivity to CO_2 is the usual reason for performing CO_2 response tests in pulmonary patients. Patients with abnormal respiratory center CO_2 sensitivity may show a greatly diminished response to exogenous CO_2. Decreased respiratory center responsiveness can be due to congenital defects or may be acquired following inflammatory or traumatic lesions of the CNS. It is important to note that chronic CO_2 retention frequently results in decreased responsiveness of the central respiratory chemoreceptors. The reason for this is that chronic CO_2 retention is accompanied by bicarbonate retention as a compensatory mechanism (see chapter 9). Consequently, the buffering capacity of the blood and tissue fluids is increased so that a given rise in CO_2 causes less of a change in hydrogen ion concentration.

The second condition affecting CO_2 response is disease of the neuromuscular system so that even normal output of the ventilatory center is insufficient to cause adequate lung ventilation. Examples are poliomyelitis, with damage to anterior horn cells, or myasthenia gravis affecting the myoneural junctions. This category of diseases will also result in decreased inspiratory work and decreased force of inspiration in response to CO_2. The presence of neuromuscular weakness can be diagnosed through tests of respiratory muscle strength (see chapter 4).

The third category for CO_2 response comprises those patients with mechanical limitations to thoracic expansion, such as obstructive or restrictive lung disease or thoracic wall deformity. In the presence of mechanical limitation, a given output from the respiratory center is likely to have decreased effectiveness in promoting ventilation. Stated another way, the respiratory center may effectively drive the respiratory muscles, but because of the altered lung mechanics the change in muscle activity is ineffective in promoting a normal increase in ventilation. Consequently, a test of CO_2 response that measures ventilation may be in error in evaluating true sensitivity of the medullary respiratory centers. However, measurement of the diaphragmatic EMG, the force of muscle contraction (P 0.1)*, or inspiratory work of breathing should provide a more definitive evaluation of respiratory center sensitivity. Many patients with severe lung mechanical dysfunction have chronic CO_2 retention, which can influence sensitivity of the respiratory center as described above.

Response to Lung Hypoxia

Clinically, evaluation of the response to alveolar hypoxia has relatively limited application. Occasionally there have been patients who have undergone surgical removal of carotid bodies and the response to alveolar hypoxia has been used to test the degree to which this procedure depressed O_2 chemosensitivity. Subjects with longstanding hypoxemia such as those born and raised at high altitude or patients with cyanotic congenital heart disease may lose much of their oxygen chemosensitivity; this possibility can be evaluated by administering low-O_2 tests, although it is mainly of research interest at present.

Patients with decreased ventilatory response to CO_2 (as, for example, those with chronic CO_2 retention) can be tested for O_2 sensitivity since their ventilation may be driven principally by hypoxemia. One can determine readily the extent to which hypoxemia is responsible for increasing or maintaining a patient's ventilation by measuring ventilation when the patient is breathing air and again when O_2 is substituted for air. In healthy individuals with normal arterial P_{O_2} and saturation, inhalation of O_2 decreases minute ventilation only slightly and only for a few breaths. In patients with depression of the central respiratory center, inhalation of O_2, by removal of the hypoxic stimulus which is relatively more important than in normal persons, may decrease ventilation markedly. Thus, in a patient suffering from emphysema and pulmonary insufficiency (arterial P_{O_2} 40 mm Hg), inhalation of O_2 was followed by a decrease in minute volume from 4.6 to 2.2 L/min; the patient's arterial blood became well saturated with O_2 (because of the

*P 0.1 is the negative pressure developed at the mouth 0.1 seconds after the initiation of inspiration against a closed shutter. It should be independent of the resistance of the lungs and thoracic cage and provide a measure of the neural drive from the respiratory centers, assuming normal nerve and muscle function.

high PO_2 in inspired gas), but arterial PCO_2 rose to 120 mm Hg and pH decreased to 7.06. A change of this severity occurs only seldom during O_2 therapy; however, it is important to recognize that it can occur and to be prepared to combat the hypoventilation by mechanical aids.

E. PULMONARY VENTILATION DURING EXERCISE

The cardiopulmonary system of a healthy young adult at rest need supply only about 250 ml of O_2 to the body tissues each minute; during the most vigorous muscular exercise, it must supply very much more (as high as 5,500 ml/min—a 22-fold increase). It accomplishes this by a great increase in cardiac output per minute and by a tremendous increase in alveolar ventilation; the latter maintains alveolar and arterial PO_2 at normal levels despite the considerable increase in blood flowing past the alveoli each minute and the huge quantities of O_2 that must be added to each milliliter of blood. Increased activity of skeletal muscle lowers tissue PO_2, raises tissue PCO_2, increases tissue temperature, and lowers tissue pH; all of these favor dissociation of HbO_2 and delivery of O_2 to the tissues and therefore lower the venous O_2 content far below the familiar levels given for the resting individual (see p. 240).

Figure 40 (p. 120) shows that the minute volume of breathing during maximal, but brief, exercise in healthy young men may exceed 100 L/min. This is about 50 L/min *less* than that attainable by maximal *voluntary* hyperventilation but very much more than the ventilation forced on the same men by inhalation of high concentrations of CO_2 or of low concentrations of O_2 or by a decrease in pH.

Since there is no significant change in arterial PO_2, PCO_2, or pH during moderate muscular exercise in a healthy individual, an increased "chemical drive," acting centrally or reflexly on systemic arterial chemoreceptors, does not exist and cannot be held responsible for the increase in ventilation. Many different theories have been proposed to explain this hyperpnea in the face of normal arterial PO_2, PCO_2, and pH. These include (1) increased "sensitivity" of the medullary respiratory center to normal arterial PCO_2 levels, possibly caused in part by liberation of adrenergic mediators; (2) bombardment of the respiratory center by impulses from the motor cortex en route to the exercising muscles; (3) an unidentified X-substance formed during muscle contraction and acting on the respiratory center; (4) a rise in blood temperature; (5) reflexes from the exercising muscles, originating in either stretch receptors or chemoreceptors; (6) conditioned reflexes: (7) reflexes originating from receptors in the central venous system or pulmonary circulation. No single theory proposed to date is adequate, and it is likely that multiple factors are responsible.

Exercise tests are often used in the evaluation of pulmonary function, even though the cause of the respiratory response is known only incompletely. Measurements can be made during mild, moderate, or maximal exercise (treadmill, stationary bicycle, or steps) and again during the recovery period. Some of the measurements made are as follows*;

1. Respiratory rate, tidal volume, minute volume, physiologic dead space, and alveolar ventilation.
2. Oxygen consumption and CO_2 output.
3. Pulmonary diffusing capacity.
4. Arterial O_2 saturation, PO_2, PCO_2, and pH.

These are certain generalizations that are useful in the interpretation of changes in pulmonary function with exercise:

1. In normal exercise, arterial PO_2 generally rises slightly and arterial PCO_2 decreases slightly, indicating ventilation in excess of metabolic requirements. However, in exhausting muscular exercise, arterial PO_2 may actually decrease and PCO_2 rise. In patients who have a limitation to ventilation, mild exercise may produce these same chemical changes; this is because their ventilation cannot keep pace with the demands for O_2 uptake and CO_2 elimination.
2. The diffusing capacity normally increases and can double with the heavy exercise (see chapter 8). Failure of diffusing capacity to increase generally indicates a restricted pulmonary capillary bed.
3. The physiologic dead space ventilation as a fraction of total ventilation (V_D/V_T) decreases indicating a relative increase in effective (alveolar) ventilation. Increased V_D/V_T during exercise indicates an abnormal increase in ventilation-perfusion mismatching.
4. Arterial pH is maintained at normal or slightly alkalotic values compatible with hyperventilation. A decrease in pH with decreased serum HCO_3^- can indicate acidosis from excess production of lactic acid by exercising muscles. The work level at

*Additional measurements related to cardiovascular performance (e.g. blood pressure, ECG, and cardiac output) are also commonly made during exercise.

which acidosis develops has been called the "anaerobic threshold" on the assumption the tissue hypoxia may be responsible in part for the excess lactate production (see chapter 9). Since increased acid production increases CO_2 generation from HCO_3^- but will not affect O_2 consumption, acidosis also increases the respiratory exchange ratio (R).

There are still gaps in our knowledge that must be filled before we can utilize fully the data from exercise tests. First, it is uncertain what normal data should be used as a basis for comparison. Responses differ in trained athletes, in healthy nonathletes, and probably again in older men and women, and in sedentary or convalescent individuals—all without pulmonary disease. Many patients with pulmonary disease have voluntarily restricted their activity for long periods because of dyspnea; the data obtained in this group may overestimate the pulmonary factors because of the changes that have occurred in the cardiovascular system and in the limb (and respiratory) muscles. Second, a very mild exercise that overtaxes some patients with severe pulmonary disease might not be sufficient to test the capacity of other patients; for this reason, there is no single standard test that can be applied to everyone. Third, brief exercise does not permit a "steady state" to develop, but some ill patients cannot exercise for longer periods. Fourth, exercise pushed beyond certain limits—to determine the capacity of the pulmonary system—may be dangerous in some patients because arterial O_2 saturation may decrease at the very time that cardiac work increases. Venous and tissue O_2 decrease still more. Consequently, exercise tests are most useful in patients with relatively mild disease that is not detected by pulmonary function tests at rest or with otherwise unexplained cardiopulmonary symptoms.

A common reason for exercise tests is to evaluate dyspnea on exertion. Possible findings in these patients include the following:

1. Decreased Pa_{O_2} and a small or no increase in diffusing capacity indicating diffusion impairment as in interstitial lung disease;
2. Increased Pa_{CO_2} and limited increase in minute ventilation indicating a mechanical limitation to thoracic expansion, abnormal respiratory center, or weakness of respiratory muscles;
3. Increased V_D/V_T suggesting an abnormality in the pulmonary vasculature such as embolism or occlusive vascular disease;
4. Low "anaerobic threshold" indicating a cardiovascular abnormality with decreased O_2 delivery to tissue;
5. Acute and reversible airway obstruction compatible with exercise-induced asthma.

The results of pulmonary function studies can provide objective evidence to correlate with the symptoms of dyspnea on exertion, although they may not in themselves "explain" the sensation of breathlessness.

F. REGULATION OF VENTILATION DURING SLEEP

During sleep in normal healthy patients, there is a physiologic reduction in the ventilatory drive from the CNS centers; arterial P_{CO_2} rises, CO_2 is retained in the body, arterial P_{O_2} and arterial oxyhemoglobin saturation fall. In patients the normally slight reduction in ventilatory drive may be greatly exaggerated, in some cases to such an extent that chronic CO_2 retention occurs along with the sequela of chronic hypoxemia.

Normal sleep is not a homogeneous state but includes several stages that have different electroencephalographic (EEG), behavioral and physiologic changes that affect the control of breathing. Sleep begins with a *quiet* or *slow-wave stage* in which the EEG shows slow 2- to 7-cycle/sec waves that increase in amplitude and become even slower as sleep progresses. Both tidal volume and frequency of breathing decrease, arterial P_{CO_2} rises, and the sensitivity of the medullary centers to increased arterial P_{CO_2} falls (the line relating the minute ventilation to arterial [alveolar] P_{CO_2} in Figure 41 is shifted to the right). This stage is followed in about 60 to 90 minutes by REM sleep, which is characterized by rapid eye movement and low-amplitude EEG waves of mixed frequencies with occasional sawtooth waves. Breathing is irregular and fails to increase with an increased arterial P_{CO_2} as much as it does when the patient is awake. REM sleep is associated with dreaming, and presumably chaotic respiratory movements are related to dream experiences. In contrast to the decrease in sensitivity to arterial CO_2, which is regulated by the medullary central regions, a decrease in arterial P_{O_2} continues to stimulate minute ventilation in all stages of sleep, attesting to the continued function of the peripheral chemoreceptors.

The most common abnormality of the regulation of respiration during sleep is the appearance of apneic episodes—"sleep apnea." A second abnormality is the development of a lack of coordination between the contractions of the accessory muscles of respiration in the upper airway with those of the diaphragm and thorax. The vocal cords may be closed during inspiration or expiration, the tongue may become flaccid and fall back in the pharynx, or the soft tissues may collapse, blocking the airway during an attempt to inspire or expire.

Pulmonary function studies on the awake patient are generally of little help in diagnosing sleep dysfunctions, and measurements should be made while the patient is asleep. Several contributory tests can be made that do not prevent the patient from sleeping:

1. EEG leads are placed on the head to permit differentiation of the different stages of sleep and to be sure that the patient is actually asleep during function tests.
2. Electromyographic electrodes are placed laterally to the orbit of the eye, in order to detect rapid eye movements, and other electrodes placed under the chin or near the larynx to detect contractions of the tongue and of the accessory muscles of respiration in the upper airway.
3. An oximeter (chapter 9) is placed on the earlobe to follow changes in the oxyhemoglobin saturation of blood in order to evaluate the extent, if any, of arterial hypoxemia.
4. Thermocouples or thermistors are placed in the nares or in front of the mouth to provide a semiquantitative indication of air flow. Air flow is better measured with a pneumotachograph provided the patient can sleep with a mask on.
5. Pneumographs are placed across the chest and possibly across the abdomen as well, to monitor respiratory movements of the thorax and abdominal muscles. An esophageal balloon is used if the patient will tolerate it.

If the patient develops apneic periods there will be a lack of air movement at the nose and mouth, as indicated by the temperature recording devices at these orifices, the absence of simultaneous chest and abdominal movements, as shown by the pneumographic records, and a lack of muscular contraction of the accessory muscles of the upper airway, as shown by the EMG records. The severity of the apnea can be judged by the depth of hypoxemia indicated by the oximeter on the ear. The EEG and the ocular EMG demonstrate the stage of sleep in which the patient was at the time of the studies. If no signs of apnea develop we must be sure that the patient was actually asleep.

If airway obstruction occurs during sleep, the lack of or reduction of airflow would be monitored at the mouth and nose but increased movements of the thorax and/or abdomen will be seen, indicating that the centers of respiratory regulation in the CNS are attempting to increase the ventilation. The severity of the period of reduced ventilation can again be judged by the reduction in arterial HbO_2 saturation shown by the oximeter. The extent of participation and relative timing of the accessory muscles of the respiration in the upper airway, the laryngeal, pharyngeal, and genioglossus (tongue) groups, can be used to tell whether the obstruction is a result of improper excitation of the muscles.

G. FATIGUE OF THE RESPIRATORY MUSCLES

It is now recognized that fatigue of the respiratory muscles (principally the diaphragm and external intercostal muscles) may contribute to ventilatory failure in some patients with primary lung or neuromuscular diseases. Immaturity in infants, weakness of old age, increased resistance to breathing, or stiff lungs or chest wall can contribute to such fatigue. Lack of oxygen or lack of nutrients for the muscle interfere with the metabolic energy source required by the breathing muscles and hasten the onset of their exhaustion. The inspiratory muscles can sustain about 40% of maximum force exerted for indefinitely long periods, but can maintain two thirds of their maximal force for only a ten-minute period. The duration prior to signs of muscular fatigue can be prolonged, or the maximal force strengthened about 50%, by bouts of training, repeated every day over a few weeks. This can then allow a person whose exercise capacity is limited owing to respiratory exhaustion, brought on by exercise, to accomplish more work before this limit is reached. However, if exercise is limited by other factors, such training would not be of help.

When the contraction of a muscle is sustained, or the muscle produces about 40% of its maximal force, the blood flow through it becomes diminished due to the pressure outside its blood vessels. Then, lactic acid is generated and fatigue sets in. The breathing muscles can be rested, and recovery begun, if mechanical assistance is provided by a respirator. However, too many days of such assistance, by resting the breathing muscles, may weaken them, just as bed rest often weakens the leg muscles. A period of retraining may restore their strength.

Although respiratory muscle fatigue can frequently be suspected on clinical grounds, objective assessment of respiratory muscle function may be useful in the diagnosis of the early stages or in charting the course of recovery. Unfortunately, most of the tests are still in the experimental stage. Some of the tests that have been proposed are as follows:

1. Electrical activity of the diaphragm (EMG) measured with electrodes positioned in the esophagus. Calculation of the power spectrum from the EMG may give the earliest indication of impending fatigue.
2. Force generated by the diaphragm muscles calculated from the difference between intrapleural (esophageal) and intra-abdominal (gastric) pressure. This requires the assumption that muscles of the abdominal wall are unaffected.
3. Mean inspiratory flow rate calculated from the tidal volume (V_t) and the inspiratory time (t_i).
4. The "duty cycle" of respiration calculated as the inspiratory time (t_i) divided by the total time for each respiratory cycle (t_{tot}).

Experimentally, diaphragmatic electrical activity, diaphragmatic force, and mean inspiratory flow (V_t/t_i) decrease with fatigue while the "duty cycle" (t_i/t_{tot}) increases. Maximum inspiratory and expiratory pressures measured at the mouth against an occluded airway and the intrapleural pressure during a maximal inspiration (see chapter 4) can also be used as tests to evaluate muscle strength. The specific utility of these tests should become clearer in the next several years.

H. SUMMARY

The respiratory control system normally maintains arterial blood P_{CO_2} and P_{O_2} at constant levels. Abnormalities of respiratory control can be assessed by measuring the ventilatory or neuromuscular response to increased CO_2 or decreased O_2.

6

The Pulmonary Circulation

The pulmonary circulation has a pump (the right ventricle), a distributing system (arteries and arterioles), a gas exchange mechanism (the capillary bed) and a collecting system (venules and veins). The functional part of the pulmonary circulation is the capillary bed. It is a remarkable structure.* Normally, at any single moment, it contains only 75 to 100 ml of blood, but this is spread out in a multitude of thin-walled vessels (0.1 μ thick) that have a surface area estimated at 50 sq m, or 30 times the body surface area. It is a readily expansible bed: as much as 30 L of blood can be pumped through it each minute without the pressure rising high enough to cause pulmonary edema.

In an evaluation of pulmonary function, these measurements of the pulmonary circulation are important:

- I. Hemodynamic properties
  - A. Pressures
    - 1. Intravascular
    - 2. Transmural
    - 3. Driving
  - B. Resistance
  - C. Flow
  - D. Volume

*The pulmonary capillary bed sometimes is described as if the red blood cells were flowing between two sheets, permeable to gas, resembling an underground parking garage with posts separating the floor from the ceiling.

II. Distribution of flow
III. Lung water content
IV. Metabolic function

I. PHYSICAL PROPERTIES

A. Pressures

Three different pressures may be measured: (1) *Intravascular pressure,* the actual blood pressure in the lumen of a vessel at any point, relative to atmospheric. (2) *Transmural pressure,* the difference between the pressure in the lumen of a vessel and that of the tissue around it; it is the pressure which tends to distend the vessel (according to its compliance, see p. 66). The pressure around the pulmonary arteries and veins is approximately intrapleural pressure. The pressure around the capillaries is approximately intra-alveolar pressure. The pressure around the smaller vessels (arterioles, venules) is neither intra-alveolar nor intrapleural pressure, but something in between. (3) *Driving pressure,* the difference in pressure between one point in a vessel and another point downstream; it is the pressure which overcomes frictional resistance and is responsible for flow between these points.

It is important to think clearly about these three different pressures. For example, the driving pressure for the total pulmonary circulation is the difference between the intravascular pressure at the beginning of the pulmonary circulation (the pulmonary artery) and that at the end of the pulmonary circulation (the left atrium); serious error may be introduced if the left atrial pressure is not measured but assumed to be normal. If mean pulmonary arterial pressure is 15 mm Hg and mean left atrial pressure is 5 mm Hg, the driving pressure is 15 − 5, or 10 mm Hg. If, as a result of mitral stenosis or left ventricular failure, the mean left atrial pressure rises to 20 mm Hg and the mean pulmonary arterial pressure rises to 30 mm Hg, calculations of pulmonary driving pressure are in serious error if one *measures* pulmonary arterial pressure and *assumes* that left atrial pressure is 5 mm Hg; actually, the driving pressure is 30 − 20, or again 10 mm Hg. In this example, although the driving pressure is the same in both cases, the circulation is not the same: in the second case the pulmonary arterial pressure, and hence right ventricular work, is increased twofold; in addition, the transmural pressure at each point in the pulmonary circulation is increased (assuming that no change occurred in extravascular pressures).

Why is this distinction important? There are two important effects of increased pulmonary vascular pressure. The first is the formation of pulmonary edema. When transudation of fluid occurs, it occurs across the pulmonary *capillary* walls—not across the arterial or venous walls. Fluid leaves the capillaries to enter the alveoli or interstitial tissues when *transmural* capillary pressure exceeds the transmural colloidal osmotic pressure. Capillary (intravascular) pressure (measured as left atrial pressure) may be greater than transmural colloidal osmotic pressure without evidence of gross pulmonary edema in some patients with mitral stenosis; presumably in these cases an elevated pericapillary *tissue* pressure reduces transmural pressure to safe levels.

The second important effect of increased pulmonary vascular pressure is right ventricular strain, hypertrophy, and possibly failure. An increase in right ventricular pressure does not mean that the right ventricle *must* fail, any more than left ventricular failure necessarily follows systemic arterial hypertension, but failure is more likely to occur than if pressure remained normal. Right ventricular failure occurs more frequently when the pulmonary hypertension is associated with anoxemia, since this reduces the O_2 concentration in coronary blood.

The pressure may be extremely high in the pulmonary artery and normal in the pulmonary capillaries; in such a case, there must be unusual resistance to flow through the artery or arterioles. It is obvious that knowledge of the pulmonary *arterial* pressure alone provides no information about the pulmonary *capillary* pressure; there may be severe right ventricular strain and failure without any tendency to transudation across the capillary bed. On the other hand, an increase in pressure in the capillaries of only 20 to 25 mm Hg may cause fulminating pulmonary edema and death, even though this same increment of pressure usually would not impose severe strain on the right ventricle if it occurred only in the *pre*capillary part of the circulation (between the right ventricle and the pulmonary capillaries).

The intravascular pressures in the pulmonary circulation are pictured in Figure 42. It is possible to place catheters in the main pulmonary artery, the right and left pulmonary artery branches, the pulmonary veins, and the left atrium and to make pressure measurements at these specific points. It is *not* possible to measure intracapillary pressure directly. Obviously, since blood flows from the pulmonary arterioles through the capillaries to the pulmonary venules, the capillary pressure must be less than the arteriolar and higher than the venular pressure. "Capillary" pressure is estimated by wedging a cardiac catheter as far as it can go into the finest branch of the arterial system and measuring the pressure there; this pressure is approximately equal to pulmonary venous pressure if there is no prevenular obstruction. "Capillary" pressure is sometimes estimated from measurements of left atrial pressure.

Pulmonary arterial pressure may rise because of (1) elevation of the level of pressure beyond the pulmonary circulation (in the left atrium), (2) increase in resistance to flow somewhere in the pulmonary circulation (blood flow remaining constant), (3) increase in blood flow (left atrial pressure and pulmonary vascular resistance remaining constant), or (4) combination of these.

If the level of pressure is increased beyond the pulmonary circulation (e.g., mitral stenosis with elevated left atrial pressure; left ventricular failure with increased end-diastolic ventricular pressure and left atrial pressure), the driving pressure must be restored to normal if the right ventricle is to maintain normal blood flow. This requires an increase in pulmonary arterial pressure, and this in turn requires an increase in right ventricular work. The pulmonary arterial pressure does not rise "because" the left atrial pressure increased; it rises because something influences the right ventricle to work harder. The mechanism involved is probably that described by Starling in his "law of the heart": initially, because the ventricle must beat against a higher pressure, it does not empty normally in diastole; the diastolic size of the right ventricle is thus increased, and this leads to increased energy of muscular contraction on the next beat.

In this type of pulmonary hypertension, intracapillary pressure must also rise, as must transmural pressure unless there is an increase in extracapillary pressure.

The other causes of pulmonary hypertension will be discussed below under "Resistance" and "Flow."

B. RESISTANCE TO FLOW IN PULMONARY CIRCULATION

Vascular resistance is usually calculated from an equation similar to Ohm's Law governing resistance, current flow, and electromotive force (emf) in electrical circuits.

$$\text{In an electrical circuit, Resistance} = \frac{\text{emf}}{\text{current flow}}$$

$$\text{In the vascular system, Resistance} = \frac{\text{driving pressure}}{\text{blood flow}}$$

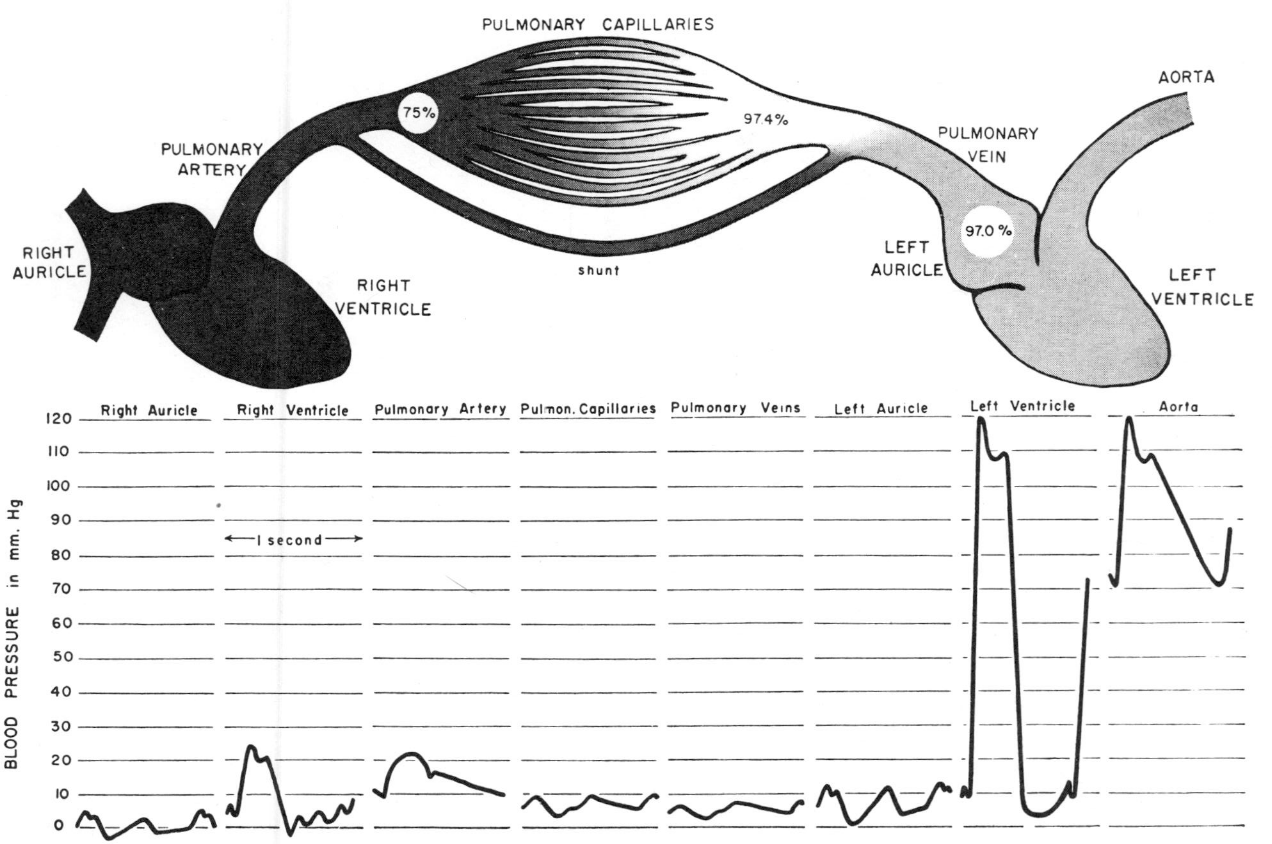
PULMONARY CAPILLARIES
AORTA
75%
97.4%
PULMONARY VEIN
PULMONARY ARTERY
97.0 %
RIGHT AURICLE
shunt
LEFT AURICLE
LEFT VENTRICLE
RIGHT VENTRICLE
Right Auricle
Right Ventricle
Pulmonary Artery
Pulmon. Capillaries
Pulmonary Veins
Left Auricle
Left Ventricle
Aorta
BLOOD PRESSURE in mm. Hg
120
110
100
90
80
70
60
50
40
30
20
10
0
1 second

Fig 42.—Pressure pulse curves obtained by catheterization techniques in man, shown for each part of the intrathoracic cardiovascular system. Venous blood which flows past well-ventilated alveoli becomes arterialized. Some venous blood does not come in contact with ventilated alveoli and some flows past poorly ventilated alveoli; this blood is not arterialized or is incompletely arterialized ("physiologic shunt"). The numbers 75%, 97.4%, and 97.0% *(in white circles)* refer to the (percent) saturation of hemoglobin with O_2 in each region.

In classic physical terms, pressure is measured in units of dynes/cm^2 (force per unit area). Blood flow is measured as cm^3/sec. Pressure/flow becomes $\frac{\text{dynes/cm}^2}{\text{cm}^3\text{/sec}} = \frac{\text{dynes} \cdot \text{sec}}{\text{cm}^5} = \text{dynes} \cdot \text{sec} \cdot \text{cm}^{-5}$. Since this is a cumbersome term, some physiologists prefer to use simpler "resistance units," using pressure as mm Hg instead of dynes/cm^2 and L/min (L for liter) instead of cm^3/sec.

$$\begin{matrix}\text{Resistance} \\ \text{(in resistance units)}\end{matrix} = \frac{\text{mm Hg (driving pressure)}}{\text{L/min}}$$

To calculate resistance, one must know values for driving pressure (not merely pulmonary arterial pressure) *and* flow. If the driving pressure remains the same while flow doubles, the resistance has been reduced to one half; if the driving pressure doubles but flow also doubles, the resistance has remained the same.

A normal value for resistance in the whole pulmonary circulation is:

$$\begin{aligned}&\text{Resistance} \\ &= \frac{\text{mean pulmonary arterial pressure} - \text{mean left atrial pressure}}{\text{pulmonary blood flow}} \\ &= \frac{14 - 5 \text{ mm Hg}}{5 \text{ L/min}} = \frac{9}{5} = 1.8 \text{ resistance unit}\end{aligned}$$

The limitations of this calculation of pulmonary vascular resistance are discussed on page 153.

The resistance in the pulmonary circulation is about one tenth that in the systemic circulation of a healthy adult. Since it is so small, small errors in the measurement of the pulmonary arterial and left atrial pressures can produce large errors in calculated resistance; a 2-mm Hg error in each could give the following:

$$\frac{12 - 7}{5} = \frac{5}{5} = 1 \text{ resistance unit}$$

Similar uncertainties apply to the partition of resistance in the pulmonary circulation. If the mean pulmonary arterial pressure were 14 mm Hg, the mean capillary pressure 7 mm Hg, and the mean pulmonary venous pressure 5 mm Hg, the resistance across the arterioles would be $\frac{14 - 7}{5}$, or 1.4 unit, and that across the venules only $\frac{7 - 5}{5} = 0.4$ unit. However, if the venules were restricted and pressures proved to be 14, 10, and 5, respectively, the arteriolar resistance would be $\frac{14 - 10}{5} = 0.8$ and the venous resistance $\frac{10 - 5}{5} = 1$ unit.

Until recently, it was believed that there was little physiologic regulation of the pulmonary resistance vessels and that the caliber of the resistance vessels changed passively with changing transmural pressure. Certainly, no striking changes in resistance are noted following stimulation of efferent pulmonary nerves, sympathetic or parasympathetic. Furthermore, many drugs with definite vasodilator or vasocontstrictor actions on systemic vessels produce little change in the normal pulmonary circulation. However, it now seems certain that there is some control over the pulmonary resistance vessels. Some of the evidence is as follows: (1) Oxygen lack appears to cause vasoconstriction. (2) The raised left atrial pressure present in mitral stenosis is followed by increased pulmonary arteriolar resistance which is, at least in part, reversible. (3) In some patients with pulmonary hypertension, acetylcholine injected into the pulmonary artery causes a decrease in pulmonary arterial pressure by a direct vasodilator effect (the acetylcholine is destroyed by blood cholinesterase before the acetylcholine reaches the systemic circulation, where it would otherwise cause bradycardia, vasodilation, and hypotension).

Total pulmonary vascular resistance may increase in many pathologic conditions, and in these the increased resistance may be in the artery, arterioles, capillaries, venules, or veins. Among the causes of increased resistance are (1) intraluminal obstructions, such as thrombi and emboli (blood clots, parasites, fat cells, air, tumor cells, white blood cells, platelets); (2) disease of the vascular wall, such as sclerosis, endarteritis, polyarteritis, and scleroderma; (3) obliterative or destructive diseases of vessels, such as emphysema and interstitial pulmonary restrictive disease; (4) arteriolar or venospasm; (5) critical closure of small vessels during and after a period of severe hypotension; (6) compression of vessels by masses or infiltrative lesions; (7) release of some chemical substances such as histamine, serotonin, and prostaglandin F_2; and (8) compression of capillaries by increased alveolar pressure.

The effects of increased resistance depend in part on its location. If it is in the venules or veins, intravascular and transmural pulmonary capillary pressures rise and pulmonary edema may result; if it is in the arteries or arterioles, pulmonary capillary pressure does not rise. In any location, an increase in vascular resistance is followed by increased right ventricular pressure and right ventricular strain, if pulmonary blood flow does not decrease.

It has been possible to compare resistance of the different segments of the entire length of the pulmonary vascular bed experimentally by continuously recording the perfusion pressure while a small bolus of saline solution is carried by the blood through a lung segment. As the low-viscosity bolus reaches the vessels of high resistance, the perfusion pressure decreases. After the bolus passes, the perfusion pressure rises again. This method shows that the arterioles have a higher resistance to blood flow than the capillaries or the veins.

Another method to judge resistance in the vascular bed of a perfused lobe depends on an abrupt occlusion of either the inflow or outflow vessels while following the time course of pressure change at the point of occlusion, either at the time of occlusion or following its release.

C. FLOW

Blood flow may be measured by many methods, including (1) the direct Fick method, (2) indicator dilution methods, and (3) inert gas uptake methods.

Direct Fick Method

The direct Fick method is based on mass balance for O_2 and requires measurements of O_2 uptake per minute and the O_2 concentration of arterial and mixed venous blood. Total O_2 uptake can be measured by comparing mixed expired gas with inspired gas, measuring the difference in O_2 concentration and multiplying by the ventilation. O_2 uptake equals the pulmonary blood flow times the O_2 difference between pulmonary artery and vein, or:

$$\text{Blood flow (L/min)} = \frac{O_2 \text{ uptake (ml/min)}}{\text{A-V difference for } O_2 \text{ (ml/L)}}$$

The pulmonary venous O_2 content is estimated by analysis of blood from a systemic artery. Pulmonary arterial O_2 content is estimated by analysis of blood obtained by catheterization of the right heart. Analysis of blood O_2 content is done by Van Slyke apparatus or calculated from the oxygen-hemoglobin equilibrium curve and a measured Po_2 (see chapter 9).

Indicator Dilution Methods

This technique can be used to calculate the volume rate of blood flow, and in addition give an estimate of the volume of blood between the injection and the sampling points. There are a number of possible different indicators, but they all must be confined to the vascular system, not be metabolized, and have no toxic effects in the blood.

A variety of indicators are available: dyes, such as T-1824 (Evans blue)* and the most widely used today, indocyanine green; radioisotopes; or heat, hot or cold saline. This last has the advantage that it can be repeated many times.

The procedure is to inject (and flush) a measured amount of indicator into the pulmonary artery through a cardiac catheter. Blood is drawn slowly and at a constant rate from a peripheral artery, or the left heart, through an analyzer that continuously records the blood concentration of the indicator. A record of indicator concentration in blood against time is plotted on ordinary graph paper as illustrated in Figure 43, using indocyanine green as an example.

The basic principle of the calculation of blood flow from this curve is that the total amount of indicator recovered from the outflowing blood must equal the quantity injected upstream since it is not metabolized. That is, the quantity injected (mg) equals blood flow rate (L/min) × mean indicator concentration (mg/L) × time over which the sample was collected (min). This relation can be rearranged to give the following equation:

$$\text{Blood flow (L/min)} = \frac{\text{Quantity injected (mg)}}{\text{Mean concentration (mg/L)} \times \text{time (min)}}$$

The product mean concentration × time of collection equals the area under the indicator dilution curve but corrected for recirculation (as in Fig 43) (see Appendix)

A major technical difficulty with the indicator dilution method is that after 10 to 30 seconds recirculation of blood containing the indicator occurs, and this dye should not be included in the computation of the total amount leaving the heart and lungs as it has already been counted once. Therefore, it is necessary to subtract the concentration contributed by this recirculated dye. When the blood is well mixed, as in the heart and great vessels, it can be assumed that the washout curve is exponential. (This is not always entirely true; deviations can be expected in abnormalities of the circulation, but this can usually be recognized by the slope of the curve.) The first appearance of recirculating indicator can be recognized on the dilution curve (shown by the arrow in Fig 43,A) and the measured concentrations beyond this point are discarded. To make this correction we plot the values of dye concentration from just after the peak to the start of recirculation, on a semilogarithmic graph (Fig 43,B). This gives a straight line since this

*The problem with T-1824 is that its absorption spectrum overlaps with that of reduced hemoglobin.

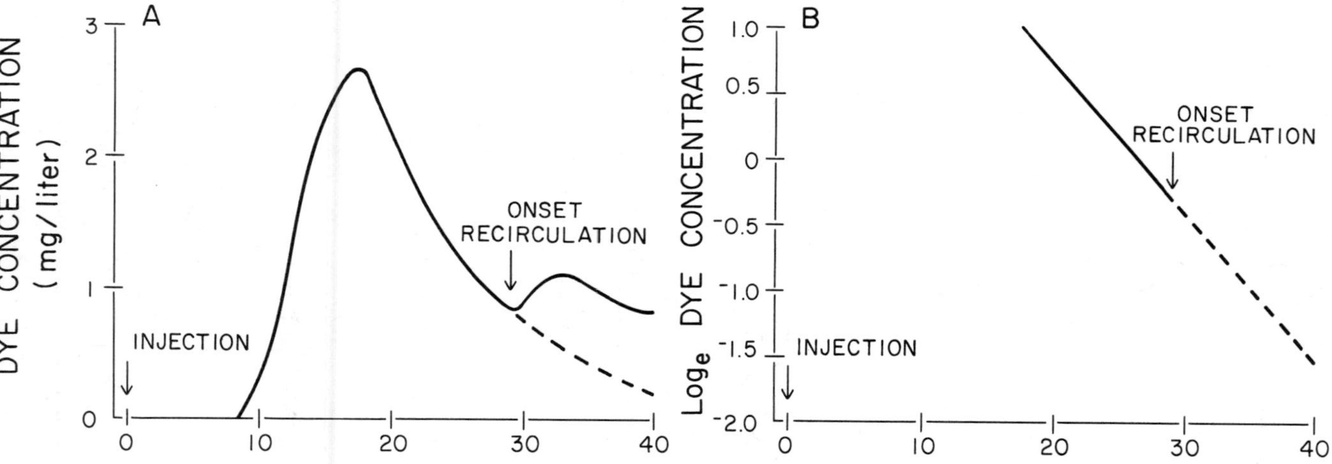

Fig 43.—An indicator dilution curve for measuring pulmonary blood flow. A dye tracer that is confined to the vascular bed, such as indocyanine green, is injected in the peripheral veins, right heart, or pulmonary arteries, and samples are collected from the peripheral arteries and analyzed for its concentration. In panel **A,** is a graph of the dye concentration vs. time. The injection took place at the arrow, time zero. The onset of recirculation of the dye is recognized by the rise, or sharp change in rate of fall, of the venous dye concentration curve. The dotted line represents the exponential extrapolation of the falling concentration curve. In panel **B,** is a semilogarithmic plot of venous dye concentration from peak concentration to the onset of recirculation, extrapolated as the dashed line.

washout process is exponential, and the original curve can be extrapolated by extending the line (shown as a dotted line in Fig 43,B). This provides the extrapolated curve shown on a dotted line in Figure 43,A. The area under this corrected curve can be computed graphically or algebraically (see Appendix), by hand, or automatically by computer.

In the example in Figure 43,A, 3 mg of indocyanine green was injected. The area under the curve was found to be 0.5 mg × min, so

$$\text{Pulmonary blood flow} = \frac{3}{0.5} = 6 \text{ L/min}$$

Inert Gas Methods

These methods all depend on the fact that the partial pressure of an inert gas, which by definition does not react chemically with blood (or tissue for that matter), is the same in blood leaving the alveolar capillary as in the alveolar gas (see chapter 8, "Diffusion"). Therefore

$$\left\{\begin{array}{c}\text{Rate of absorption of inert}\\ \text{gas in the lungs}\end{array}\right\} = \left\{\begin{array}{c}\text{Alveolar partial pressure of the gas}\\ \times \text{ its solubility in blood } \times\\ \text{pulmonary blood flow}\end{array}\right\}$$

The different inert gas techniques vary in the method by which the rate of uptake of the inert gas in the lungs is obtained. In the "single-breath method" the rate of uptake is calculated from the change in alveolar concentration during breath-holding × the effective alveolar volume. The patient makes a single large inspiration of a gas mixture containing a low (nonexplosive) concentration of acetylene and holds this breath for 2 to 20 seconds, during which time some acetylene dissolves instantly in the lung tissue and some is carried away by the blood. At the end of the breath-holding period, the patient breathes out rapidly and an alveolar gas sample is collected (after the dead space gas is washed out) and analyzed for acetylene and helium. The greater the blood flow, the more acetylene is carried away. Helium, which does not react with either blood or lung tissue and which is very insoluble in both, is included in the inspired gas in order to be able to calculate the initial concentration of acetylene in the alveolar gas sample (see Fig 44).

A graph of expired alveolar acetylene concentration after different times of breath-holding is shown in Figure 44. The alveolar acetylene disappears in two steps; there is an instantaneous decrease to about 90% of the initial value, after which the concentration falls exponentially (linearly on a semilogarithmic plot). From 20 to 30 seconds of breath-holding there is increasing deviation from linearity as a result

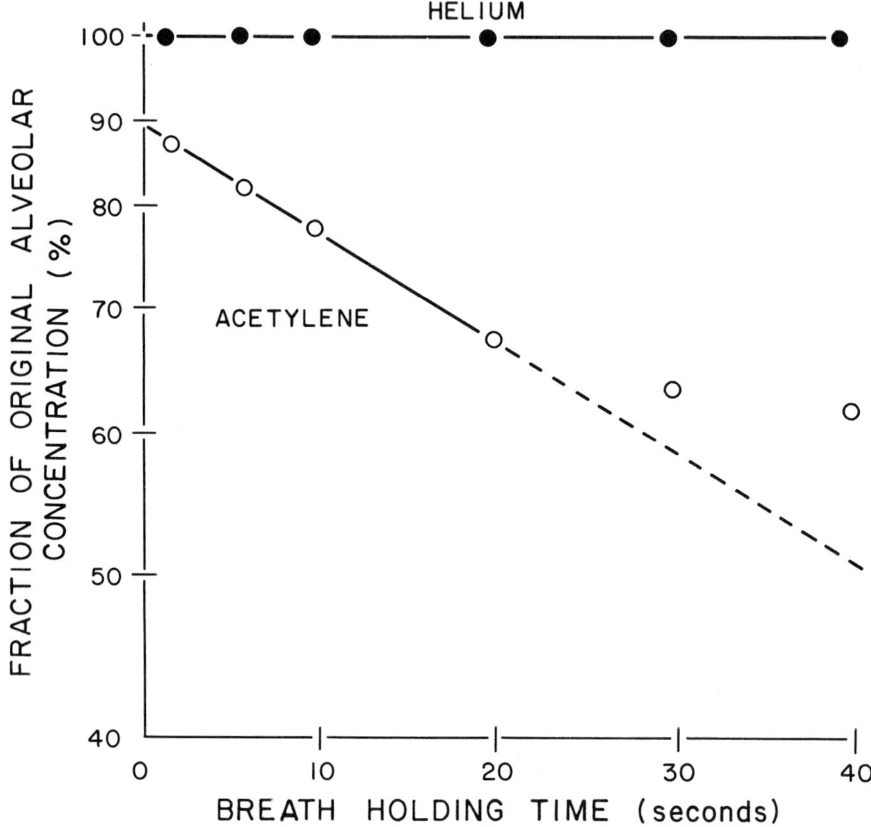

Fig 44.—The disappearance of acetylene from alveolar gas during breath-holding. The patient made a maximal inspiration of a gas mixture containing 0.5% acetylene, 10% helium, 20% O_2, and the remainder N_2. He then held his breath from two to 40 seconds, rapidly breathed out, and an alveolar sample was collected. (The first liter of the expired gas was discarded.) Many patients will not be able to hold their breath as long as 40 seconds, but much shorter times will suffice. The alveolar samples were collected and analyzed for helium and acetylene concentration. No detectable helium was lost in the blood or dissolved in the lung tissue. Therefore the acetylene concentration in each expired alveolar sample was expressed as a fraction of the original acetylene in that sample by the following calculation:

$$\text{Fraction original acetylene} = \frac{\text{expired alveolar acetylene \% x inspired He \%}}{\text{inspired acetylene \%} \times \text{expired alveolar He \%}}$$

Note that the expired alveolar acetylene ceases to disappear exponentially after about 20 seconds, the presumed onset of significant recirculation of the blood.

of the recirculation of blood containing acetylene. The initial drop is produced by the solution in a lung tissue of 10% of the acetylene that initially was in the alveolar gas.

During the linear phase the loss of acetylene from alveolar gas and acetylene that dissolved in lung tissue equals that carried away by the blood. This loss from alveolar gas equals the change in alveolar acetylene concentration × the effective lung volume. The rate at which the blood carries away acetylene is equal to the pulmonary blood flow × the alveolar acetylene concentration × the solubility of acetylene in blood. Both pulmonary blood flow and the volume of pulmonary tissue in diffusion equilibrium with alveolar gas can be calculated from the data in Figure 44 using an exponential equation given in the Appendix.

This method requires patient cooperation but provides a value of pulmonary blood flow in reasonable agreement with measurements by other methods and does not require blood samples. It has the disadvantage that the breath-holding procedure must be done at least twice in order to obtain the rate of change of alveolar acetylene concentration after the initial drop. The other side of the coin is that the method in addition to blood flow provides a measure of lung tissue volume. The value of pulmonary blood flow obtained represents an average over the entire period of breath-holding, and measurements must be restricted to the period before recirculation occurs.

In the *body plethysmographic method,* the absorption of a soluble inert gas, usually N_2O* is continuously registered by a decrease in pressure, providing a measure of instantaneous flow through the pulmonary capillaries, whereas the other methods yield values for average blood flow over minutes or seconds. The principle is shown in Figure 45. The patient sits in an air-tight chamber about the size of a telephone booth; pressure around the subject is measured continuously by a sensitive electrical manometer (Fig 45,*1*). On request, the patient inhales 80% N_2O–20% O_2 from a bag into his alveoli (Fig 45,*2*); as N_2O leaves the gas phase to dissolve in blood flowing through the pulmonary capillaries, the total gas pressure in the chamber decreases, and this change is registered continuously by the manometer (Fig 45,*3*). The same procedure, but after inspiration of air, provides a 'control' record that must be subtracted from the N_2O record. Knowing alveolar N_2O pressure, solubility of N_2O in blood and alveolar volume (also measured plethysmographically), the pulmonary capillary blood flow can be cal-

*Acetylene cannot be used for the plethysmographic method because the concentrations required would be explosive.

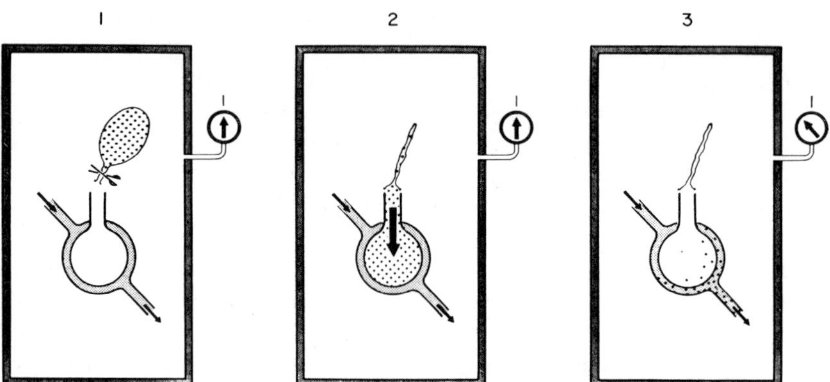

Fig 45.—Measurement of pulmonary capillary blood flow: body plethysmograph technique. The rectangle is the same air-tight body plethysmograph pictured in Figure 5. Here, the "patient" is a little more complete: in addition to alveoli and conducting airway, he also has pulmonary capillary blood flow *(stippled channel surrounding alveoli).* The circle with pointer is a sensitive gauge that continuously records pressure within the plethysmograph (around the patient). The bag with black dots (N_2O molecules) represents an anesthesia bag filled with 80% N_2O–20% O_2. When N_2O molecules leave the alveolar gas and dissolve in the pulmonary capillary blood, these no longer occupy space; because the total number of molecules of gas in the alveoli, airway, and body plethysmograph is less, pressure falls. Control measurements must be made while the patient breath-holds after inhalation of air; this is followed by inhalation of the N_2O–O_2 mixture and breath-holding for 10 to 15 seconds (see text).

culated instant by instant throughout the cardiac cycle and the nature of the capillary volume pulse can be recorded. This method involves no catheterization, no injections, and no collections of blood samples but is difficult to use when a patient is exercising because of the increased heat and water vapor production.

Pulmonary blood flow may increase in many conditions, such as exercise, hyperthyroidism, fever, anemia, anoxemia, and arterial-to-venous shunts (including left-to-right shunts associated with septal defects and patent ductus arteriosus).* Since *flow = driving pressure/resistance,* one would expect that to increase flow through the pulmonary circulation there must be a corresponding increase in driving pressure. However, measurements in normal persons have shown that pulmonary vascular pressures do not necessarily rise and certainly do not double when pulmonary blood flow is doubled by exercise. This means that pulmonary vascular resistance must decrease, either by dilatation of existing channels or by opening of new channels, or both. These measurements suggest that all available vascular channels are not in use during rest.

The total pulmonary tissue may be reduced by lobectomy or pneumonectomy without any great increase in pulmonary vascular pressures. Pneumonectomy performed in a young patient for strictly unilateral disease usually does not lead to any appreciable increase in pulmonary vascular pressures, even though the remaining vascular bed now conducts twice its former flow. It is more likely to rise in older patients because the aging process alone appears to reduce the size and distensibility of the pulmonary vascular bed. The pressure is apt to rise more if disease of the remaining lung has already destroyed, compressed or restricted part of its vascular bed. It is possible before operation to catheterize the pulmonary artery of the lung to be removed and to occlude it by inflation of a cuff around the catheter. This forces the whole right ventricular output to flow through the lung to be spared. If the pressure in the main pulmonary artery rises only transiently, the vascular bed in that lung is expansible; if it rises sharply and remains elevated, the surgeon may anticipate that the patient will have high pulmonary arterial and right ventricular pressures after pneumonectomy. Radiopaque contrast media, radioactive isotopes, and scanning methods have largely replaced occlusion by a balloon on a catheter as a means of judging adequacy of circulation in the undiseased lung prior to a resection of a diseased lung.

D. VOLUME

Pulmonary blood volume is the volume of blood between the beginning of the pulmonary artery and the end of the pulmonary veins; in a healthy adult, it is about 900 ml. It can be calculated from the pulmonary venous dilution curve of an intravascular indicator (Fig 43,A) injected into the pulmonary artery as explained in the Appendix.

Pulmonary capillary blood volume is the volume of blood in the capillary bed at any given moment. It can be estimated from measurements of the diffusing capacity for CO when the patient breathes gas of a high and a low O_2 concentration (see p. 216). The values for pulmonary capillary blood volume obtained are reasonable ones (75 to 100 ml in the resting adult); they increase as anticipated during exercise, hypervolemia, and pulmonary congestion, and decrease in patients with destructive lesions of the pulmonary parenchyma. This measurement may provide useful information regarding the absolute volume of the capillary bed and its ability to enlarge its capacity.

When the measurements of capillary blood volume obtained from the diffusing capacity for CO are compared with potential capillary volume estimated from morphometry, it appears that not all the capillaries are open all the time. To some extent the capillary bed fills during systole and empties during diastole.

Just as pulmonary arterial pressure may be changed without any change in pulmonary capillary pressure, so total pulmonary vascular blood volume may change without comparable changes in capillary blood volume.

II. DISTRIBUTION OF PULMONARY CAPILLARY BLOOD FLOW

In chapter 3, we defined uniform and nonuniform distribution of inspired air to the alveoli, listed some causes of nonuniform distribution of gas and discussed several tests which identify nonuniform distribution of gas. We shall now define nonuniform distribution of pulmonary capillary blood flow and mention some of its causes and effects and several ways of identifying it.

Capillary blood flow may be considered uniform (1) when blood flow is the same to every unit of alveolar volume (anatomic uniformity) or (2) when blood flow is distributed to each alveolus in proportion to its ventilation (physiologic uniformity).

In this section we will consider only the former; uniformity of pulmonary capillary blood flow in relation to alveolar ventilation will be considered in chapter 7.

A. CAUSES OF UNEVEN CAPILLARY BLOOD FLOW

Physiologic Causes

Just as there is some nonuniformity of *gas* distribution in healthy persons, so there is also some unevenness of capillary blood flow in erect healthy individuals (Fig 46). The latter occurs in part because of the effect of gravity. The lesser circulation is acted upon by four pressures: (1) The pulsatile intravascular pressure produced by the work of the heart; (2) the hydrostatic pressure produced by the column of blood in the lung vasculature; (3) the markedly different pressures surrounding the pulmonary vessels (from intrapleural to alveolar); and (4) possible

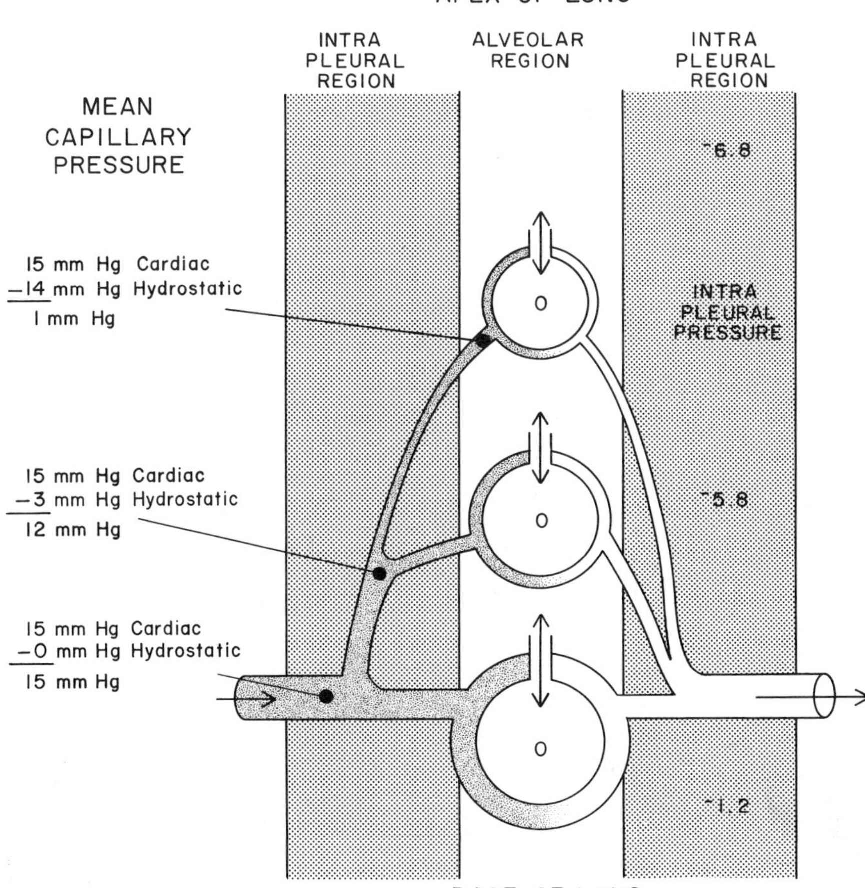

Fig 46.—Diagram showing the transmural pressure of the pulmonary capillaries at the apex, mid-level and base of the lung. Transmural pressure = mean capillary pressure − alveolar pressure (which is zero). Mean capillary pressure = mean pressure produced by the cardiac pulse-hydrostatic pressure of the column of blood in the vessels, referred to the height of the pulmonary vein (right auricle) as zero. The hydrostatic pressure of the total blood column in the lung was considered 30 cm water or 21.7 mm Hg. Intrapleural pressure is measured in reference to atmospheric pressure and its value at end expiration in mm Hg is indicated by the numerals in the *shaded* (pleural) *region* on the right-hand side. Its value was 5.6 mm Hg more negative at the apex than at the base of the lung owing to the force of gravity acting on the lung-pleural system. Its value at the mid lung level at end expiration was considered −5.8 mm Hg. The intrapleural pressure at all levels decreases with inspiration (about 2 mm Hg for a 0.5 L tidal volume). Transcapillary pressure is considerably less at the apex than in the base and is not sufficient to keep these vessels open during the entire cardiac and respiratory cycles.

large absolute changes in intravascular pressure. The lesser circulation has a relatively low pulse pressure produced by the work of the heart, so that the extravascular and hydrostatic pressures have a significant effect on its hemodynamics.

While there is neural and humoral regulation of the resistance of some larger vessels, the smaller vessels, and particularly the capillaries, are regulated largely by transmural pressure; they have no muscle and little rigidity. For this reason the pressure drop along the pulmonary capillary bed can be the largest component of the pumonary vascular resistance. The pulmonary capillary transmural pressure equals the intravascular pressure minus extravascular pressure, both in relation to atmospheric pressure as 0. That is:

Transmural pressure = Pressure produced by the heart −
height of the column of blood above the heart − alveolar pressure

Normally the pulmonary artery has a systolic pressure of 25 mm Hg, a diastolic of 10 mm Hg, and a mean pressure of 15 mm Hg, all compared to the pressure within the right auricle, which is considered 0. The blood in the lung vessels represents a column about 30 cm high, so the pressure in the vessels at the base is 21.5 mm Hg (density of mercury is 13.5 times that of blood) higher than at the apex. With the right auricle as our zero reference (which is higher than the base of the lung), this means the apical blood vessels will have a hydrostatic pressure of 17.0 mm Hg less than the right auricle.

In Figure 46, on the lefthand side, the mean pressure produced by the heart and the hydrostatic pressure are summated to give the net pressure difference across the alveolar capillary walls. Intra-alveolar pressure exactly equals atmospheric pressure when there is no air flow and the glottis is open. During normal breathing in a healthy patient, it changes less than 1 to 2 mm Hg. The transmural pressure difference of alveolar capillaries at the level of the right auricle is 15 times that of capillaries at the apex, so the apical capillaries are much narrower.

This calculation does not take into account variations in two additional pressures. The first is the pulsatile nature of the pulmonary arterial pressure, which is about 5 mm Hg less than the mean during diastole and 10 mm Hg greater than the mean at peak of systole. Therefore during diastole the transmural pressure in the apical capillaries will be *less* than atmospheric (alveolar).

Second, the variations in intrapleural pressure will be transmitted to the heart and great vessels as the intrapleural pressure region encloses them within the thoracic cage. Intrapleural pressure at a given height becomes more negative with inspiration, going from an average of −4 mm Hg at end normal expiration to −8 at the end of inspiration (see chapter 4 on mechanics of breathing). Intrapleural pressure at the same lung volume also increases as one moves down from the apex of the lung to the base because part of the weight of the lung bears on the intrapleural space. Intrapleural pressure is about 5 mm Hg higher at the base than at the apex. These effects are summated on the right-hand side of Figure 46 where the numbers represent intrapleural pressure at end expiration at different heights.

The effect of the pulsatility of pulmonary arterial blood pressure and the changes in intravascular pressure produced by swings in intrapleural pressure with inspiration and expiration is to produce greater transient changes in capillary pressure than would be concluded from considerations of hydrostatic and mean arterial pressure alone.

When capillary luminal pressure becomes less than alveolar pressure, the capillaries collapse and flow ceases. Thus, the effect of all of these pressure variations is to produce a lower capillary blood flow in the apical alveoli than in the bases. Because the influence of gravity is most important, this nonuniformity of capillary blood flow is most extreme in the erect position, but is present to some degree in the horizontal positions as well. An increase in pulmonary blood flow, as in exercise, raises the general level of capillary pressure, reducing the proportion of alveolar capillaries that collapse and, therefore, reducing the nonuniformity of pulmonary capillary blood flow.

This discussion does not mean that only capillary pressure controls pulmonary blood flow distribution. If the capillaries are open the flow limiting vascular resistance is elsewhere in the path. If they are shut, this means that the capillary resistance is infinite, and therefore controlling.

Pathologic Causes

Uneven capillary blood flow occurs in many pathologic conditions affecting the lungs and circulation. Some of these are:

1. Embolization or thrombosis of parts of the pulmonary circulation by blood clots, fat, gas, parasites, or tumor emboli.
2. Partial or complete occlusion of one pulmonary artery or some of the arterioles by arteriosclerotic lesions, endarteritis, collagen disease, or congenital anomalies.
3. Compression or kinking of large or small pulmonary vessels by masses, pulmonary exudates, or pneumothorax or hydrothorax.

4. Reduction of part of the pulmonary vascular bed by destruction of lung tissue or by fibrotic obliteration of pulmonary vessels.
5. Regional congestion of vessels such as occurs in some types of heart failure.
6. Closure of some pulmonary vessels, such as appears to occur when circulating blood volume is greatly reduced during severe hypotension and circulatory shock.
7. Anatomic venous-to-arterial shunts such as pulmonary hemangiomas; in such shunts, however, the distribution of blood that is flowing to *capillaries* may be uniform, the abnormality being that some mixed venous blood bypasses capillaries completely to empty directly into pulmonary venules or veins.

B. TESTS FOR UNEVEN DISTRIBUTION OF PULMONARY CAPILLARY BLOOD FLOW

Intravascular Impaction

Radiolabeled nontoxic degradable microemboli (over 10 μ in diameter), such as aggregated human-albumin, are injected into the venous circulation and impact in the pulmonary capillaries, where their distribution can be determined by measuring the radioactivity by scanning the surface of the chest. In normal lungs, less than 1% of the capillaries are occluded and they are rechanneled in hours. It can be assumed that the injected emboli are well mixed in the right heart so that the concentration of emboli in a volume of lung tissue, which is proportional to the measured radioactivity, is a measure of relative pulmonary blood flow. Geometric and other technical factors make the interpretation of the scans only qualitative, However, this technique is useful in the diagnosis of gross changes of the pulmonary vascular bed.

Inert Insoluble Radioactive Gas

A gas, such as radioactive xenon dissolved in saline, is injected into the venous circulation. When the blood reaches the alveoli, the inert gas equilibrates with the alveolar gas and, being highly insoluble, almost all ends up in the gas phase on passage of the blood. Since we assume the inert gas is mixed in the pulmonary artery blood the radioactivity at a given point is proportional to pulmonary blood flow. The radioactivity can be detected on the surface of the chest by radioactive scanning instruments, and the output calibrated quantitatively by inspiring the radioactive gas until equilibrium is reached (as described under "Distribution of Inspired Gas," p. 59). The radiolabeled gas, once deposited in the alveolar gas, is more slowly carried away by the blood in the same manner as acetylene (see Fig 44 and Appendix, p. 280), since the gas equilibrates between the alveolar gas phase and the capillary blood. This process provides a quantitative measure of pulmonary blood flow/(alveolar volume plus effective tissue volume) without any additional calibrations. The measures can be combined with measures of the spatial distribution of inspired radioactive inert gas to give alveolar ventilation and pulmonary blood flow in the same region—in other words, to determine the physiologically important alveolar ventilation/blood flow (see chapter 7 on Nonuniformity of Alveolar Ventilation/Blood Flow).

O_2 Uptake by Individual Lungs

Using the technique of bronchospirometry (see p. 60), the physiologist can separate the gas to and from the right and left lungs and measure the volume and composition of each of the streams. If he finds that only 50 ml of O_2 is absorbed from the right lung each minute, while 200 ml is being absorbed from the left lung, it may be surmised that only one fifth of the total pulmonary blood is flowing past alveoli in the right lung while four fifths of the total is flowing through the left lung. This test is usually performed by giving O_2 to breathe to eliminate possible effects of diffusion limitation. The test has been generally supplanted by the radioactive gas and embolization methods.

III. LUNG FLUID

A. Normal Water Balance of the Lung

Pulmonary edema, defined as an increased water content of the lung, is a common event in lung disease and represents an imbalance of the normal processes of fluid formation and removal. There is normally constant filtration of fluid into the lung interstitial space from the capillary blood and removal by the pulmonary lymphatics and cellular pathways. The pulmonary capillary endothelium presents only a partial barrier to filtration of macromolecules, and the concentration of albumin in the lung interstitial fluid has been estimated as not 0% but approximately 50% that of plasma.

The classic application of the Starling Hypothesis of the net exchange of fluid across the pulmonary capillary endothelium is given in the following equation:

$$\text{Rate of lung fluid formation} = \begin{array}{l}\text{(Transmural capillary pressure difference} - \\ \text{transmural oncotic pressure difference)} \times \\ \text{permeability of the capillary endothelial} \\ \text{barrier to water}\end{array}$$

Recent evidence has indicated that the alveolar epithelium may actively absorb fluid and electrolytes from the alveolar space and thereby help to regulate the water content of alveoli.

While the pulmonary edema of left ventricular failure presumably results from increased capillary blood pressure, it is usually not possible in man to measure these forces accurately enough to be of help to the clinician. Tests can be performed that measure the lung water content.

B. TESTS FOR ABNORMAL LUNG WATER CONTENT

Indicator Dilution Method

The indicator dilution technique for the calculation of pulmonary blood flow uses a label confined to the vascular tree (indocyanine green) as described on page 144 and illustrated in Fig 43,A. If we include a second tracer, such as tritiated water (Fig 47) that diffuses into and reaches equilibrium with the extracellular and intracellular water of the lung, we can calculate a volume for lung water. On the rising limb of the dye dilution curve (sampled in left atrium or systemic artery), the concentration of tritiated water at each moment on the venous outflow curve is reduced below that of the impermeable tracer dye because the labeled water distributes to the extravascular water volume, while the dye cannot. As the dye curve passes through its peak value and falls, the tritiated water in the tissues diffuses back into the blood and the venous tritiated water values rise above those of the dye. The greater the volume of tissue water around the capillaries, the lower the venous tritiated water dilution curve becomes and the further its peak value is displaced to the right in time.

This relative lag of the venous tritiated water dilution curve in relation to the indocyanine green dye dilution curve is a measure of the lung water volume. To be more exact, we calculate the extracellular water volume as the difference between the mean transit time of the molecules of labeled water through the lung and the mean transit time of the indicator dye times pulmonary blood flow. (This is described in detail in the Appendix.) If radiosodium is injected, along with indocy-

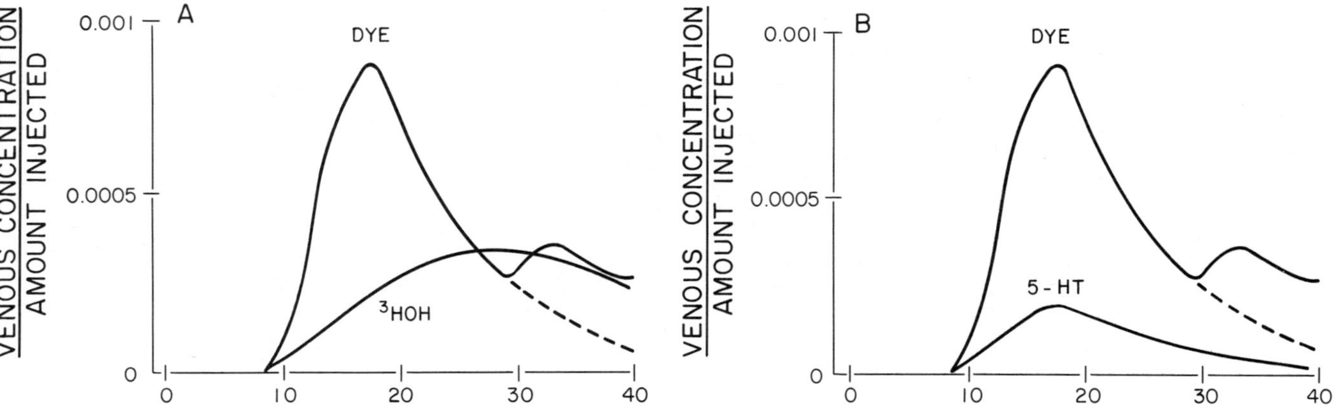

Fig 47.—Double indicator dilution curves for the pulmonary circulation. **A,** intravascular tracer *(dye)* and tritiated water (^{3}HOH) were injected in the right atrium and samples collected from a peripheral artery. The labeled water diffuses out of the capillaries into the lung tissues, lowering its concentration in the venous blood in relation to the dye tracer. The labeled water appears in the venous outflow, but delayed in time. By calculating the mean transit time of the labeled water (on the assumption that the tritiated water is in diffusion equilibrium with the lung tissue water), we can calculate the distribution volume (lung water volume) from this result (see Appendix). **B,** intravascular tracer *(dye)* and 14-C labeled 5-hydroxytryptamine (5-HT) were injected in the right atrium, and samples were collected from a peripheral artery. Approximately 60% of the 5-HT was taken up in the lung vascular bed and was not returned to the venous blood. Thus, the venous 5-HT concentration curve has the same shape as the vascular indicator curve except that it is reduced by about 60%; the shape is not shifted in time. This test provides a measure of the ability of the lung, probably of the lung capillary endothelium, to take up 5-HT.

anine green and tritiated water, the difference between its mean transit time and that of any impermeable vascular dye in the same way provides a measure of extracellular fluid volume because the sodium is permeable through the capillary wall but cannot permeate the cell walls (in a reasonable time).

The indicator dilution technique has been used to study changes in lung water volume in patients. Unfortunately, in pulmonary edema focal areas of the lung may be underperfused so that the method underestimates the total volume of lung water.

Soluble Inert Gas Method; Nuclear Magnetic Resonance

Total lung water can also be estimated by the breath-holding soluble inert gas technique (acetylene) method used to measure pulmonary capillary blood flow (Fig 44). The instantaneous (extrapolated) decrease in alveolar acetylene as compared to helium represents a solution of the acetylene in lung tissues exposed to alveolar gas. The greater the volume of lung water in relation to alveolar volume, the greater the decrease in the acetylene time zero intercept. Knowing the solubility of acetylene in the lung tissue, tissue volume can be calculated (see Appendix).

This technique is limited by the errors inherent in the breath-holding test for pulmonary blood flow, with the additional problem that there is nonuniform delivery of the inspired acetylene to poorly ventilated areas of the lung found in pulmonary edema as well as in other lung diseases.

The water content of the lung can be detected and imaged by the use of nuclear magnetic resonance techniques, which depend on measuring nuclear magnetic resonance of the water protons. However, at present there is no acceptable method for the calibration of the image in terms of absolute water mass or volume.

IV. LUNG METABOLIC FUNCTIONS

While the main function of the lung is as an organ of gas exchange, it has important metabolic functions, some of which may be disturbed in disease and can be tested. Normally, the entire cardiac output passes through the pulmonary circulation, which places the pulmonary endothelium in a unique position to modify the chemical composition of the arterial blood. While the capillary and alveolar epithelia are considered as a passive and permeable (to gas) membrane separating alveolar gas from capillary blood, the pulmonary capillary bed presents a large endothelial surface for rapidly processing blood components. Many vasoactive substances such as 5-hydroxytryptamine (5-HT or serotonin), norepinephrine, and prostaglandins are inactivated by uptake and metabolism in the lungs, while others, such as angiotensin I, are activated. The indicator dilution technique can be used to measure the binding, chemical reactions, absorption, and excretion of these compounds.

An example of a metabolic function of the lung is the catabolism of 5-HT, a vasoconstrictor liberated by thrombocytes, to inactive 5-hydroxyindoleacetic acid. This chemical reaction takes place inside the endothelial cells of the pulmonary capillaries, not on the surface, and a specific transport system exists to carry the 5-HT from the capillary blood into the cell. A test for 5-HT uptake is performed by injecting a bolus of 5-HT and a nonmetabolized, nontoxic tracer that is retained in the vascular system, such as indocyanine green or radioactively labeled dextran, collecting serial peripheral arterial samples, and analyzing them for the two species. The arterial concentration of each chemical as a fraction of the amount injected is graphed against time in Figure 47,B. The fraction of injected 5-HT that is removed from the blood is proportional to the difference between the amount of impermeable tracer that flows out in the arterial blood and the amount of serotonin that flows out. The difference between the two curves is a measure of the fraction of the injected dose of 5-HT that was taken up by the endothelial cells. The procedure determines 5-HT uptake, not its catabolism in the cells, which is much slower. There are several different methods of calculating the extraction of 5-HT; all require some approximation (see Appendix).

Another important substance that is metabolized in the lung is angiotensin I, a decapeptide that is converted by an enzyme on the surface of the capillary endothelium to an octapeptide, angiotensin II, which is an important vasoconstrictor and regulates the secretion of aldosterone by the adrenals. This converting enzyme also degrades bradykinin, a nonapeptide vasodilator, to a biologically inactive form. Converting enzyme function can be studied by the double indicator dilution method (in a similar fashion to 5-HT), analyzing for reaction products in arterial blood.

Tests of lung metabolic function are not widely used yet, but represent a type of test that is potentially very useful. Damage to the endothelium, as in oxygen toxicity, alters specific metabolic functions of the pulmonary capillary bed. The concentrations of the substrates can be varied and estimates of the binding characteristics, Km, and turnover number of the functional enzymes obtained. Unfortunately, these tests are influenced not only by lung metabolic activity but also by uneven distribution of capillary blood in the lung. While the tests require a catheter in the right side of the heart and in a peripheral artery, these are often already present for patient care in pulmonary conditions that are of particular interest, such as adult respiratory distress syndrome.

V. SUMMARY

The functional parts of the pulmonary circulation are the pulmonary capillaries. The right ventricle, pulmonary arteries, and arterioles represent a distributing system and the venules and veins a collecting system for the pulmonary capillary blood. The pressure and resistance to flow in the pulmonary capillaries is normally low and must remain so to prevent transudation of fluid into the intermembrane spaces or into alveoli. The pressure and resistance to flow in the pulmonary artery and arterioles is normally low and must remain so to prevent right ventricular strain and hypertrophy and possibly failure. Normally, all mixed venous blood in the pulmonary arteries is distributed uniformly to the alveolar capillaries, in relation to the ventilation of alveoli; when it is not, hypoxemia results unless there is hyperventilation.

Tests of pulmonary function can measure pressures, blood flow, vascular resistance, and distribution of blood flow in the pulmonary circulation; they can indicate the presence of venous-to-arterial shunts, vascular occlusion, diminution in pulmonary capillary volume and, in some instances, locate the specific area involved.

Tests are being developed to evaluate lung water and metabolic function of the pulmonary endothelium; these will provide information with respect to cellular integrity of the pulmonary vasculature.

7

Distribution of Ventilation and Blood Flow

In discussing both the nonuniform distribution of inspired gas in chapter 3 and the nonuniform distribution of capillary blood flow in chapter 6, we postponed discussion of the effects of uneven distribution of inspired gas on arterial O_2 and CO_2. This is because, other factors being normal, the O_2 and CO_2 in blood leaving the lungs is determined not only by ventilation and not just by blood flow as individual factors, but also by the various ratios of the ventilation of different alveoli to their capillary blood flow. The effects of uneven ventilation/blood flow on arterial blood P_{O_2} and P_{CO_2} will be discussed in detail in the following sections.

I. EFFECTS OF UNEVEN RATIOS ON ARTERIAL BLOOD P_{O_2}

Figure 48 shows the ideal relationship: Inspired air (all of the same composition) is distributed uniformly so that all alveoli have the same end-inspiratory P_{O_2} and the same end-inspiratory P_{CO_2}. Mixed venous blood (all of the same composition) is distributed uniformly to all of the pulmonary capillaries in relation to the ventilation of each group of alveoli. Alveoli *A* receive 2 L/min of ventilation and 2.5 L/min of capillary blood flow; alveoli *B* (which have a gas volume equal to that of alveoli *A*) also receive 2 L/min of ventilation and 2.5 L/min of capillary blood flow. This results in an alveolar and arterial O_2 tension of

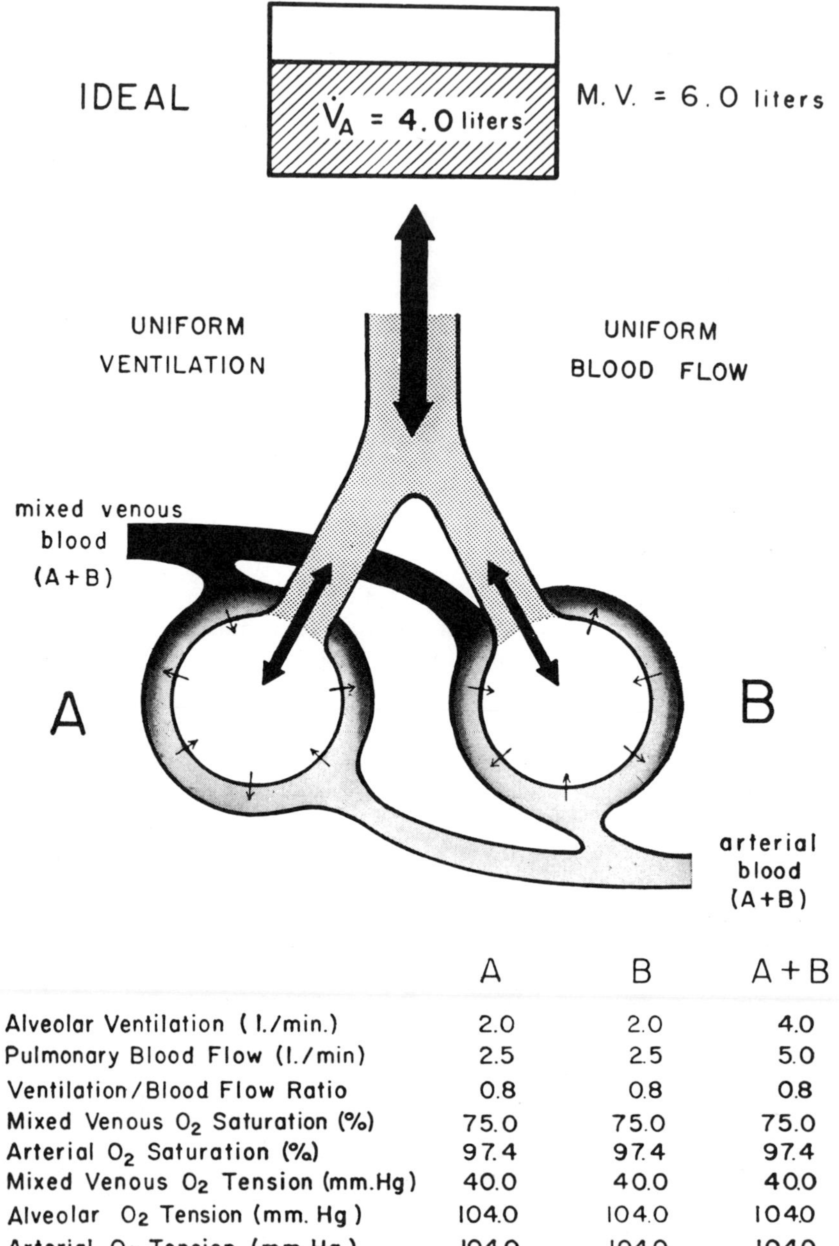

	A	B	A+B
Alveolar Ventilation (l./min.)	2.0	2.0	4.0
Pulmonary Blood Flow (l./min)	2.5	2.5	5.0
Ventilation/Blood Flow Ratio	0.8	0.8	0.8
Mixed Venous O_2 Saturation (%)	75.0	75.0	75.0
Arterial O_2 Saturation (%)	97.4	97.4	97.4
Mixed Venous O_2 Tension (mm.Hg)	40.0	40.0	40.0
Alveolar O_2 Tension (mm. Hg)	104.0	104.0	104.0
Arterial O_2 Tension (mm.Hg)	104.0	104.0	104.0

Fig 48.—Ideal case with uniform ventilation and uniform blood flow to all parts of the lungs. Total area of the rectangle signifies minute volume of ventilation, and shaded area,

104 mm Hg (it is assumed here that there is no barrier to diffusion of O_2) and arterial O_2 saturation of 97.4%.*

Does nonuniformity of the ratios of ventilation to blood flow throughout the lung make any difference if the total alveolar ventilation is normal (let us say 4 L/min) and the total capillary blood flow also is normal (5 L/min)? It does, because such a condition must produce a decrease in arterial PO_2 (arterial hypoxemia) and a slight increase in arterial PCO_2 (CO_2 retention). Indeed, uneven ventilation in relation to blood flow is the commonest cause of hypoxemia in clinical medicine. A number of cases will be presented to illustrate this.

An extreme case is illustrated in Figure 49; although it is an impossible situation in a living person, it serves to prove the point. In Figure 49 alveolar ventilation is normal in *volume* (4 L/min) and capillary blood flow is normal in *volume* (5 L/min). However, all of the ventilation goes to the left lung, which has *no* blood flow, and all of the blood flows to the right lung, which has *no* ventilation. Minute *volumes* of alveolar ventilation and capillary blood flow are normal, but the patient would be dead of asphyxia caused by uneven distribution of alveolar gas and capillary blood flow.

The left side of Figure 49 represents pure "alveolar" dead space ventilation such as might occur with left pulmonary arterial occlusion: the ratio alveolar ventilation/capillary blood flow = 4/0 = infinity. The right side represents a complete venous-to-arterial shunt such as might occur with complete bronchial obstruction: the ratio, alveolar ventilation/capillary blood flow = 0/5 = 0. These two extreme cases are dis-

---

alveolar ventilation/min. Mixed alveolar gas *(A + B)* has the same PO_2 as gas in alveoli *A* and *B*. Mixed capillary blood *(A + B)* has the same PO_2 as blood in capillaries *A* and *B*. There is no alveolar-arterial PO_2 difference. (For the sake of simplicity, mixed blood from pulmonary capillaries *A* and *B* is called *arterial blood;* this is true only when there is no anatomic shunt from right to left. This applies also to Figures 50, 51, 52, and 53.)

*An equation has been developed for the calculation of ventilation/blood flow ratios (see Appendix, p. 284). To make this calculation, one must know the concentration of O_2 in inspired and alveolar gas and the concentration of O_2 in mixed venous and pulmonary venous blood. Using values obtained in normal men under basal conditions, the ventilation/blood flow ratio is found to be 0.8 for the whole lung. It is sometimes convenient to think of the 0.8 ratio as a 4:5 ratio because alveolar ventilation in resting adult man is about 4 L/min and pulmonary blood flow is about 5 L/min. In this "ideal" situation, the ratio is 0.8 for alveoli *A* (2:2.5), 0.8 for alveoli *B* (2:2.5), and 0.8 for the whole lung, alveoli *A* and *B* (4:5).

This ratio is often called the $\dot{V}_A/\dot{Q}_C$ ratio ($\dot{V}_A$ = alveolar ventilation in L/min; $\dot{Q}_C$ = pulmonary capillary blood flow in L/min) or the ventilation/perfusion ratio. Because the term *perfusion* often brings to mind an isolated organ and a pump, we prefer the term *blood flow*. The correct term *alveolar ventilation/pulmonary capillary blood flow ratio* is cumbersome, and we shall therefore use *ventilation/blood flow ratio*.

cussed in greater detail on pages 180, 183, and 184. There may also be a continuous spectrum of alveoli *between* these extreme situations—alveoli that have ratios between zero and infinity. These alveoli have both ventilation and blood flow, but some will have too much ventilation in relation to blood flow and some too little.

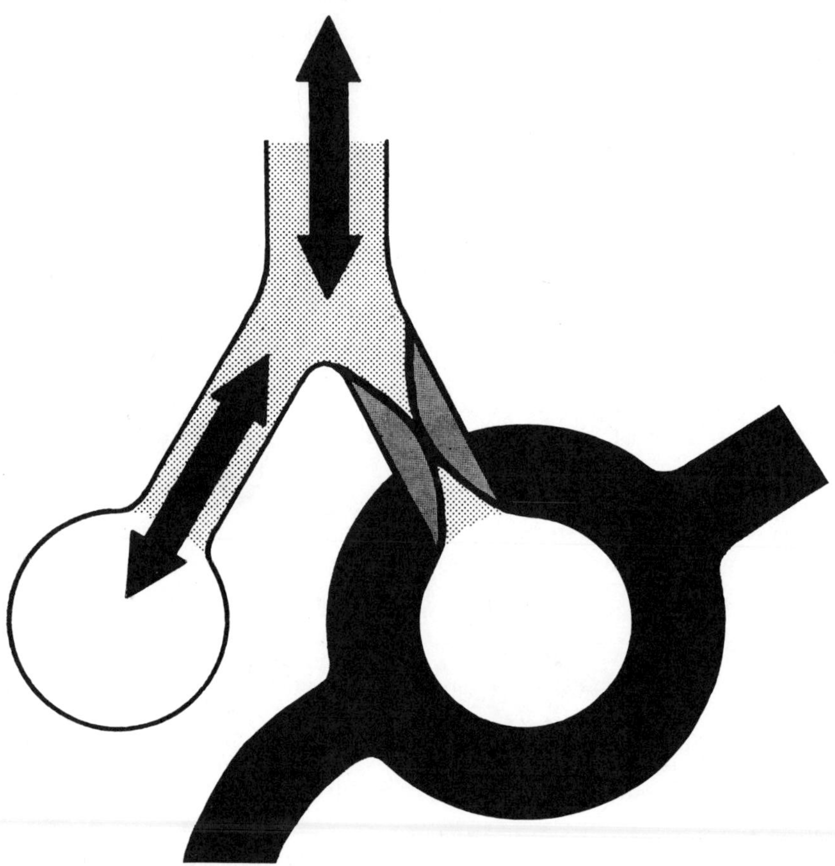

Fig 49.—Extreme case of uneven ventilation and uneven blood flow. Here and in Figures 48 to 55 circles represent groups of alveoli with their pulmonary capillary blood flow. Stippled areas represent the conducting airway (anatomic dead space). Size of arrows represents volume and distribution of alveolar ventilation; thickness of blood channels signifies volume of pulmonary capillary blood flow/min. Dark *gray* indicates poorly oxygenated blood; in the figures that follow, very light gray denotes well-oxygenated blood. This figure represents the extreme (and impossible) situation in which total ventilation and total blood flow are normal but all the blood flow goes to nonaerated alveoli and all the ventilation to alveoli with no blood flow. In this case the pulmonary capillary flow is 100% shunt and the ventilation is all dead space, physiologic dead space (see Chapter 3). The anatomic dead space is stippled and the alveolar dead space is clear.

Figure 50 illustrates a very common type of uneven distribution of gas in relation to blood flow. Here, as in Figures 48 and 49 *total* alveolar ventilation is normal ($A + B = 4$ L/min) and *total* blood flow is normal ($A + B = 5$ L/min). The only abnormality is uneven distribution of inspired gas; blood flow is evenly distributed to the alveoli. However, this results in uneven ratios: 3.2/2.5 in alveoli A (hyperventilation in relation to blood flow) and 0.8/2.5 in alveoli B (hypoventilation in relation to blood flow). Oxygen tension and saturation must decrease in blood leaving hypoventilated alveoli B; and O_2 saturation must rise in blood leaving the hyperventilated alveoli A, but because of the nature of the HbO_2 dissociation curve (see p. 224), this is not enough to compensate for the decrease effected in alveoli B. The mixed arterial blood has a Po_2 of 84 mm Hg (an O_2 saturation of 95%) instead of 104 mm Hg (an O_2 saturation of 97.4%), as in the "ideal" case (Fig 48, p. 164); therefore, uneven ratios have resulted in anoxemia.†

In this connection it should be pointed out that the volume of the alveoli has nothing to do with the O_2 saturation of the blood leaving them. An alveolus may be very poorly ventilated compared to its volume, and this will be shown by a very slow washout of the N_2 in this alveolus when O_2 is breathed for a long time. This, however, tells us nothing about the effectiveness of this alveolus in oxygenating the blood. An alveolus with little ventilation and a large volume can be perfectly effective in oxygenating the blood if it has a very small blood flow. What matters for the blood is the ventilation/blood flow ratio, but what determines the rate of N_2 washout is the ratio of ventilation to alveolar volume.

Figure 51 shows the slight degree of uneven ventilation existing in "normal" man; this prevents him from having the maximal value for arterial Po_2 of the man with the "ideal" lung; because of uneven ventilation, he has a Po_2 of only 100.2 mm Hg (an oxyhemoglobin saturation of 97.1%) instead of 104 mm Hg (97.4% saturation). Uneven blood flow may also exist in normal man (especially in the sitting or standing position); only uneven ventilation is pictured in Figure 51 for purposes of clarity.

In the case pictured in Figure 52, total alveolar ventilation and

†The arterial Po_2 saturation would rise to normal if a patient with this abnormality could hyperventilate enough to provide 2.0 L of ventilation to alveoli B per minute. However, the abnormality could still be detected by the existence of a considerable alveolar-arterial blood Po_2 difference that is not present in the "ideal" case; for a discussion of the alveolar-arterial Po_2 difference, see page 176. In the examples presented, we have held alveolar ventilation at the normal level in order to illustrate clearly the effect of uneven ratios, uncompensated by increased total ventilation or vasomotor or bronchomotor changes.

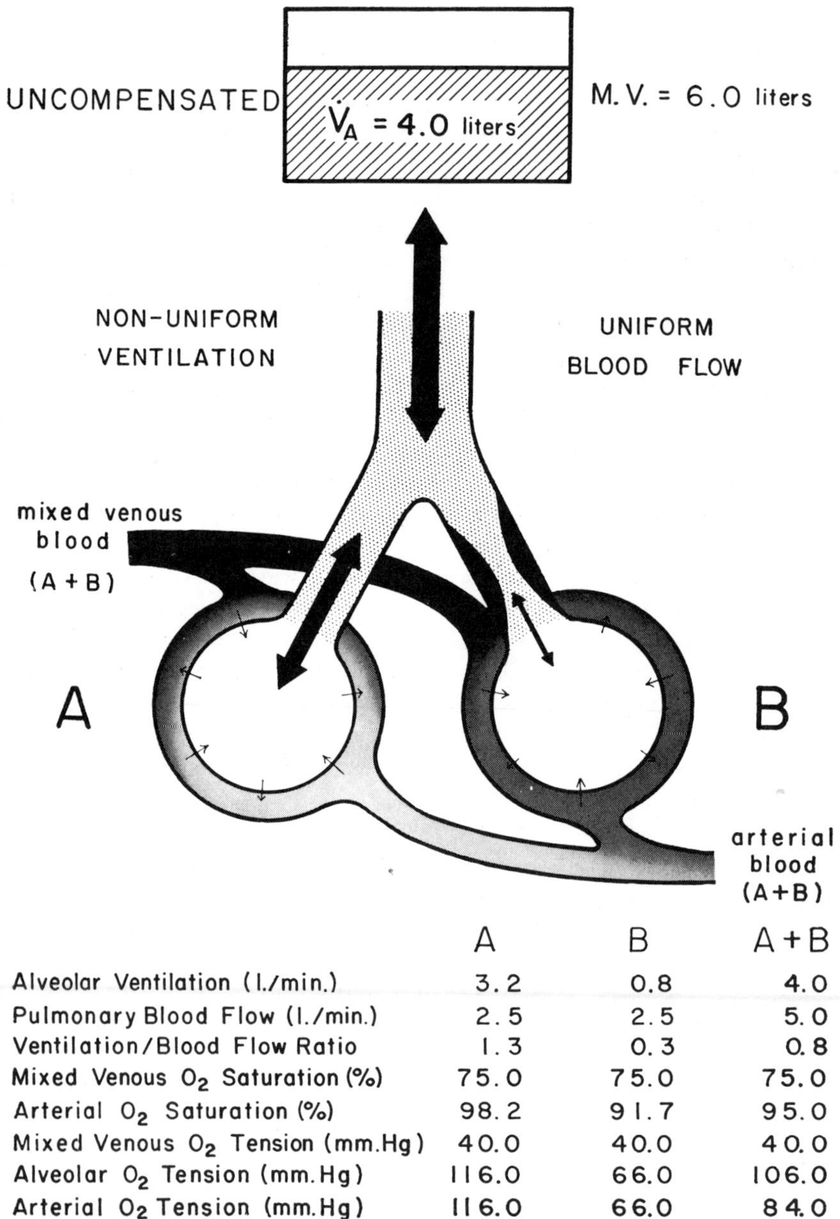

	A	B	A+B
Alveolar Ventilation (l./min.)	3.2	0.8	4.0
Pulmonary Blood Flow (l./min.)	2.5	2.5	5.0
Ventilation/Blood Flow Ratio	1.3	0.3	0.8
Mixed Venous O_2 Saturation (%)	75.0	75.0	75.0
Arterial O_2 Saturation (%)	98.2	91.7	95.0
Mixed Venous O_2 Tension (mm.Hg)	40.0	40.0	40.0
Alveolar O_2 Tension (mm.Hg)	116.0	66.0	106.0
Arterial O_2 Tension (mm.Hg)	116.0	66.0	84.0

Fig 50.—Effect of nonuniform distribution of air in a patient with uniform blood flow, such as might occur in asthma. It differs from the "normal" (Fig 51) in extent of uneven ventilation. Here the uneven ventilation results in an alveolar-arterial Po_2 difference of 22

blood flow are, once more, normal (4 and 5 L/min, respectively), but here pulmonary capillary blood flow is uneven, being 4 L/min to alveoli *A* and 1 L/min to alveoli *B*. Although alveolar ventilation is uniform (2 L/min to *A* and 2 L/min to *B*), the ratios are uneven because of non-uniform blood flow. In *B*, the ratio is 2:1 (hyperventilation in relation to blood flow), and in *A* it is 2:4 (hypoventilation in relation to blood flow). The result again is a lowering of the arterial Po_2: 90 mm Hg instead of 104 mm Hg (arterial O_2 saturation of 96.2% instead of 97.4%).‡

We stated previously that the most common cause of clinical hypoxemia is uneven ventilation/blood flow ratios. In some patients, uneven ratios may be caused only by uneven ventilation (see Fig 21); in others, they may be solely or predominantly by uneven blood flow (see Fig 46). In the majority, both uneven ventilation and uneven blood flow exist and cause even more hypoxemia.

It is possible theoretically to have both uneven ventilation and uneven blood flow and no reduction in arterial Po_2 (even without compensatory hyperventilation) because either chance or perfectly functioning compensatory mechanisms maintain the same ratios in all parts of the lungs. Figure 53 represents such a hypothetical case: ventilation is 3 L/min and blood flow 3.75 L/min in alveoli *A;* ventilation is 1.0 L/min and blood flow 1.25 L/min in alveoli *B*. The ratio is 0.8 for alveoli *A,* 0.8 for alveoli *B,* and 0.8 for the whole lung, and the arterial Po_2 is as high as it can be: it equals the alveolar Po_2, and the blood is well oxygenated (saturation = 97.4%). Such a situation apparently can exist in some cases of bronchopneumonia, or of pneumothorax in which arterial O_2 saturation remains normal.

It is believed that the lungs have mechanisms that decrease blood flow to poorly ventilated regions by increasing vascular resistance, and increase ventilation to well-perfused areas by decreasing airway resis-

---

mm Hg and a reduction of arterial O_2 saturation from the "ideal" value of 97.4% to 95.0%. Hyperventilation of alveoli *A* raises saturation of blood *A* to only 98.2%; this cannot compensate completely for the low O_2 saturation (91.7%) of blood coming from hypoventilated alveoli *B*. Values given for arterial blood (really mixed pulmonary capillary blood) represent the *immediate* effect of mixing equal volumes of blood from *A* and *B;* final "steady-state" values will differ from these, depending upon cardiovascular and respiratory adjustments. Again, it is assumed that no anatomic shunts exist.

‡Again, the anoxemia will in general be corrected by the patient increasing his alveolar ventilation so that alveoli *A* receive 3.2 L/min. However, again there will be a considerable alveolar-arterial Po_2 difference, instead of none as in the "ideal" lungs.

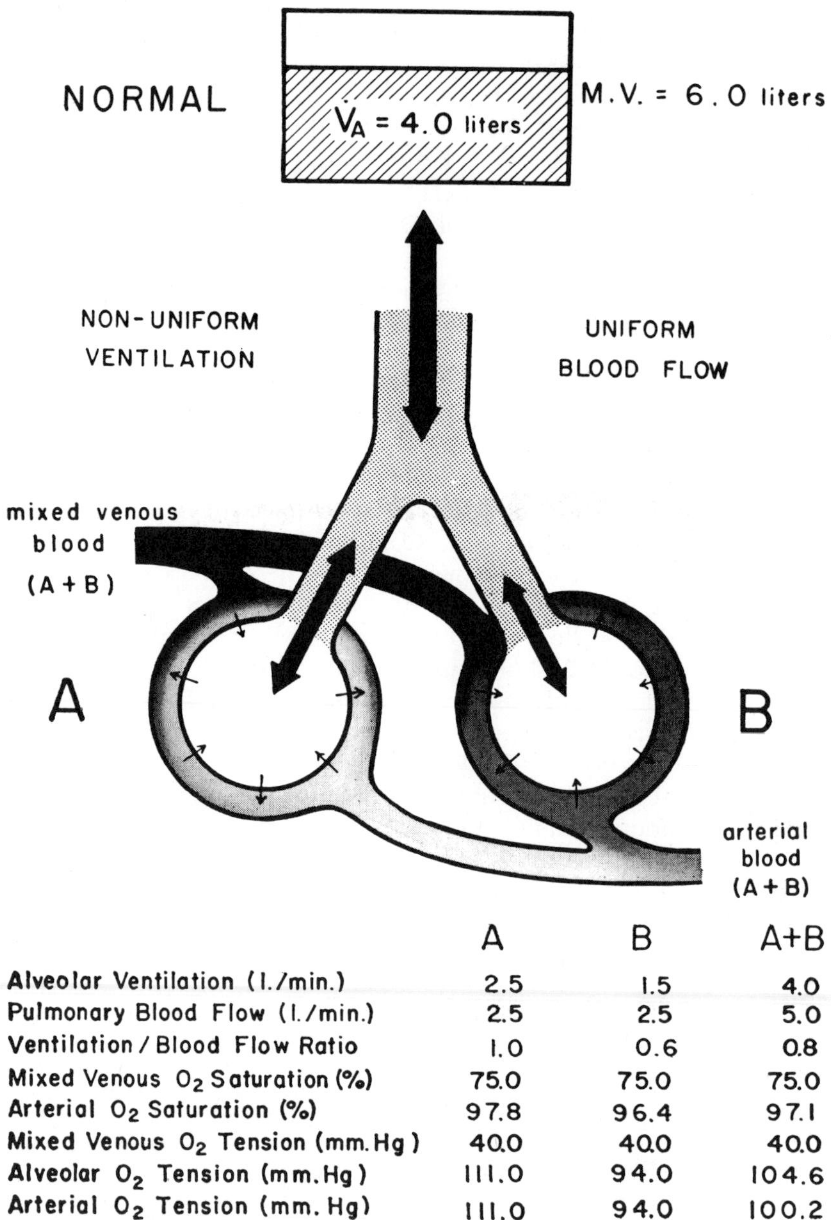

	A	B	A+B
Alveolar Ventilation (l./min.)	2.5	1.5	4.0
Pulmonary Blood Flow (l./min.)	2.5	2.5	5.0
Ventilation / Blood Flow Ratio	1.0	0.6	0.8
Mixed Venous O_2 Saturation (%)	75.0	75.0	75.0
Arterial O_2 Saturation (%)	97.8	96.4	97.1
Mixed Venous O_2 Tension (mm. Hg)	40.0	40.0	40.0
Alveolar O_2 Tension (mm. Hg)	111.0	94.0	104.6
Arterial O_2 Tension (mm. Hg)	111.0	94.0	100.2

Fig 51.—This differs from the "ideal" in that there is some uneven ventilation. Blood flow may also be uneven in normal individuals. The degree of uneven ventilation present is responsible for an alveolar-arterial P_{O_2} difference of about 4.4 mm Hg; the remainder of

tance. Regulatory mechanisms of this type can be demonstrated experimentally at the level of individual lobes. It is assumed that physiologic regulation of this nature must take place in smaller domains to bring about the remarkable exchange function of the lungs in the face of known nonuniformity of both alveolar ventilation and capillary blood flow.

So far we have discussed two causes of hypoxemia: alveolar hypoventilation (chapter 3), and now uneven ventilation/blood flow ratios. The two may coexist. The ideal lung (see Fig 48) has ratios of 0.8 in alveoli *A* and *B,* and the blood is maximally arterialized for this amount of ventilation. If the "ideal" lung were hypoventilated but still had uniform ventilation/blood flow ratios (let us say, 0.6), there would be hypoxemia, but the blood would be maximally arterialized for that amount of ventilation (2.4 L of ventilation for 4 L of blood flow). However, when the ventilation/blood flow ratios vary throughout the lungs, the blood cannot be maximally arterialized for whatever volumes of ventilation and blood flow exist. In other words, even if total alveolar ventilation and total pulmonary blood flow are normal and diffusion is unimpaired, arterial hypoxemia will occur if the ratio of ventilation/blood flow is not the same everywhere in the lungs. If total alveolar ventilation is less than normal, so that there is arterial hypoxemia on that account, *the addition of uneven ratios to overall hypoventilation will further aggravate the hypoxemia.*

II. EFFECTS OF UNEVEN RATIOS ON ARTERIAL BLOOD P_{CO_2}

When the ventilation/blood flow ratios are the same throughout the lung, the P_{CO_2} must also be equal in blood and gas in *A, B,* and *A* + *B*. However, when the ratios differ in *A* and *B,* the alveolar P_{CO_2} will also be different in *A* and *B*.

It is generally agreed that, because of the rapid rate of diffusion of CO_2 across body membranes, there is no detectable difference between the P_{CO_2} in the gas of any alveolus and its capillary blood (see chapter 8). The fact that there is equality of gas tensions for the gas and blood *of any single alveolus* has led some to a misconception, namely, that a

---

the normal P_{O_2} difference (Table 10, p. 214) is due to anatomic shunts, which are ignored in this illustration (arterial blood assumed to be identical to mixed blood from the pulmonary capillaries).

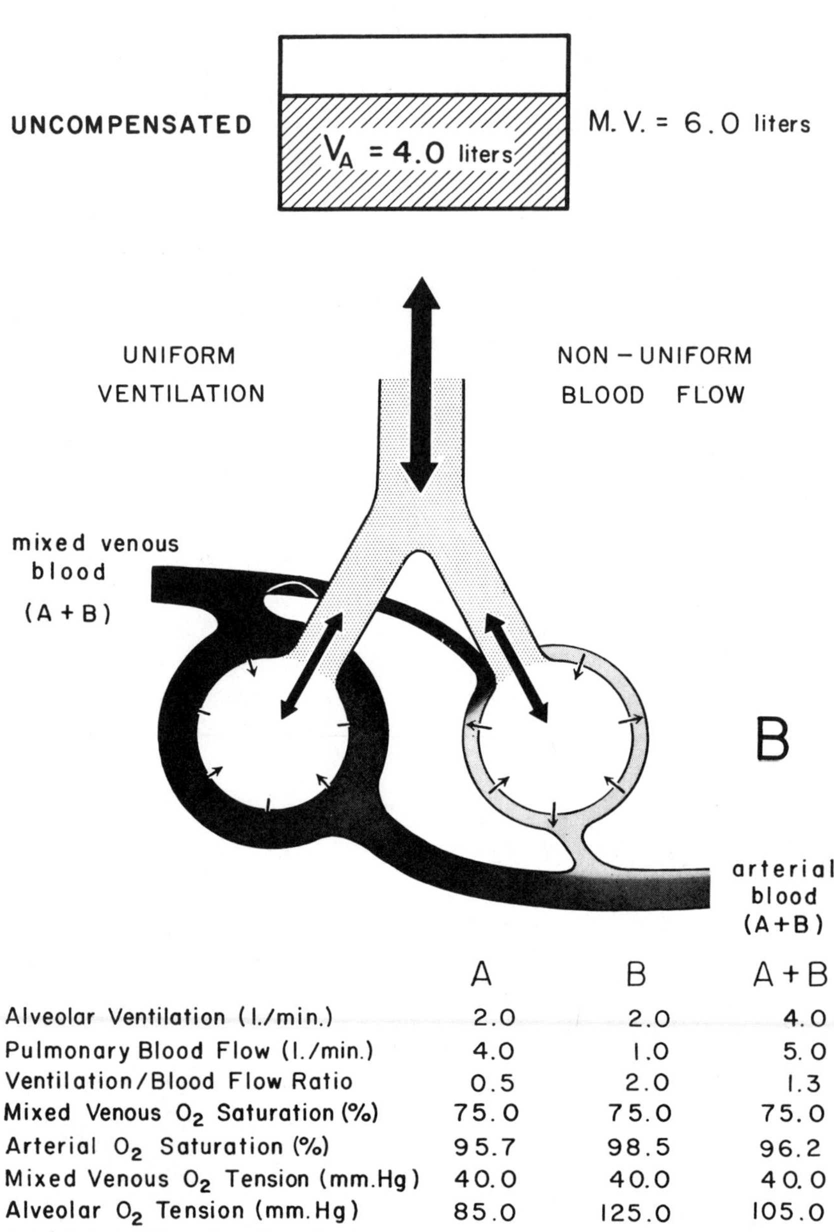

	A	B	A + B
Alveolar Ventilation (l./min.)	2.0	2.0	4.0
Pulmonary Blood Flow (l./min.)	4.0	1.0	5.0
Ventilation/Blood Flow Ratio	0.5	2.0	1.3
Mixed Venous O_2 Saturation (%)	75.0	75.0	75.0
Arterial O_2 Saturation (%)	95.7	98.5	96.2
Mixed Venous O_2 Tension (mm.Hg)	40.0	40.0	40.0
Alveolar O_2 Tension (mm.Hg)	85.0	125.0	105.0
Arterial O_2 Tension (mm.Hg)	85.0	125.0	90.0

Fig 52.—Effect of nonuniform distribution of blood in a patient with uniform distribution of air, as might occur following partial obstruction of a right or left pulmonary artery. Alveoli *A* receive a "normal" amount of ventilation, but this is insufficient to arterialize 4.0

difference in CO_2 tension cannot exist between *mixed* end-capillary blood and mixed alveolar gas. Actually, such a difference can exist in several conditions; one of these is when there are uneven ventilation/blood flow ratios. Calculations show that a difference must exist under conditions such as those in Figure 50 (p. 168). For example, the P_{CO_2} in alveoli *A* might be 39 mm Hg and that in alveoli *B* might be 47 mm Hg. Assuming that the P_{CO_2} of end-pulmonary capillary blood is equal to that of alveolar gas (for each alveolus), the P_{CO_2} of mixed blood from *A* and *B* would be $(39 + 47)/2 = 43$ mm Hg, since regions *A* and *B* contribute an equal volume of blood to the "arterial" blood.* However, alveoli *A* contribute 3.2 L to the expired alveolar gas and alveoli *B* contribute only 0.8 L; the true mean P_{CO_2} of expired alveolar gas is therefore $[(3.2 \times 39) + (0.8 \times 47)]/4 = 40.8$ mm Hg. Thus, a P_{CO_2} difference of $43 - 40.8$, or 2.2 mm Hg, exists in this particular condition.† The P_{CO_2} difference is much less than the P_{O_2} difference in the same circumstances, in part because the difference between venous and arterial tensions is less for CO_2 and partly because the dissociation curve for CO_2 is almost linear over the physiologic range, whereas that for O_2 is not (Fig 65, p. 225). Therefore, for CO_2, regions with a high ventilation/blood flow ratio tend to compensate for those with a low ventilation/blood flow ratio.

We know that *hypoventilation* of the whole lung must lead to increase in alveolar and arterial P_{CO_2}. It is now clear, for reasons just given, that even though there is a *normal volume* of alveolar ventilation,

---

L of mixed venous blood per minute; alveoli *B* also receive a "normal" amount of ventilation, but they are in fact *hyper*ventilated because alveoli *B* receive only 1.0 L of mixed venous blood per minute. The result of uneven ventilation/blood flow ratios (*total* ventilation and blood flow held constant) is again anoxemia.

Occlusion of one pulmonary artery results in low P_{CO_2} in alveoli previously supplied by it and this causes local bronchiolar constriction and a considerable shift of ventilation to the alveoli with unoccluded vessels; operation of such a mechanism would change this *un*compensated illustration to or toward a compensated picture (Fig 53).

*This calculation assumes that the slope of the blood CO_2 content against P_{CO_2} is precisely linear. This is only approximately true. The correct arterial P_{CO_2} can be calculated by obtaining the CO_2 content of blood leaving alveoli *A* and *B* from this dissociation curve and the known P_{CO_2}'s, averaging these CO_2 contents to obtain arterial CO_2 content, and then reading the P_{CO_2} of this arterial blood from the dissociation curve.

†The point that uneven ventilation/blood flow in the lung produces an arterial-expired alveolar partial pressure difference even for CO_2 whose concentration in blood increases approximately linearly with partial pressure over the usual physiological range, and for gases that only physically dissolve (such as N_2) is also discussed in connection with the urine-atmospheric P_{N_2} (p. 188) difference and the multiple inert gas tests (p. 183) for nonuniformity of ventilation/blood flow.

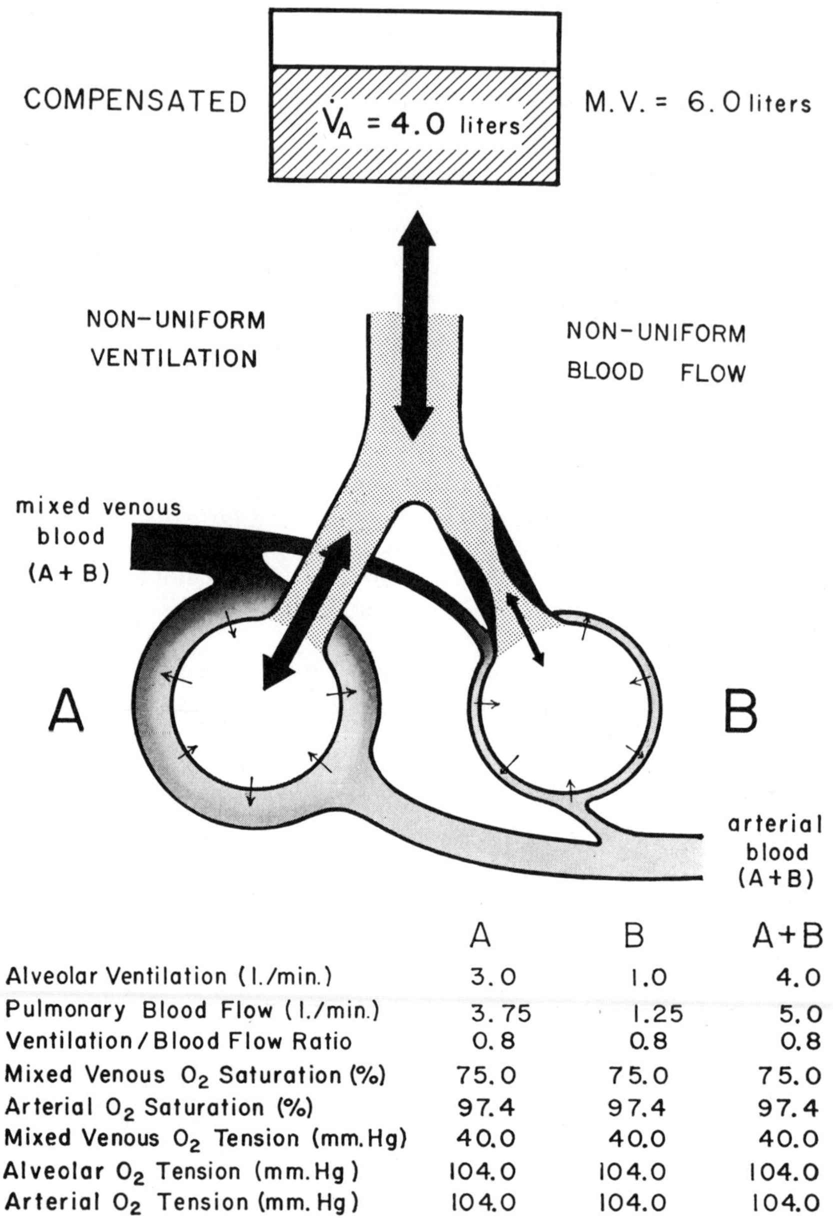

	A	B	A+B
Alveolar Ventilation (l./min.)	3.0	1.0	4.0
Pulmonary Blood Flow (l./min.)	3.75	1.25	5.0
Ventilation/Blood Flow Ratio	0.8	0.8	0.8
Mixed Venous O_2 Saturation (%)	75.0	75.0	75.0
Arterial O_2 Saturation (%)	97.4	97.4	97.4
Mixed Venous O_2 Tension (mm.Hg)	40.0	40.0	40.0
Alveolar O_2 Tension (mm.Hg)	104.0	104.0	104.0
Arterial O_2 Tension (mm.Hg)	104.0	104.0	104.0

Fig 53.—Both ventilation and blood flow are nonuniform, but ventilation and blood flow are increased in proportion to each other in alveoli *A* and decreased in proportion to each other in alveoli *B*. Despite the nonuniformity, there is no alveolar-arterial P_{O_2} difference because ventilation/blood flow ratios are equal through the lungs.

there must be a difference in CO_2 tension between alveolar gas and arterial blood if ventilation/blood flow ratios are uneven throughout the lungs. However, this does not necessarily mean that arterial P_{CO_2} must be greater than normal. Many patients with pulmonary disease hyperventilate, and their arterial P_{CO_2} may be normal, increased, or decreased depending on whether their hyperventilation has compensated, not compensated or overcompensated for the wasted ventilation that results from uneven distribution.

III. CAUSES OF UNEVEN VENTILATION IN RELATION TO BLOOD FLOW

Causes of variations in capillary blood flow have been discussed (p. 152), and those in alveolar ventilation on p. 60. The mechanisms that produce these variations in blood flow and ventilation do not necessarily alter them proportionately so as to keep alveolar ventilation/blood flow constant, except by chance. It is presumed that additional mechanisms in the vascular tree and airway smooth muscle normally regulate blood flow and ventilation to keep their ratio even and that nonuniformity occurs when the regulatory mechanisms break down or are overwhelmed.

Uneven alveolar ventilation/blood flow can occur between large regions of relative uniformity; an example would be a lobe that has blood flow reduced by obstruction in an artery, or airflow reduced by obstruction in an airway. Uneven ventilation/blood flow more commonly occurs diffusely in chronic diseases, where there is unevenness within the subdivisions of the lung as a result of widespread pathologic processes that destroy the capillary bed, the structure of the airways of the regulatory mechanisms, or both.

IV. TESTS OF UNEVEN VENTILATION IN RELATION TO BLOOD FLOW

We have described several tests of uneven distribution of inspired air to the alveoli (p. 53) and of uneven alveolar capillary blood flow (p. 156). These tests per se do not provide the information needed to determine uneven ratios of ventilation to blood flow because they cannot tell whether the nonuniformity in one compensates for the nonuniformity in the other, or actually exaggerates it. For these reasons, it is important to detect and to measure nonuniformity of ventilation/blood flow ratios.

The only techniques available for the direct measurement of the uniformity of the ratio of ventilation to blood flow in the lung (as contrasted to independent measurements of uniformity of ventilation/alveolar volume and of blood flow/alveolar volume are measurements of O_2, CO_2, or inert gas exchange. The calculations require steady-state conditions—that is, the alveolar partial pressure is constant and the amount of gas deposited in the lung by the blood at any instant equals that washed out of the lung by the ventilation. If the alveolar partial pressure is changing, some gas must be removed or deposited in the lung gas or tissue and the rate of transport by the blood will not equal the rate of transport by alveolar ventilation. In the case of O_2 exchange we must measure arterial P_{O_2}, arterial P_{CO_2}, inspired P_{O_2} and expired P_{O_2} to obtain (alveolar P_{O_2} $-$ arterial P_{O_2}). In the case of CO_2 we must measure arterial and expired P_{CO_2}. For the inert gas (the multiple inert gas method) we need to know the partial pressures of inert gas in expired gas, and arterial and mixed venous blood.

It is also possible to measure the ratio of ventilation to blood flow indirectly. The procedure is to measure the distribution of alveolar ventilation/alveolar volume in different regions of the lung fields by one radioactive gas technique and the distribution of pulmonary blood flow/alveolar volume by another radioactive gas technique and then compute ventilation/blood flow for different regions. Of course, the resolution of these methods is limited to the resolution of a given projected area on a lung field, while for the steady-state techniques the measured gas concentration is directly dependent on ventilation/blood in each alveolus.

A. TESTS USING ALVEOLAR-ARTERIAL P_{O_2} DIFFERENCES

The tests in this group are based on the very large increases in alveolar-arterial P_{O_2} differences produced by uneven ventilation/blood flow. Alveolar P_{O_2} is calculated from the alveolar air equation (chapter 3), using measured values of arterial P_{CO_2} and inspired P_{O_2}. Nonuniform ventilation/blood flow can increase alveolar-arterial P_{O_2} difference by the following two mechanisms.

Variation in Contributions to Mixed Expired Alveolar Air and Arterial Blood with Ventilation/Blood Flow.

Alveoli with low ventilation/blood flow will have a low P_{O_2} and on the average will contribute a smaller fraction of alveolar gas with a low P_{O_2}

to the expired air, but a larger fraction of blood with a low P_{O_2} to arterial blood. This tends to lower arterial P_{O_2} in reference to expired gas. The opposite is the case for alveoli with a high ventilation/blood flow and a high P_{O_2}, which contribute on the average more to expired gas and less to arterial blood, acting to raise expired gas P_{O_2} in relation to arterial blood P_{O_2}. The result is an increased alveolar-arterial P_{O_2} difference.

This mechanism will produce an alveolar-arterial P_{O_2} difference even if the increase in blood O_2 content is a linear function of P_{O_2} (as it is at P_{O_2} above about 150 mm Hg). This mechanism will also produce an alveolar-arterial partial pressure difference for CO_2, whose blood content is more nearly linear against P_{CO_2}. Similarly, it will produce alveolar-arterial pressure differences for inert gases that only dissolve in blood so the blood content of inert gas is proportional to its partial pressure. (See multiple inert gas method for estimating nonuniformity of ventilation/blood flow.)

Exaggeration of Variations in Contribution to Mixed Expired Alveolar Air and Arterial Blood With Ventilation/Blood Flow Because of the Shape of the Oxygen-Hemoglobin Equilibrium Curve

In a patient breathing air, the normal alveolar P_{O_2} is about 100 mm Hg and the oxyhemoglobin saturation is about 98%. Hyperventilation (as in alveoli with a high ventilation/blood flow) will increase alveolar P_{O_2}, but cannot increase oxyhemoglobin saturation much over 98%. In contrast, alveoli that are hypoventilated have a lower P_{O_2}, and because of the curvature of the hemoglobin-oxygen equilibrium curve, blood leaves those alveoli with a reduced oxyhemoglobin saturation. This less oxygenated blood from alveoli with lower ventilation/blood flow ratios will contribute relatively more to the arterial blood. For both reasons, arterial oxyhemoglobin saturation and arterial P_{O_2} will be lowered. In contrast, the mixed expired alveolar gas P_{O_2} will be the average of gas from the different alveoli weighted by their ventilation. The alveoli with the greater ventilation/blood flow and the higher P_{O_2} contribute more, those with the lower ventilation/blood flow contribute less. The net effect is to raise alveolar P_{O_2} in respect to arterial P_{O_2}, so there is a significantly increased alveolar-arterial P_{O_2} difference. This effect of uneven ventilation/blood flow on alveolar-arterial P_{O_2} differences at different alveolar P_{O_2} is seen in Figure 54.

The magnitude of the alveolar-arterial partial pressure difference depends on the degree of curvature of the oxygen-hemoglobin equilibrium curve. If alveolar P_{O_2} is lowered to the linear part of the equilibrium curve, the alveolar-arterial P_{O_2} difference produced by a given

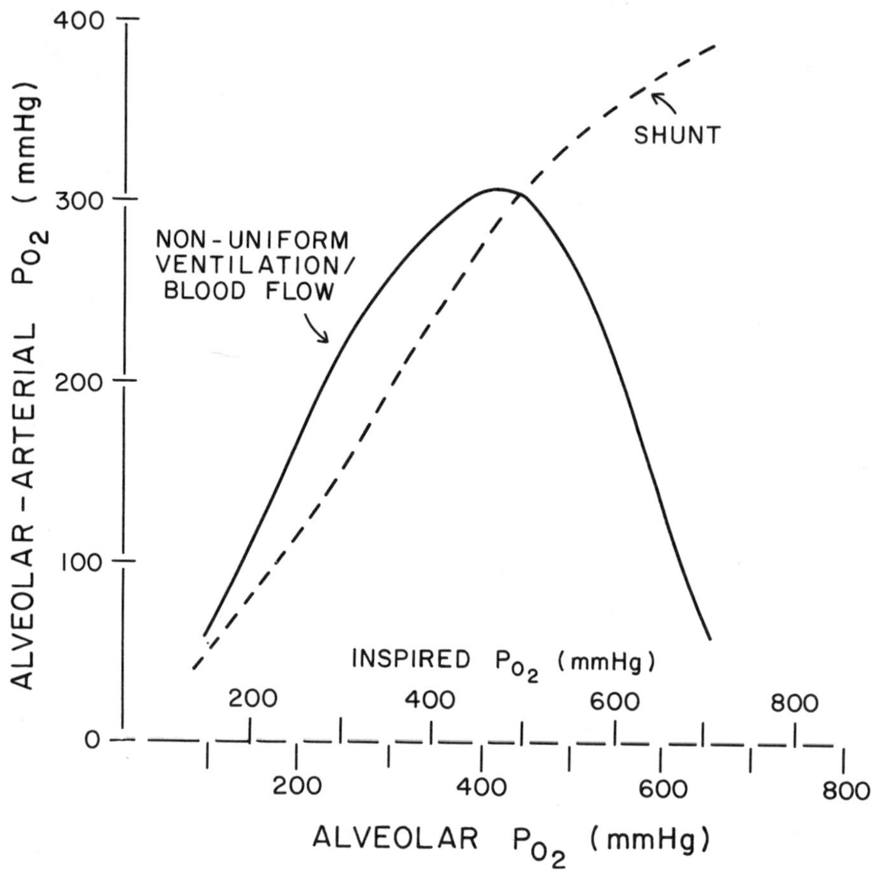

Fig 54.—The variation in alveolar-arterial P_{O_2} with increasing alveolar P_{O_2} (and inspired P_{O_2}) for *(solid line)* nonuniform distribution of alveolar ventilation/capillary blood flow (logarithm normal distribution of ventilation/blood flow with a standard deviation of 2.0) and *(dashed line)* 20% right to left shunt. Arterial blood O_2 content, 20 ml/100 ml of blood; mixed venous O_2 content, 15 ml/100 ml of blood.

nonuniformity of ventilation/blood flow is small. This is the reason for measuring the alveolar-arterial P_{O_2} difference at low P_{O_2} in the analysis of venous admixture and pulmonary diffusing capacity for O_2 of Riley et al. (see Appendix); it decreases the effect of nonuniform ventilation/blood flow.

Alveolar-arterial P_{O_2} difference increases with increasing alveolar P_{O_2}, in large part because the upper part of the oxygen-hemoglobin equilibrium curve is concave downward, but this difference reaches a maximum and then decreases at higher P_{O_2} (see Fig 54). The reduction of alveolar-arterial Po_2 difference occurs because when alveolar Po_2 exceeds 350 to 450 mm Hg it becomes more uniform despite the nonuniformity of ventilation/blood flow. With increasing alveolar Po_2, alveolar N_2 partial pressure falls, leaving only O_2 and CO_2 in alveolar gas. Alveolar Pco_2 can vary only over a narrow range. Pco_2 can be no higher than mixed venous, normally about 46 mm Hg, and even a fourfold increase in ventilation/blood flow would only reduce it to 12 mm Hg. Therefore, the Po_2 of all alveoli must lie within this same narrow range.

In those alveoli with a very low ventilation/blood flow, less than 0.05, the blood absorbs oxygen more rapidly than it can be replaced by the ventilation, particularly at the increased Po_2. This reduces total pressure, causing additional inspired gas to be pulled into the alveoli, effectively increasing their alveolar ventilation and rendering Po_2 more uniform throughout the lung. If the nonuniformity is due to high airway resistance and fresh gas cannot flow into the alveoli fast enough, it will collapse (become atelectatic).

The bell-shaped curve of alveolar-arterial Po_2 difference shown in Figure 54 must be borne in mind when interpreting alveolar-arterial Po_2 differences as a measure of nonuniformity of ventilation/blood flow in patients breathing high concentrations of oxygen.

Use of Alveolar-Arterial Po_2 Difference (A-a gradient) as a Measure of Ventilation/Blood Flow Uniformity

The alveolar-arterial Po_2 difference is extremely sensitive to nonuniformity of ventilation/blood flow ratios (see Fig 54) and thus is a useful test of lung function in patients. Arterial Po_2 can be measured by electrode on blood samples but we must use the alveolar air equation to calculate alveolar Po_2.* In many circumstances inspired oxygen concentration is greater than in air but less than 100% because it is varied by requirements of patient management. Thus, alveolar N_2 is not negligible; therefore, arterial Pco_2 must also be measured (with an electrode), and inspired Po_2 measured directly in order to use the alveolar air equation (p. 267). Often, as in an intensive care unit, alveolar-arterial Po_2 difference is measured serially, and any increase interpreted as an index of increasing nonuniformity of ventilation/blood flow ratios; its absolute values are then less critical.

*If the patient is breathing 100% oxygen and the N_2 has been washed out of his lungs, the correction factor in the alveolar air equation (chapter 3) becomes unity and can be neglected.

Calculation of Venous Admixture

The alveolar-arterial PO_2 difference breathing high (air) and low (about 14%) inspired O_2, can be analyzed to give quantitative measures of nonuniformity of ventilation/blood flow and the effectiveness of O_2 diffusion between alveolar gas and alveolar capillary blood (see Appendix). At the low inspired O_2 the contribution to the alveolar-arterial gradient produced by nonuniform ventilation/blood flow is minimized (see Fig 54) but the contribution from the failure of alveolar O_2 to equilibrate with capillary blood (the *end capillary gradient*) is increased (see chapter 8 on diffusion). Breathing air the reverse is true; the contribution of nonuniform ventilation/blood flow to the alveolar arterial PO_2 difference is increased and the end-gradient decreases. From the alveolar-arterial PO_2 difference at the higher PO_2 we can calculate *venous admixture*, a hypothetical venous-arterial shunt that has the same effect in reducing alveolar-arterial gas exchange as existing ventilation/blood flow nonuniformity. It is simply a method of expressing the effect of nonuniform ventilation/blood flow and anatomic shunt upon gas exchange and is about 6% of pulmonary blood flow in a normal adult. Largely from the alveolar-arterial PO_2 difference at low PO_2 we can also calculate the alveolar-end capillary PO_2 difference, and from this the diffusing capacity of the lung for O_2 (see Appendix).

The effect of a shunt on the alveolar-arterial PO_2 difference is not the same as that of nonuniform ventilation/blood flow (see Fig 54), and the value of venous admixture really only applies at a given PO_2.

Test for Anatomic Venous-to-Arterial Shunt

Shunting of mixed venous blood around alveolar capillaries and directly into the pulmonary venous or systemic arterial blood, either in the lungs or heart can be measured quantitatively by an O_2 test.

If an individual with such a shunt breathes pure O_2, there is no opportunity for the shunted blood to be exposed to the O_2 in the alveoli, and the venous blood passes into the pulmonary veins without any increase in its O_2 content. However, mixed venous blood flowing to ventilated alveoli would become equilibrated with the high alveolar PO_2. This PO_2, some 640 mm Hg* greater than mixed venous blood, transports O_2 into the capillary blood and saturates the hemoglobin

*N_2 has been practically all removed by rebreathing pure O_2. Therefore, alveolar $PO_2 = P_{barometer} - P_{water} - PCO_2$, or choosing normal values, 760 mm Hg − 47 mm Hg − 40 mm Hg = 673 mm Hg.

quickly. Further O_2 added to the blood dissolves in it. This process is completed in a brief additional time period. Thus, the capillary blood leaving each alveolus contains maximally saturated hemoglobin plus an additional 2 ml of dissolved O_2 in each 100 ml of blood (673 mm Hg $\times$ 0.003 ml O_2 per 100 ml of blood per mm Hg of PO_2) (chapter 9). This is true even for poorly ventilated alveoli, because if the patient breathes O_2 long enough (10 to 20 minutes), N_2 will be eliminated even from these and the O_2 concentration will rise maximally. This is also true if there is impairment of diffusion for O_2 between alveolar gas and capillary blood. Whenever a patient with an anatomic shunt breathes pure O_2, his systemic arterial blood cannot be oxygenated maximally because a stream of mixed venous (poorly oxygenated) shunted blood merges in the pulmonary veins with fully oxygenated blood from the alveolar capillaries. The size of the shunt can be calculated using the following equation:

$$\text{Shunt as a fraction of blood flow} = \frac{\text{end capillary } O_2 \text{ content} - \text{arterial } O_2 \text{ content}}{\text{end capillary } O_2 \text{ content} - \text{mixed venous } O_2 \text{ content}}$$

End capillary blood is blood as it leaves an alveolar capillary, before it has mixed with shunted blood in the pulmonary vein or right heart. It is assumed to have a PO_2 equal to that in the alveolar gas. Mixed venous blood oxygen content is determined by analyzing a sample that can only be obtained by right ventricular catheterization.* Alternatively a value of arterial-mixed venous O_2 content difference, which is relatively constant among patients, is generally assumed from normal data to be 5 ml/dl. The difference between end capillary and arterial O_2 content can be calculated from alveolar PO_2, arterial PO_2, and the normal oxygen-hemoglobin equilibrium curve.

When the shunt is small† and the arterial blood is fully saturated with oxygen, the difference between end capillary and arterial blood oxygen content can be calculated as the product:

$$(\text{alveolar } PO_2 - \text{arterial } PO_2) \times \text{solubility of oxygen in blood}$$

namely, 0.003 ml/dl for each mm Hg of PO_2. The shunt equation then becomes:

*Rebreathing and breath-holding methods can be used to obtain partial pressures of gases in mixed venous (pulmonary arterial blood), but require patient training and cooperation and are not practical.

†Healthy individuals have a small amount of "anatomic shunt" because some venous blood normally drains into the pulmonary veins, left atrium, or left ventricle (some bronchial and coronary blood flow).

$$\text{Shunt as a fraction of pulmonary blood flow} = \frac{(\text{alveolar } P_{O_2} - \text{arterial } P_{O_2})\ 0.003}{(\text{alveolar } P_{O_2} - \text{arterial } P_{O_2})\ 0.003 + \text{assumed (arterial-mixed venous) } O_2 \text{ content}}$$

The 100% O_2 test can rule out a shunt as a cause of hypoxemia. The O_2 test does not determine the location of a shunt, which may be intracardiac or intrapulmonary; intrapulmonary shunts include any condition in which pulmonary blood continues to flow through regions with no alveoli or nonaerated alveoli, such as pulmonary atelectasis or arteriovenous malformations.

Alveoli with a low ventilation/blood flow ratio may collapse completely if they are ventilated with 100% oxygen because the O_2 is absorbed by the blood faster than fresh gas is added by ventilation. Once collapsed they can lead to an overestimation of the anatomic shunt as they shunt pulmonary venous blood around the alveoli.

B. INCREASES IN PHYSIOLOGIC DEAD SPACE

Computation of physiologic dead space is based on the assumption that arterial P_{CO_2} equals alveolar P_{CO_2} (page 39). However, uneven ventilation/blood flow increases the normal difference between mixed expired P_{CO_2} and arterial P_{CO_2} and increases the computed value of physiologic dead space, which can thus be used as a measure of nonuniform ventilation/blood flow. This occurs because those alveoli with a high ventilation/blood flow ratio have a low P_{CO_2}, both in alveolar gas and in effluent capillary blood, and these contribute a greater proportion of total expired gas, but a lesser proportion of capillary flow to mixed arterial blood. The converse is true for those alveoli with a low ventilation/blood flow ratio. They have a higher P_{CO_2} and contribute less to the mixed expired gas and more to arterial blood, again making expired P_{CO_2} less than arterial P_{CO_2}. This is similar to the effect of nonuniform ventilation/blood flow in producing an increased alveolar-arterial P_{O_2} difference (p. 176).

If the alveolar-arterial P_{O_2} difference is significantly increased, the only possible physiologic causes are nonuniform ventilation/blood flow or anatomic venous to arterial shunt, or diffusion impairment. Anatomic shunt can be diagnosed by the 100% O_2 test and diffusion impairment by measuring the diffusing capacity of the lung.

Increasing pulmonary blood flow normally does not affect arterial P_{CO_2}, P_{O_2}, or oxyhemoglobin saturation; the lung capillary bed handles the increased blood flow by expanding; the hemodynamic resistance does not rise for moderate increases in flow, and gas exchange is unaffected. It is therefore somewhat surprising that increased pulmonary blood flow tends to reduce the nonuniformity of ventilation/blood flow and lower alveolar-arterial P_{O_2} difference.

An extreme example of the effect of nonuniform ventilation/blood flow on the arterial-mixed expired P_{CO_2} difference is shown in Figure 55. The respiratory center will increase tidal volume in order to keep arterial P_{CO_2} constant at 40 mm Hg. It is assumed for simplicity that respiratory frequency remains constant, as does anatomic dead space and, of course, CO_2 output. Tidal volume will be 733 ml and the P_{CO_2} of the mixed expired breath 19 mm Hg. Inserting these data in the Bohr equation (p. 39) the physiologic dead space is as follows:

$$733 \text{ ml } (40 \text{ mm Hg} - 19 \text{ mm Hg})/40 \text{ mm Hg} = 384 \text{ ml}$$

The presence of uneven ventilation/blood flow has produced an increase in the size of the physiologic dead space despite the fact that there is no P_{CO_2} difference between alveolar gas and end capillary blood. However, the increases in the alveolar-arterial P_{O_2} are so much greater and more reliable that the physiologic dead space is not often relied upon to diagnose nonuniformity of ventilation/blood flow ratios.

C. COMBINED RADIOACTIVE MEASUREMENTS OF DISTRIBUTION OF INSPIRED GAS AND PULMONARY CAPILLARY BLOOD FLOW

We can determine the distribution of inspired gas in relation to alveolar volume as described in the discussion of distribution of ventilation (chapter 3), using a relatively insoluble radioactive inert gas, such as xenon.^{133} We can determine regional blood flow independently in a second procedure by injecting a solution of xenon^{133} intravenously as described in the section on Distribution of Pulmonary Capillary Blood Flow (chapter 6). The results of these two techniques can be combined to give alveolar ventilation/capillary blood flow ratios for observed regions of the lung.

D. MULTIPLE INERT GAS METHOD FOR ESTIMATING DISTRIBUTION OF VENTILATION FLOW RATIOS

A saline solution of low concentrations of six different chemically inert gases, such as SF_6, ethane, cyclopropane, halothane, diethyl ether, and

PULMONARY ARTERY LIGATION

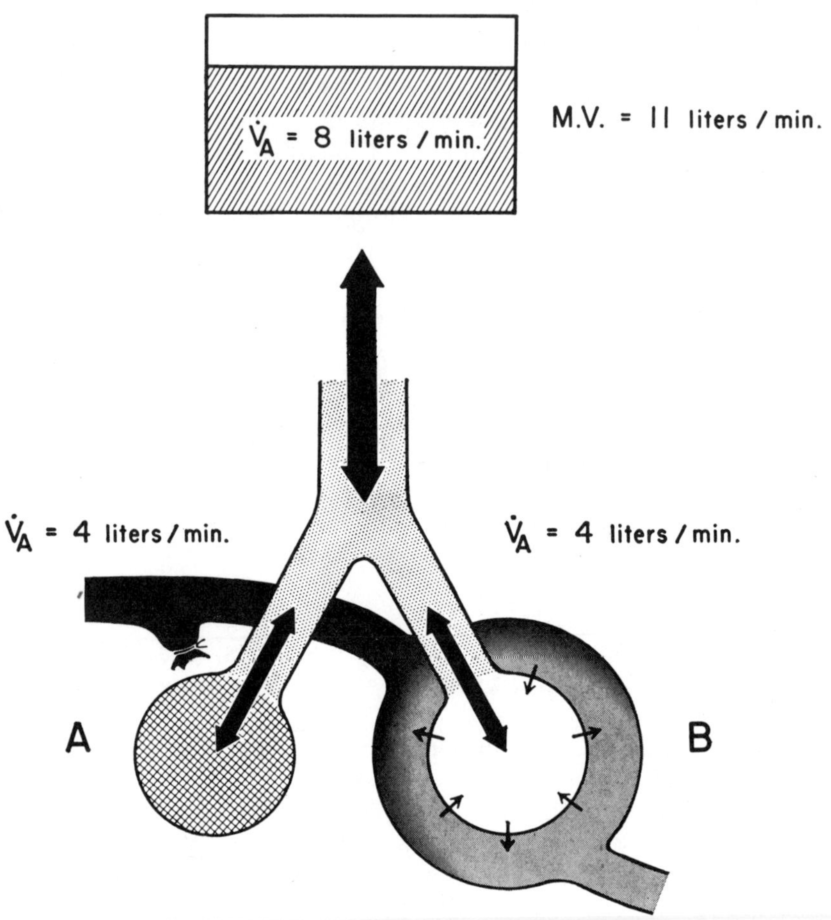

$\dot{Q}_C$ = 0 liters / min.

$\dot{Q}_C$ = 5 liters / min.

$\dot{V}_A / \dot{Q}_C = 0.8$

Fig 55.—Ventilation of alveoli *A* contributes nothing to arterialization of the venous blood and is therefore "dead space ventilation." Normal arterial O_2 saturation is maintained by hyperventilation so that the $\dot{V}_A/\dot{Q}_C$ ratio of alveoli *B* is 0.8. In fact, some increase in airway resistance occurs in *A*, and more than half of the total alveolar ventilation goes to *B*. The total $\dot{V}_A$ of 8 liters/min in the shaded box is calculated as frequency (tidal vol-

acetone, with solubilities varying from 0.0085 to 28.5 ml gas (STPD)/ml blood per atmosphere are slowly infused into a patient's peripheral vein for about 20 minutes, to reach a steady state of secretion from the lungs. At this time simultaneous samples of arterial and mixed venous blood and expired gas are collected and analyzed for the six inert gases, and total ventilation and cardiac output are measured, the latter by the indicator dilution method. Partial pressure of inert gas in arterial blood/mixed venous blood (called *retention*) and of expired gas/mixed venous blood (called *excretion*) are calculated for each inert gas used and graphed against blood solubility. The concentrations of the inert gases are all well below the levels at which effects on the central nervous or circulatory systems appear. The computations are based on the following physiologic considerations. Because there is a steady state,* the rate of elimination of the inert gas by ventilation must equal its rate of removal from the blood passing through the lungs. Therefore, for a single alveolus

Alveolar ventilation (ml STPD/min) × alveolar gas concentration (fractions of atmosphere) = pulmonary blood flow (ml/min) × mixed venous concentration (ml gas STPD/ml blood)
− end capillary concentration (ml STPD/ml blood

The partial pressure of the inert gas in the blood at the end of the capillary will be equal to that in the alveolar gas.
Therefore, taking acetylene (C_2H_2) as an example,

C_2H_2 concentration in blood (ml STPD $\times$ ml blood^{-1} $\times$ atmosphere^{-1}) = $\alpha \times$ alveolar partial pressure of C_2H_2 (mm Hg)

Where α is the solubility of the C_2H_2 gas in blood at 37°C given in milliliters of gas STPD in a milliliter of blood at a partial pressure of 1 atmosphere. Combining these two equations, we obtain the equation that states how ventilation/blood flow and C_2H_2 solubility (α) determine the end capillary and alveolar partial pressures of C_2H_2 in a single alveolus. (It is most convenient to express these pressures in relation to the inert gas partial pressure in mixed venous blood, which is the same for all alveoli.)

---

ume – anatomical dead space volume) and clearly includes the ventilation of alveoli *A* (see text for discussion). Frequency is 20/min; anatomical dead space 0.15L.

*The retained inert gases recirculate so there is a slow buildup of inert gas partial pressure in the mixed venous blood. However, this does not invalidate the equation over the short periods of observation.

$$\frac{\text{End capillary } P_{C_2H_2}}{\text{Mixed venous } P_{C_2H_2}} = \frac{1}{\dfrac{\text{Alveolar ventilation}}{\alpha\text{-Capillary blood flow}} + 1} = \frac{\text{Alveolar } P_{C_2H_2}}{\text{Mixed venous partial pressure}}$$

Figure 56 is a graph of alveolar (or end capillary) for the least soluble inert gas generally used, SF_6, and for the most soluble gas used, acetone, against ventilation/blood flow. Ventilation/blood flow is presented in a log scale on the abscissa to cover the range of values present in the lungs of patients. The important result for the measurement of ventilation/blood distribution in the whole lung is that the alveolar partial pressure of an inert gas varies in an inverted "s"-shaped manner with ventilation/blood flow, and that at a given value it can be extremely sensitive to the solubility of the inert gas. Alveoli with a ventilation/blood flow of 1.0 eliminate all SF_6, while they retain all acetone.

Expired alveolar inert gas concentration will equal its concentration in each alveolus times its proportional contribution to the mixed expired alveolar gas, namely $\dot{V}_A$, of the particular alveolus/$\dot{V}_A$ of the lung. Likewise, the contribution of each alveolus to the arterial, or mixed end capillary partial pressure of inert gas equals the end capil-

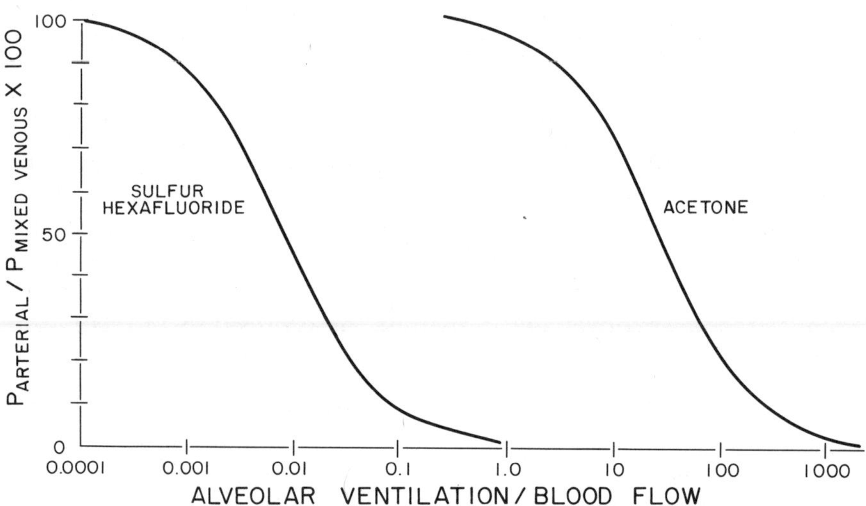

Fig 56.—Variation in arterial partial pressure/mixed venous partial pressure with alveolar ventilation/capillary blood flow for the chemically inert gases, sulfur hexafluoride and acetone with gas to blood partition coefficients of 0.0085 and 140, respectively. Alveolar ventilation/capillary blood flow is considered uniform throughout the lung.

lary partial pressure times the contribution of that alveolus to arterial blood, namely $\dot{Q}$c of the alveolar capillary blood/$\dot{Q}$c of the lung.

While the partial pressure of the inert gas in each alveolus equals that in its end capillary blood, the partial pressure of each inert gas in arterial blood is always greater than that in expired alveolar gas, because of nonuniformity of ventilation/blood flow that is always present to some degree, even in healthy normal persons.

The distribution of alveolar ventilation/blood flow (in other words, the number of alveoli for each $\dot{V}$A/$\dot{Q}$c) affects $P_{expired\ alveolar\ gas}/P_{mixed\ venous}$, or excretion and $P_{arterial}/P_{mixed\ venous}$ or retention, differently; both vary independently with solubility of the inert gas. The contribution of each alveolus to the arterial blood equals the end capillary partial pressure as defined by the equation above, multiplied by the blood flow from that particular alveolus. Similarly, the contribution of each alveolus to the expired gas will be the alveolar partial pressure (which equals the end capillary pressure) but multiplied by the ventilation of that alveolus. Alveoli with a greater ventilation/blood flow have a lower inert gas partial pressure, and will have greater alveolar ventilation and thus will contribute proportionally more to the expired gas, lowering the expired inert gas partial pressure. Similarly, alveoli with a lower ventilation/blood flow have a higher inert gas partial pressure, and will contribute proportionally more to arterial blood so the average partial pressure of inert gas in the blood will be raised. Thus, an inert gas partial difference has been produced between mixed expired alveolar gas and arterial blood, despite the fact that in each alveolus diffusion is complete and the inert gas partial pressure in the alveolar gas equals that in the end capillary blood and that the concentration of inert gas in blood is linearly related to its partial pressure. This difference in partial pressure of inert gas between arterial blood and expired alveolar gas produced by nonuniform ventilation/blood flow does not result from an asymptotic equilibrium curve, as in the case of oxyhemoglobin-O_2 (see Fig 65), since the curve of inert gas concentration against partial pressure is strictly linear (Henry's law, p. 293), but because of the varying contributions of alveoli with different ventilation/blood flow to expired gas and arterial blood.

The aim of the technique, or of any technique for measuring ventilation/blood flow is to calculate a distribution curve of the number of alveoli with each ventilation/blood flow, from the measurement of $P_{alveoli}/P_{arterial}$. Many distributions of ventilation/blood flow among the alveoli can be assumed that will produce the values of retention and excretion found experimentally for one inert gas (the number of distributions could approach the total number of alveoli). When experimental data from a second inert gas are included, the number of distributions that fit is reduced. Although we cannot obtain an exact, correct distribution without a prohibitive number of different inert gases, by the use of six gases, with a wide range of solubilities, each of which is influenced differently by the existing distribution of ventilation/blood flow, reasonable results can be obtained.

E. ATMOSPHERIC–BODY FLUID P_{N_2} DIFFERENCE

There is more O_2 than CO_2 eliminated in the lung, the respiratory exchange ratio is less than one, so the volume of inspired air shrinks in the alveoli, concentrating the N_2. Therefore, the arterial blood leaving the lung should have a P_{N_2} greater than moist air (wet at 37° C). In the presence of nonuniformity of ventilation/blood flow, those alveoli with a low ventilation/blood flow will also have a low respiratory exchange ratio (see Fenn-Rahn diagram in Appendix), therefore a lower CO_2 output/O_2 absorption, and a greater shrinkage of inspired air and thus a higher P_{N_2}. These alveoli with higher P_{N_2} contribute proportionally more to the arterial blood, tending to raise its mixed P_{N_2}. Those alveoli with a higher ventilation/blood flow and thus a lower P_{N_2} will, on the other hand, contribute less to that arterial blood. Thus, the body fluid P_{N_2} will rise in the presence of nonuniformity of ventilation/blood flow.

Because N_2 is not consumed under steady-state conditions, the N_2 partial pressure should be the same in all body fluids. Urine is a convenient fluid of large volume, but must be collected anaerobically to prevent changes in its P_{N_2}. The P_{N_2} in air (wet 37° C) is 570 mm Hg, and arterial blood P_{N_2} is normally 22 mm Hg greater, increasing of the order of 10 to 20 additional mm Hg in disease. It is technically difficult to measure such small changes. Because of this difficulty, the test is not widely used.

V. SUMMARY

Ventilation/capillary blood flow in each alveolus determines its P_{O_2}, and thus its end capillary P_{O_2} and P_{CO_2}. Alveolar volume, alveolar ventilation/alveolar volume, or capillary blood flow/alveolar volume are by themselves unimportant. The maintenance of a uniform ventilation/blood flow in different alveoli of the lung requires regulation of vasculature and of the airways at the finest architectural level. Nonuniformity of alveolar ventilation/blood flow produces an inefficiency in the overall function of the lung as an exchanger; the mixed expired alveolar gas PO_2 becomes less than mixed arterial blood, despite the fact that they may be equilibrated in each alveolar unit. Since capillary blood flow/lung volume and alveolar ventilation/lung volume vary widely throughout the lung independently, and since arterial PO_2 is normally only 10 mm Hg less than mixed alveolar PO_2—a remarkable although not perfect adjustment of ventilation/perfusion—some regulatory processes must be modulating ventilation and blood flow to maintain the ventilation/blood flow at uniform values.

Nonuniform alveolar ventilation/blood flow is an important and common dysfunction in pulmonary disease, particularly in chronic lung disease. Pulmonary function tests are available to measure distribution of capillary blood flow/lung volume and alveolar ventilation/lung volume. These can be combined to detect differences in alveolar ventilation/blood flow among large regions of the lung. A limited number of useful tests can measure the effects of diffuse microscopic nonuniformity of alveolar ventilation/blood flow directly; these involve primarily measuring the alveolar-arterial PO_2 difference, the physiologic dead space (equivalent to measuring the alveolar-arterial PCO_2 difference) or multiple inert gas excretion.

8

Diffusion

Once blood has been brought to the pulmonary capillaries and fresh air to the alveolar gas, the exchange of O_2 and CO_2 takes place by diffusion. The efficacy of the lung as an organ for diffusion exchange decreases in some diseases, and this decrease can be detected by measuring the diffusing capacity of the lung (D_L) (in the United Kingdom called the *transfer factor*), which is expressed in units of milliliter of gas* STPD transferred per minute for each mm Hg of pressure difference between alveolar gas and capillary blood. The better the lung is as an aerator of blood, the greater the rate of O_2 exchange for a given mean pressure difference between alveolar gas and the blood in the alveolar capillaries, and the larger the diffusing capacity of the lung.

These physiologic tests of diffusion require the use of gases that combine reversibly with hemoglobin (see p. 197), i.e., O_2 and CO. They measure the quantity of O_2 or CO that is transferred in a minute from alveolar gas to blood in the pulmonary capillaries. Figures 57 and 58 indicate the various processes involved in the transfer. First, O_2 or CO must diffuse across the alveolar-capillary membranes; the rate of diffusion here depends on (1) the difference between the partial pressure of O_2 or CO in the alveolar gas and that in the plasma, (2) the thickness of the tissues, (3) the surface area available for diffusion of gas, and (4) the physical characteristics of the tissues. Second, the gas must diffuse in the plasma until it meets a red blood cell. Third, it must pass across

*Carbon monoxide (CO), because of its high affinity for hemoglobin, is the best gas with which to measure D_L, and so diffusing capacity of the lung is generally defined as milliliters of CO diffusing per minute per mm Hg.

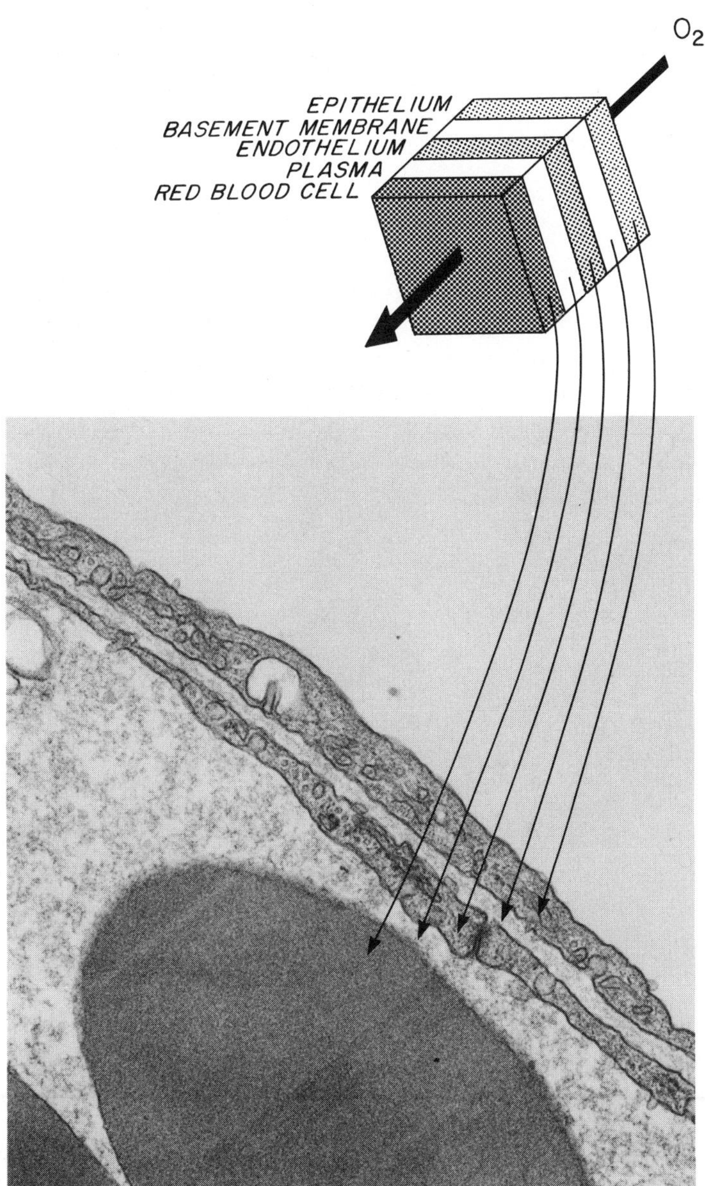

Fig 57.—Electron microphotograph of rabbit lung. The photograph (×50,000) illustrates the tissues through which O_2 must pass from the gas phase in the alveolus until it combines with hemoglobin within the red blood cell. No attempt has been made in the schema to portray relative thickness of the different tissues. (Photograph courtesy of J. Gil.)

DIFFUSION

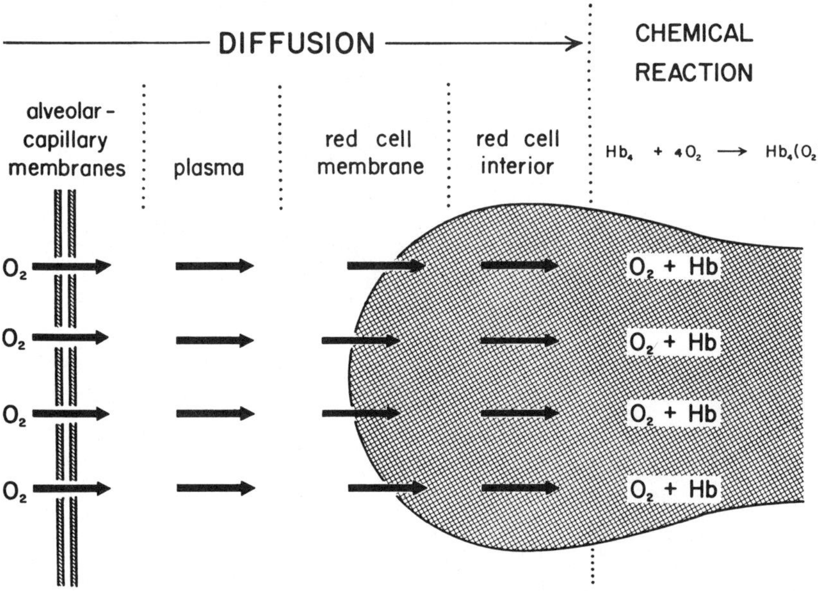

Fig 58.—Schematic representation of passage of O_2 molecules from alveolar gas to pulmonary capillary blood. From left to right are shown the *diffusion* of O_2 molecules (1) across the alveolar-capillary membranes (and normal or pathologic interstitial fluid or tissues), (2) through the plasma, (3) across the red blood cell membrane, and (4) within the erythrocyte, and finally the *chemical reaction* within the erythrocyte whereby O_2 becomes associated with hemoglobin.

the red cell membrane. Fourth, it must diffuse within the red cell and meet and combine chemically with Hb molecules; this is dependent on the chemical reactions of O_2 or CO with Hb.

It was originally considered that the first step in Figure 58, diffusion across the alveolar-capillary membrane, was the only important and rate-limiting process and that once the gas reached the blood the second, third, and fourth steps were instantaneous. Impaired diffusion, or impaired exchange, in a patient was thought to result from thickening of the pulmonary membrane, as can be seen in microscopic sections of a fibrotic lung, for example, or a decrease in total capillary surface area such as that caused by destruction of alveolar septa in some types of emphysema. The rate of uptake of CO by the red blood cells in the pulmonary capillary bed is not instantaneous but normally limits the overall rate of CO uptake in the lungs to the same extent as does diffusion across the alveolar-capillary membrane.

A. FACTORS INFLUENCING DIFFUSING CAPACITY OF THE LUNG

The factors that may alter the diffusing capacity are presented in two parts: first, those that affect diffusion through alteration of the alveolar-capillary membrane, and second, those that affect diffusion and gas uptake in the capillary red cells.

Factors Influencing Transport Across the Alveolar Membrane

Distance for Diffusion

Before entering the blood, molecules of O_2 or CO must first traverse the alveolar-capillary membrane, including the extracellular lining layer, the alveolar epithelium, the basement membrane, the interstitial fluid, and the capillary endothelium (shown clearly in Fig 57). Functionally, the pulmonary membrane (whose permeability is described by the diffusing capacity of the pulmonary membrane, D_M) includes the entire diffusion path from alveolar gas to the surface of the red cells in the pulmonary capillaries; this represents most of the diffusion path through the plasma to the red blood cell surface. Normally, the total path for diffusion is very short—0.1 μ—but in disease it may be very much longer; (1) the alveolar wall may be thickened; (2) the capillary endothelium may be thickened; (3) the cell layers may be separated by interstitial edema fluid and exudate, which may be replaced by fibrous tissue; (4) there may be intra-alveolar edema fluid or exudate; and (5) the intracapillary path may be increased if capillaries are dilated and contain several red blood cells abreast. Anything that lengthens the path CO must travel, decreases the rate of diffusion and the "diffusing capacity." The term *alveolar-capillary block* originated to describe this kind of interference with diffusion, namely, a block between the alveolar gas and its capillary bed, a longer pathway across the alveolar-capillary membrane.

Surface Area for Diffusion

A decrease in the number of patent capillaries or in the number of ventilated alveoli can lead to a decrease in diffusing capacity even though the length of the diffusion path is not increased at any point. It must be emphasized that the critical area for diffusion is neither that of the alveoli nor that of the pulmonary capillaries but that of the functioning alveoli in contact with functioning capillaries.

The surface area can be decreased by diseases that disrupt normal alveolar architecture (pulmonary emphysema, cysts), by diseases that decrease the functioning pulmonary capillary bed (pulmonary embolism, some types of restrictive disease, emphysema), or by diseases that cause significant block of airways and so decrease the number of alveoli available for gas exchange. In all of these conditions, the diffusing capacity is reduced, but pathologically the dominant lesion is not alveolar-capillary "block," but a decrease in effective surface area.

Physical Characteristics of the Alveolar-Capillary Membranes

Gases move from alveoli to capillaries by going from a gaseous state to a state of solution on the surface of tissues and then move through the tissue because of concentration gradients (see p. 293). Therefore, the solubility of O_2, CO, or CO_2 in the alveolar-capillary membrane is one important determinant of the diffusing capacity of the membrane, and D_M should be proportional to gas solubility in it. The membrane's composition is usually considered to be saline for this purpose, since this is the major component of the tissues. This is only an assumption, however, and the solubility of a gas in the lipid-rich cell membrane itself may be more important in determining gas movement.

A second important factor in determining D_M is the ease with which gas diffuses through the alveolar-capillary membrane itself, once it is dissolved. (This property of the material making up the membrane is generally called the *diffusion coefficient.*) Little is known about this factor. For example, it is possible that fibrotic tissue may impede gas diffusion more than normal tissue of similar thickness and area.

Factors Influencing the Uptake of CO and O_2 by Red Blood Cells in the Alveolar Capillary Bed

The velocity at which red blood cells in the alveolar capillaries can take up CO is not instantaneous but is normally a rate-limiting factor of equal importance to diffusion across the alveolar-capillary membrane (at alveolar P_{O_2} around 100 mm Hg). As a measure of the ease with which the intracapillary exchange of CO takes place in the blood, we can measure the diffusing capacity of CO between the surrounding plasma and red blood cells in the capillary bed, in units of ml CO STPD per minute per mm Hg of partial pressure of CO in the plasma around the cells. In order to do this we measure in vitro the rate at which the red cells in 1 ml of blood can pick up CO; the standard rate used is designated by the Greek letter theta (θ) and given in milliliters of gas STPD combining per minute per mm Hg of partial pressure of CO per milliliter of blood with a normal hemoglobin concentration. Thus, the diffusing capacity of the total red blood cells of the capillary bed equals the rate of uptake per milliliter of blood, θ, multiplied by the volume of the pulmonary capillary bed, V_C. The diffusing capacity of the red blood cells equals θV_C. The factors that influence the uptake of CO or O_2 by the pulmonary capillary blood can be divided into those that influence θ and those that influence the pulmonary capillary blood volume.

Factors That Influence The Rate of CO (or O_2) Uptake by a Milliliter of Blood (θ)

Only the rate of CO combination with red blood cells is of practical interest. While the speed of the reaction of O_2 with capillary red blood cells is known to influence the value of the diffusing capacity for oxygen, $D_{L}O_2$,* there is no convenient method for measuring $D_{L}O_2$ to determine the extent of these influences. Furthermore, θ for oxygen is much greater than θ for CO so that the rate of uptake of oxygen by red cells in the pulmonary capillaries is much less limiting in determining $D_{L}O_2$ than is the rate of uptake of CO in the pulmonary capillary blood in determining $D_{L}CO$. We will therefore discuss only factors that change θCO.

1. No significant variations in θ have been found for the same number of red blood cells from different individuals provided it is measured under the same chemical conditions.

2. An increase in the CO (or O_2) capacity of a milliliter of blood will increase θCO proportionally. A decrease in Hb concentration will decrease θCO, and this occurs in anemia. Therefore, the greater the hemoglobin concentration per milliliter of blood, the more rapidly CO is taken up from the alveolar gas. The in vitro measurements available show no effect of change in mean corpuscular hemoglobin concentration or cell size or θCO independent of total hemoglobin concentration (or CO capacity). Therefore, if we know the hemoglobin concentration in the pulmonary capillary blood (assumed to be that in the peripheral blood). We can calculate the θ of the pulmonary capillary blood from the following relationship:

*The capital letter *D* is used, at least in the United States, to represent "diffusing capacity." Because the diffusing capacity of the whole lung can be separated into the diffusing capacity of the alveolar membrane and the diffusing capacity of the red blood cells in the capillary bed at any instant, the subscripts *L* and *M* were added to symbolize the diffusing capacity of the whole and the diffusing capacity of the alveolar-capillary membrane alone respectively. The subscripts O_2 and CO are used to indicate the gases used in the measurements. D_L stands for the diffusing capacity of the whole lung, and D_M stands for the diffusing capacity of the alveolar-capillary membrane alone.

$$\text{Patient's } \theta\text{CO} = \frac{\text{Patient's blood } O_2 \text{ capacity (ml/ml)} \times \text{standard } \theta\text{CO}}{[O_2] \text{ (ml/ml)}}$$

3. An early experimental finding was that an increase in alveolar PO_2 produced a decrease in D_LCO. Carbon monoxide reacts only with unoxygenated hemoglobin; more properly, a CO molecule (or an O_2 molecule for that matter) can only bind onto an iron atom in a hemoglobin tetramer to a position that is not already attached to a ligand (O_2 or CO) molecule. The rate of formation of HbCO is proportional to the concentration of these unbound hemoglobin iron sites. As PO_2 is increased the number of these sites decreases and θCO decreases.

4. An increased alveolar CO_2 or decreased pH causes a slight increase in θCO, which results in an increased D_LCO.

5. A decrease in temperature will decrease θCO just as it does all chemical reactions.

Factors That Influence the Magnitude of the Pulmonary Capillary Blood Volume (V_C)

V_C is the volume of the pulmonary capillary blood in milliliters. This can be varied by hemodynamic forces; it increases with increased pulmonary blood flow,† with increased transmural pressure, or with the opening up of the previously closed capillaries. It is decreased when pulmonary blood flow decreases, when transmural pressure decreases, or when capillaries are destroyed or are closed.

Diffusing Capacity of the Lung Can Be Altered by a Combination of Factors

Just as nonuniformity of alveolar ventilation/blood flow can decrease the aeration of the arterial blood at the same total alveolar ventilation and same total pulmonary blood flow, so can nonuniformity of diffusing capacity decrease the effective diffusing capacity of the whole lung so that it becomes less than the sum of the diffusing capacities of all the different alveoli. As a reasonable approximation we would expect diffusing capacity to parallel pulmonary capillary blood flow; closure of a capillary bed would reduce both the blood flow through the region

†V_C is a volume, not a flow, but when the right ventricle contracts it thrusts blood into the pulmonary vascular bed more rapidly than it can empty into the pulmonary veins and left ventricle, which is contracting at the same time, so the pulmonary vascular bed, including the capillaries, increases in volume.

and diffusing capacity; similarly, an increase in blood flow would increase the diffusing capacity through the area. Thus there will be parallelism between nonuniformity of diffusing capacity in the lung and nonuniformity of pulmonary capillary blood flow.

Extreme values of nonuniformity of diffusing capacity throughout the lung may remain undetected by pulmonary function testing because of the great reserves of the pulmonary capillary bed. An alveolus that is filled with fluid, as in pulmonary edema, might be considered to have an extreme form of diffusion defect, but since it is not aerated it would not contribute in a measurement of total lung D_L. The intrinsic regulatory response of the capillaries would most likely decrease blood flow through the region, directing it to other parts of the lung, which would thereby have their diffusing capacity increased. Because these capillaries would probably be part of the circulatory reserve of the lung, this might not alter the total diffusing capacity of the lung. Similarly, a capillary with extreme thickening of the walls is liable to occlude completely; it would have no blood flow and would behave as an alveolar dead space. Again, however, its capillary blood flow is likely to be diverted to other parts of the lung, so the abnormal area might not be included in the measurement of total lung diffusing capacity at all.

It is important to point out here that the "diffusing capacity" can increase as well as decrease. The distance for diffusion cannot become much shorter than 0.1 μ, but the surface area can become greater by (1) an increase in the number of pulmonary capillaries with active circulation, (2) dilatation of capillaries already functioning, and (3) by increase in surface area of functioning alveoli. The capillary blood volume can increase—for instance, through congestion—and increased pulmonary capillary hemoglobin concentration will increase θCO.

B. MEASUREMENT OF PULMONARY DIFFUSING CAPACITY

General Principles

The test requires the use of a gas that is considerably more "soluble" in blood than in the alveolar-capillary membranes. As stated previously, only two such gases are known, O_2 and CO. Both of them owe this unusual pattern of "solubility" to the chemical association that occurs with hemoglobin. Both presumably measure the same process, and the diffusing capacity measured by CO can be converted to the diffusing

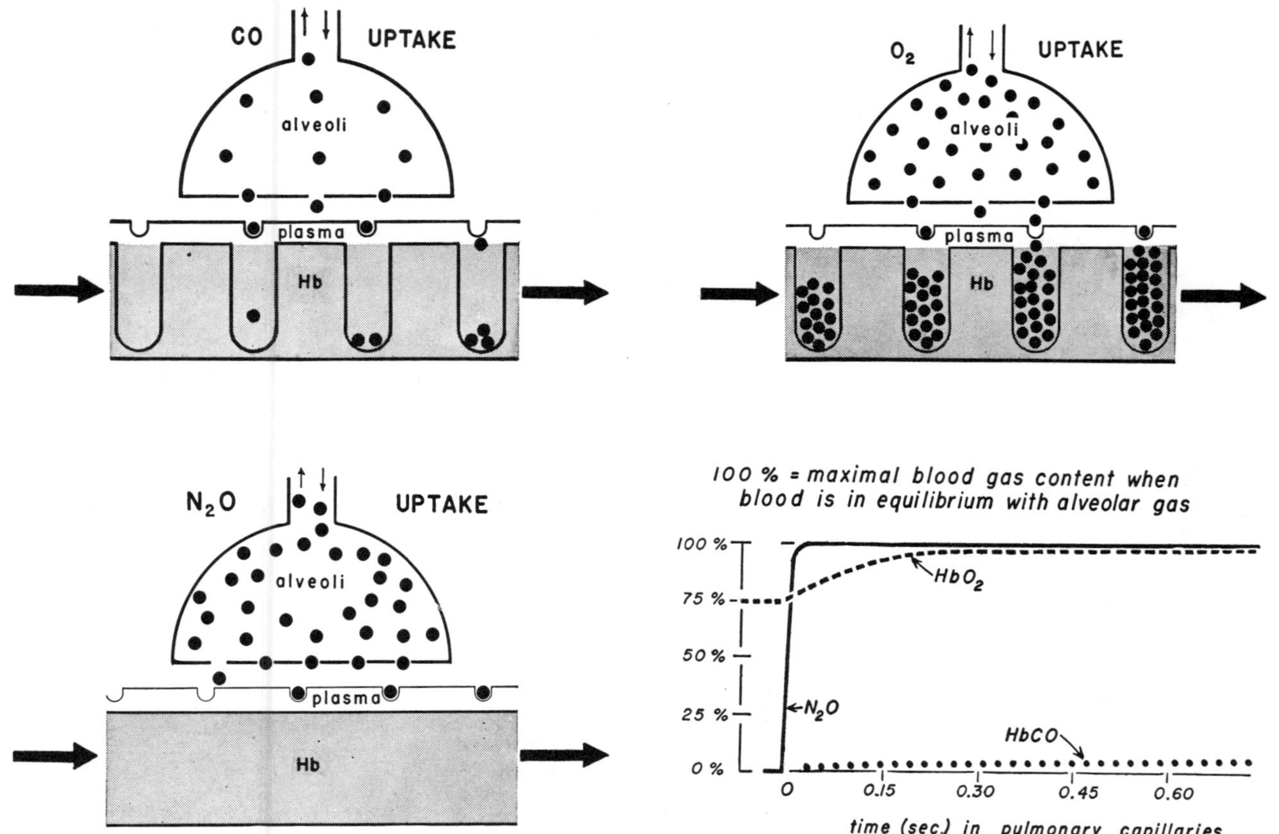

CO
UPTAKE
alveoli
plasma
Hb
O_2
UPTAKE
alveoli
plasma
Hb
N_2O
UPTAKE
alveoli
plasma
Hb
100 % = maximal blood gas content when
blood is in equilibrium with alveolar gas
100 %
75 %
50 %
25 %
0 %
HbO_2
N_2O
HbCO
0
0.15
0.30
0.45
0.60
time (sec.) in pulmonary capillaries

Fig 59.—In each *schema,* the black dots signify gas molecules. The bottom of each alveolus represents the alveolocapillary membrane with numerous pores to permit diffusion of gas molecules. Blood moves from left to right through the pulmonary capillary beneath the pulmonary membrane. The bloodstream, solely for purposes of illustration, is divided into two portions: upper portion represents plasma (and all other watery parts of the blood), with a certain number of pockets to indicate its capacity for dissolving each gas; lower portion represents hemoglobin; there are no compartments in the hemoglobin layer for N_2O because it does not combine chemically with hemoglobin, but large pockets are available for CO and O_2. Mixed venous blood enters the capillary with no CO or N_2O in the plasma and hemoglobin compartments (since these are foreign gases) but with the O_2 compartments partly full.

The *graph* presents blood gas content (ordinate) plotted against the time that the blood spends in the pulmonary capillary. The horizontal line at the top indicates maximal gas content of the blood when it is *saturated* at the gas pressure maintained in the alveoli. In the case of CO, there is only a very slight increase in HbCO concentration along the capillary; it never approaches the maximal value because of the low partial pressure of CO in the alveoli. It must be remembered that 100 ml of blood, when saturated with CO, will contain about 20 ml of CO, yet the alveolar gas at any instant contains only about 1.3 ml CO (assuming that functional residual capacity is 2000 ml and contains 0.065% CO). In the case of N_2O, the blood attains maximal concentration before it has gone 1/20 the distance along the capillary. In the case of O_2, saturation increases from 75% to 97% along the capillary.

factor for O_2 by multiplying by a factor of 1.23.* Figure 59 presents schematically the basis for the measurement of diffusing capacity, employing CO or O_2.

CO Uptake

A low concentration of CO is maintained in the alveolus† by adding about 0.2% CO to inspired air. The concentration of CO in mixed venous blood entering the pulmonary capillaries is zero for all practical purposes. Therefore, molecules of CO diffuse across the membrane and dissolve in the watery parts of blood. Carbon monoxide is a remarkable gas because of the great affinity between it and Hb; it has 210 times the affinity for Hb that O_2 does. Thus, a partial pressure of CO of only 0.46 mm Hg (equivalent to 0.065% CO) produces the same percent saturation of Hb, at equilibrium, as does a partial pressure of 100 mm Hg O_2 (equivalent to 14% O_2) (Fig 60). For this reason, any CO in the vicinity of a Hb molecule becomes bound to it, so that the partial pressure of dissolved CO stays at a very low level in the red blood cell. The Hb "compartments" for CO are so large (except when the patient has severe anemia) that they cannot possibly be filled by the number of molecules of CO that diffuse from the alveolar gas to the capillary blood at these low alveolar CO tensions. Even if pulmonary blood flow stopped, transfer of CO would continue until the "pockets" became full. Therefore, the transfer of CO is not limited by the rate of pulmonary blood flow; in normal lungs it is limited approximately equally by the rate of diffusion across the alveolar-capillary membrane and by the rate of uptake of CO by erythrocytes in the pulmonary capillary blood (including simultaneous diffusion and chemical reaction of CO with hemoglobin within the red blood cell).

On the other hand, gases such as N_2O (see Fig 59), ethyl iodide, and acetylene are soluble to an equal extent in the alveolar-capillary membranes and in blood, since they do not combine chemically with any of the components of blood. These gases diffuse across the alveolar-capillary membranes and quickly fill up all of the plasma "compartments"; since the plasma is now saturated, further diffusion is prevented until

*Derivation of this factor is given in the Appendix on p. 293.

†There is no danger in using 0.2% to 0.4% CO in these tests since the concentrations are very low and the gas is breathed for only short intervals. However, the use of higher concentrations of CO in the inspired gas can be dangerous and the CO concentration should be checked in each new tank. Carbon monoxide may be considered not a "physiologic" gas as compared to O_2. However, it is always present in the blood as it is produced in the body by the catabolism of the heme ring of hemoglobin, and many other cytochromes, at a rate greater than 0.4 ml/hr in normal males.

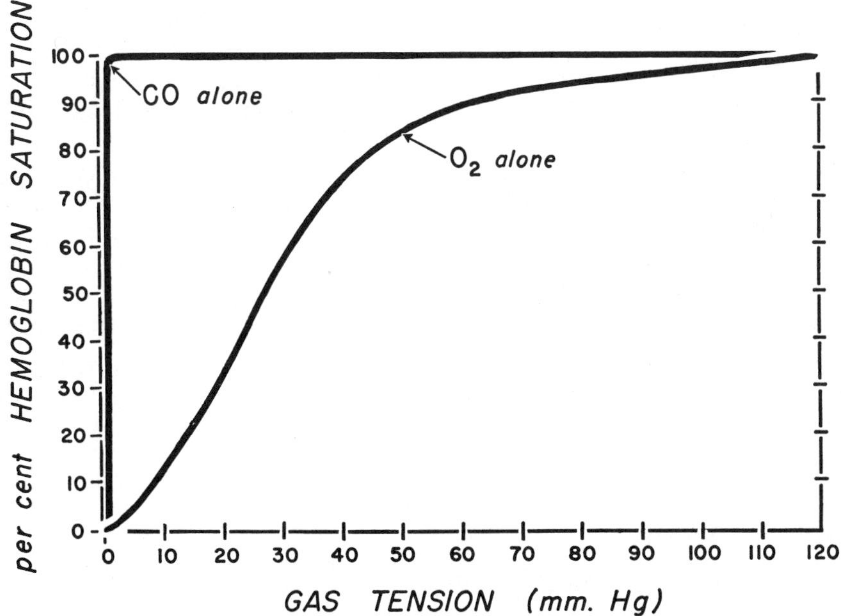

Fig 60.—Dissociation curves for HbO_2 and HbCO. Dissociation curves are plotted on the same scale. Maximal saturation of hemoglobin with O_2 is not reached until the P_{O_2} is greater than 120 mm Hg; with CO, however, maximal saturation is attained with a P_{CO} of less than 1 mm Hg.

the blood is replaced by fresh blood, with empty "compartments," entering the pulmonary capillaries. The rate of uptake of these gases is limited, therefore, by the rate at which blood enters the pulmonary capillaries rather than by the rate of diffusion of gases across the alveolar-capillary and red blood cell membranes. Actually, the first measurements of pulmonary capillary blood flow were made by Krogh and Lindhard, using N_2O as the test gas (see Fig 44). If there were no red blood cells and Hb, and only plasma flowed through the pulmonary capillaries, CO uptake would then also be "flow limited" and would measure capillary blood flow; in patients with very severe anemia and Hb deficiency, CO uptake may be partly "flow limited" and partly "diffusion limited."

In summary, the rate of CO uptake is limited by diffusion and can be used to measure the diffusing capacity; the uptake of N_2O, ethyl iodide, or acetylene is limited by the rate of pulmonary blood flow and can be used to estimate pulmonary capillary blood flow.

O_2 Uptake

Figure 59 shows O_2 diffusing across the pulmonary membranes into the plasma and then associating chemically with hemoglobin. An obvious difference between the CO and O_2 schemas is that both the plasma and the hemoglobin "compartments" are partly filled with O_2 when mixed venous blood enters the pulmonary capillaries. The rate of diffusion of O_2 into the blood depends upon the difference in pressure of O_2 in the alveolar gas and that in the blood at every point along the capillary. As O_2 is transferred across the alveolar-capillary membranes, the capillary P_{O_2} rises and the increase in capillary P_{O_2} narrows the difference between alveolar and capillary P_{O_2} and slows the rate of diffusion. This means that the blood P_{O_2} must be known at every moment along the capillary. This information can be obtained by certain measurements and a series of mathematical computations (p. 301).

Carbon Monoxide Methods for Measuring Pulmonary Diffusing Capacity

$$\text{Pulmonary diffusing capacity for CO} = \frac{\text{ml of CO transferred from alveolar gas to blood/min}}{\text{mean alveolar CO pressure} - \text{mean capillary CO pressure}}$$

Therefore, to measure the pulmonary diffusing capacity for CO, three measurements must be made:

1. Milliliters of CO transferred from alveolar gas to blood per minute
2. The mean alveolar CO pressure
3. The mean pulmonary capillary CO pressure*

There are three methods to measure CO uptake: (1) the steady-state technique, (2) the single-breath technique, and (3) the rebreathing technique. These methods provide all the data required for quantitative measurement of the diffusing capacity of the lungs. It is also possible to measure the fractional *CO uptake,* but this gives only an index of the pulmonary diffusing capacity.

Steady-State Technique

In this method the patient breathes a gas mixture containing a low concentration of CO (about 0.1% to 0.2%). After about 12 breaths, the alveolar P_{CO} reaches a plateau and the measurements are made.

*The mean capillary CO partial pressure (P_{CO}) is that in equilibrium with the Hb in the red blood cell according to the Haldane relationship (see Appendix).

The amount of CO transferred from alveolar gas to capillary blood per minute is calculated by measuring CO in the inspired and expired gas and subtracting that expired from the amount inspired. The mean capillary P_{CO} is so small that it can be neglected. The *mean alveolar* P_{CO} can be calculated if one measures the P_{CO} in *expired* gas and knows the volume of the "physiologic dead space" (p. 296). Thus, all the data necessary for the computation of the diffusing capacity for CO can be obtained.

This method has the advantages that it requires little cooperation on the patient's part, it is carried out under normal breathing conditions, and can be used during severe exercise. The analysis of CO in inspired and expired gas is usually done with physical analyzers, infrared, oxidation cell, or gas chromatograph.

The test requires arterial puncture and analysis of the arterial P_{CO_2} in order to compute mean alveolar P_{CO}. Slight errors in the analyses of CO_2 and CO can lead to large errors (as much as 40%) in the calculation of the diffusing capacity for CO.

There are other possible ways of estimating alveolar P_{CO}, such as (1) collecting an expired alveolar sample or (2) assuming a respiratory dead space and calculating alveolar P_{CO} from the inspired and expired CO concentrations. Although these methods avoid the necessity of sampling arterial blood, they are at least theoretically susceptible to considerable errors in the presence of uneven distribution of gas in the lung; (1) is subject to all the errors attendant on calling a single sample of gas representative of alveolar gas, and (2) is quite unreliable at rest because the value of dead space chosen is exquisitely critical.

Single-Breath Test Using CO

In this test, the patient inspires a gas mixture containing a low concentration of CO and a few tenths of a percent of a chemically inert insoluble gas, such as helium, then holds his breath for approximately ten seconds and delivers an expired sample, which is then analyzed for both CO and He. During the breath-holding period some CO leaves the alveolar gas and enters the blood; the larger the diffusing capacity, the greater is the amount of CO that enters the blood during the ten-second period.

Again, three values are required: (1) *milliliters of CO transferred,* which can be calculated from measurements of the percent CO in the alveolar gas in the beginning and at the end of the breath-holding period if the volume of alveolar gas (functional residual capacity plus inspired volume) is also known; (2) *the mean capillary* P_{CO}, which is so small that it can be neglected; and (3) *the mean alveolar P_{CO}.*

The percent CO in the alveolar gas sample at the beginning of the breath-holding period can be calculated from the dilution of the inspired He in the alveolar gas sample, since He is chemically inert and is not absorbed by the lung tissue or capillary blood flow. In the single-breath test, alveolar P_{CO} is not maintained at a nearly constant concentration as in the steady-state method because here the breath is held after the CO is inspired, and CO is absorbed during the period of breath-holding. Further, the mean alveolar P_{CO} is not the average of the P_{CO} at the beginning and end of the breath-holding period. However, by a special equation (p. 295), the mean alveolar P_{CO} can be calculated and the diffusing capacity measured.

The single-breath test has the advantage of requiring little cooperation from the patient, who has only to inhale and hold his breath for ten seconds. The analyses are performed with an infrared or other type of physical analyzer. No blood samples are needed. The test can be repeated a number of times in rapid succession if desired. However, a measurement of the patient's functional residual capacity is needed,† because a value for the total alveolar volume during the period of breath-holding is required in order to measure CO uptake. Furthermore, one must inhale a gas such as helium along with CO in order to correct for uneven distribution of the inspired CO. The method also has the disadvantage that breath-holding is not a normal breathing state. Finally, dyspneic patients or exercising patients may find it difficult to hold their breath for ten seconds and may not be able to inspire and deliver an alveolar sample rapidly, making it difficult to measure the exact time the CO and helium resided in the lung.

Rebreathing Technique Using CO

In this test, the patient rebreathes for about 1½ minutes from a bag containing approximately 6 L of a mixture of air and a low concentration of CO. He breathes quite rapidly (about 25/min) so that the gases in the bag are well mixed with those in the lung. The pulmonary diffusing capacity can be calculated in a manner similar to that for the single-breath technique. The change of CO concentration in the gas within the bag is measured over a portion of the rebreathing period. The total volume of the system, residual volume plus bag volume, mul-

†The total alveolar volume during the breath-holding period is often calculated from the dilution of inspired helium (see Appendix) thus:

Alveolar volume = inspired volume × inspired % of He/expired alveolar % of He

The gas concentrations are given dry and inspired volume is corrected to give alveolar volume as STPD or BTPS. Because the inspired volume is large, approximating vital capacity, the error in calculating alveolar volume from the dilution because of nonuniform distribution of inspired gas is minimized.

tiplied by the change of CO concentration gives the *volume of CO transferred. The mean capillary* P_{CO} can again be neglected. *Mean alveolar* P_{CO} is calculated from the concentration in the bag at the start and end of the period of measurement, using the same equation as that for the single-breath test (p. 295).

The relative advantages of the test are that it does not require arterial samples or breath-holding, and the rebreathing tends to compensate for uneven distribution of gas and blood throughout the lung. On the other hand, breathing at such a rapid rate requires considerable cooperation from the patient and is not natural. In addition, a measure of the functional residual capacity is needed; if a low concentration of helium is included in the original gas mixture, the lung volume can be calculated from the final helium concentration in the same manner as for the closed-circuit helium measurement of functional residual capacity (p. 16).

Fractional CO Uptake

The percentage of the inspired CO that is taken up by the blood over a period of several minutes yields an *index* of the diffusing capacity because, in general, the greater the diffusing capacity, the greater the amount of CO that will be absorbed per minute; it does not provide a measure of *diffusing capacity* in any quantitative sense.

$$\text{Fractional CO uptake (in \%)} = \frac{\text{CO absorbed/min}}{\text{CO inspired/min}} \times 100$$

This index is approximately 50% in normal subjects. Values of less than 30% generally indicate an impairment of diffusion.

This test has the advantage of relative simplicity, because the only measurements are of the CO concentration in the inspired and expired gas. If the mean alveolar P_{CO} is not estimated, a calculation of diffusing capacity cannot be made.

Fractional CO uptake is influenced by the minute volume and the frequency of breathing; the higher the minute volume, the lower the fractional CO uptake, even though the diffusing capacity is the same. Thus it is difficult to tell whether a low fractional CO uptake is the result of impairment of diffusion or of a high alveolar ventilation. It is possible to make corrections if the alveolar ventilation per minute is known.

Oxygen Method for Measuring Pulmonary Diffusing Capacity

The more difficult and time-consuming O_2 method has been largely displaced in clinical laboratories by the CO methods for measuring diffusing capacity. An account of the concepts underlying the O_2 method is presented here because the basic principles and reasoning involved in the test are fundamental to an understanding of pulmonary gas exchange.

Pulmonary diffusing capacity for O_2

$$= \frac{\text{ml of } O_2 \text{ transferred from alveolar gas to blood per minute}}{\text{Mean alveolar } O_2 \text{ pressure} - \text{mean capillary } O_2 \text{ pressure}}$$

To measure the diffusing capacity for O_2, three measurements must be made:

1. Milliliters of O_2 transferred from alveolar gas to blood/min
2. The mean alveolar O_2 pressure
3. The mean pulmonary capillary O_2 pressure

Milliliters of O_2 Transferred

This is measured easily, since it is the O_2 consumption of the patient per minute.

Mean Alveolar P_{O_2}

In chapter 3, it was emphasized that uneven distribution of inspired gas occurs frequently in pulmonary disease, and this makes it difficult to call any "spot" sample of expired alveolar gas truly representative of *all* alveolar gas. However, it is possible to calculate a value for mean alveolar P_{O_2} by use of the alveolar air equation, using a measured value of arterial P_{CO_2} instead of alveolar P_{CO_2}.

*Mean Pulmonary Capillary O_2 Pressure**

Its measurement presents a real challenge. With CO, the capillary pressure was so low that it could be neglected. With O_2, the P_{O_2} at the beginning of the pulmonary capillary is that of mixed venous blood, about 40 mm Hg; the P_{O_2} at the end of the capillary is normally very nearly the same as alveolar P_{O_2}, about 100 mm Hg (Fig 61). However, the *mean* capillary P_{O_2} is not simply the average of these values.

Fortunately, one can compute (by Bohr's integration procedure) the mean capillary P_{O_2} if one knows four things:

1. The pressure of O_2 in the blood just at the beginning of the pulmonary capillaries (mixed venous blood).
2. The pressure of O_2 in the alveoli, which establishes the pressure gradient across the alveolar capillary membranes.

*In the interest of clarity of presentation, we are ignoring the pressure gradient between the plasma and the interior of the red blood cell. "Capillary P_{O_2}" really should read "P_{O_2} within the erythrocyte in the pulmonary capillary."

3. The pressure of O_2 in the blood just at the end of the pulmonary capillaries.
4. The physiologic oxygen-hemoglobin dissociation curve.

It is possible to measure (1), estimate (2), and consult tables or graphs for (4). The measurement of the end-capillary Po_2 is more difficult, but can be accomplished.

End-Capillary Po_2

Assume for the moment that it is possible to obtain blood for analysis from the end of the pulmonary capillaries or from the pulmonary veins. However, even then, there is no method available for measuring the Po_2 in this blood with the accuracy required at normal alveolar Po_2 (100 mm Hg). Figure 61 and Table 8 show that the *mean* capillary Po_2 (calculated by Bohr's integration procedure) will be 91 if end-capillary pressure is more than 99.99 mm Hg (example *A*), 85 if end-capillary Po_2 is approximately 99.9 (example *B*), and 72.5 mm Hg if end-capillary pressure is 96 mm Hg (example *C*). Methods for measuring blood Po_2 have an error of ± 2 mm Hg, and one is not justified in measuring a 0.1 mm Hg difference with a method that has a 2 mm Hg error!

However, if the end-capillary Po_2 were considerably lower than the alveolar Po_2, the difference could be measured with reasonable accuracy. Fortunately, Lilienthal and Riley found that this end-capillary O_2 gradient can be increased, presumably without any change in the diffusing capacity of the lungs, by giving the patient a low O_2 mixture to breathe (Fig 62). When air (20.93% O_2) is breathed, the O_2 pressure gradient at the beginning of the capillary is *large* (about 60 mm Hg), the initial transfer of O_2 across the membranes is rapid, and near equilibrium with alveolar gas is reached quickly. A healthy subject has practically no alveolar to end-capillary Po_2 difference when he breathes air. When 14% O_2 is breathed, the O_2 pressure gradient at the beginning of the capillary is small (about 25 mm Hg), the initial transfer is less rapid, and a measurable pressure gradient still exists at the end of the capillary. *Therefore, decreasing the alveolar Po_2 increases the alveolar to end-capillary Po_2 difference; increasing alveolar Po_2 decreases alveolar to end-capillary Po_2 difference.* A sample calculation demonstrating this point is illustrated in Figure 61 (p. 210). The clinical measurement of the diffusing capacity of the lung for O_2 includes measurements made during the inhalation of 12% to 14% O_2 in order to provide a measurable end-capillary diffusion gradient.

It was assumed earlier that a representative sample of end-capillary blood could be obtained. Unfortunately, this cannot be done. Samples of pulmonary "capillary" blood have been obtained by the catheteriza-

ALVEOLAR-CAPILLARY DIFFUSION

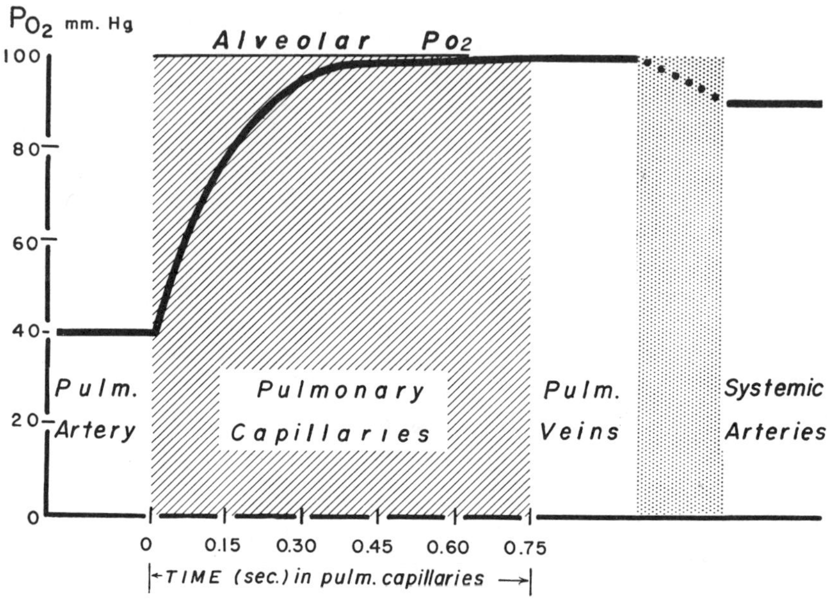

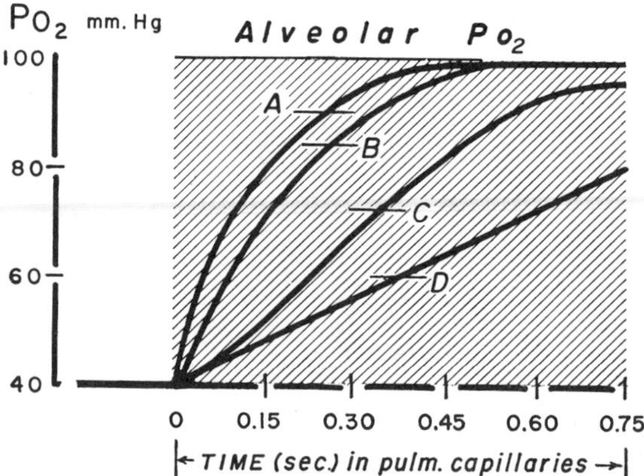

Fig 61.—*Above,* mixed venous blood enters pulmonary capillaries with Po_2 of 40 mm Hg. Blood normally requires about 0.75 sec to pass through the capillaries. At the end of this time, its Po_2 has risen to almost 100 mm Hg. The Po_2 of arterial blood is lower because of venous to arterial shunts.

tion technique, but these are not representative of all capillary blood; indeed, this is really blood with a high ventilation/blood flow ratio since it has twice passed ventilated alveoli.

On the other hand, *arterial* blood *can* be obtained and its Po_2 measured reasonably accurately. Can *arterial* blood be used as representative of end-pulmonary capillary blood? Figure 61 shows that it cannot because its Po_2 is lower than that of end-pulmonary capillary blood, owing to the existence of a "physiologic shunt" even in normal individuals (pp. 152 and 180 and Fig 42 p. 140); this "physiologic shunt" includes blood from areas with a decreased ventilation/blood flow ratio.

The Po_2 difference between alveolar gas and *arterial* blood thus includes two components: (1) an *alveolar* to *end-capillary* difference owing to incomplete equilibrium between the Po_2 of alveolar gas and that of end-capillary blood ("membrane component"), and (2) an *end-capillary* to *arterial* difference due to the "physiologic shunt" ("venous admixture"). Fortunately, the second of these can be eliminated almost entirely by giving the patient 12% to 14% O_2 to inhale.

The explanation for this depends entirely on the unique shape of the O_2 dissociation curve, which has a flat portion and a very steeply sloping portion. When the patient breathes air (20.93% O_2), his arterial

TABLE 8.—ALVEOLAR AND END-CAPILLARY Po_2 IN PATIENTS WITH NORMAL AND DECREASED DIFFUSING CAPACITIES*

EXAMPLE	DO_2	ALVEOLAR PO_2	END-CAP. PO_2	END-CAP. GRADIENT (PO_2)	MEAN CAP. PO_2	MEAN CAP. GRADIENT (PO_2)
A	>27.7	100	>99.99	<0.01	91	9
B	>16.6	100	>99.9	<0.1	85	15
C	9.1	100	96.0	4.0	72.5	27.5
D	6.4	100	81.4	18.6	61	39

*Data of Fig 61; Po_2 in mm Hg.

Below, illustrations of different rates at which venous blood may be oxygenated in pulmonary capillaries depending upon diffusing capacity of the lung (see Table 8). In each, alveolar Po_2 is 100 mm Hg; end-pulmonary capillary Po_2 is 99.99, 99.9, 96, and 81.4 mm Hg for *A, B, C,* and *D,* respectively. Although the gradients between alveolar gas and end-pulmonary capillary blood are not measurably different (by present techniques) for *A* and *B,* mean pulmonary capillary O_2 pressures calculated by Bohr's integration procedure are quite different. End-pulmonary capillary blood in *A, B,* and *C* would all have normal O_2 saturation though diffusing capacity is different in each case (only in *D* would blood O_2 saturation at the end of the capillary be reduced). If the *time* in the capillary were shortened, as by exercise, from 0.75 to 0.30 sec, O_2 saturation at this time would then be low in *B, C,* and *D.*

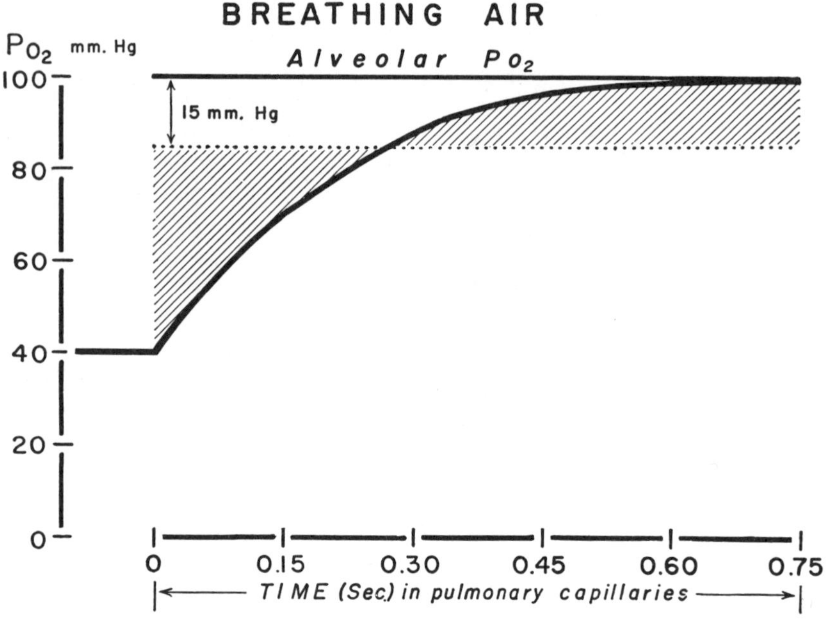

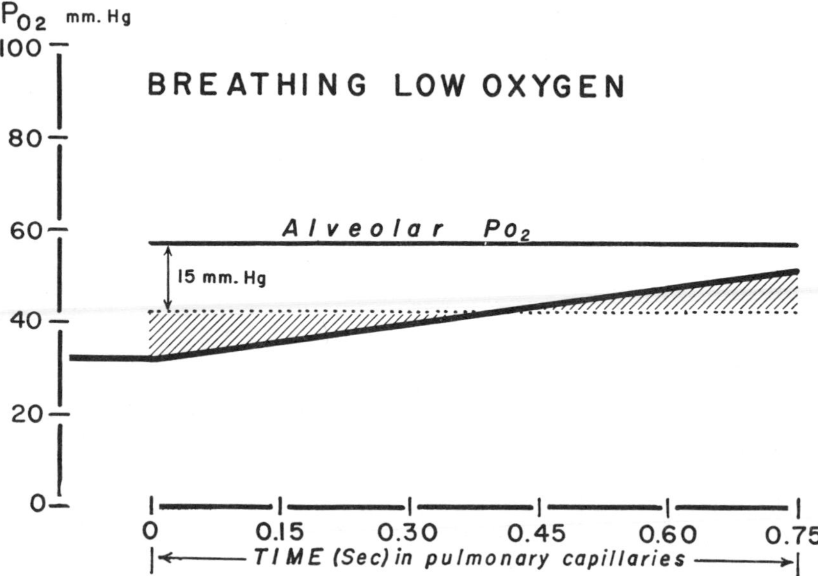

Fig 62.—When the patient breathes air (20.93% O_2), the high initial alveolo-capillary P_{O_2} gradient results in rapid transfer of O_2 so that the P_{O_2} of end pulmonary capillary blood

P_{O_2} and O_2 saturation lie on the flat part, and a small decrease in arterial O_2 saturation, caused by shunted blood, is associated with a large decrease in arterial P_{O_2}. On the other hand, when the patient breathes 12% to 14% O_2, his arterial P_{O_2} and saturation are lowered and fall on the steep slope; now the same decrease in arterial O_2 saturation, caused by the same amount of shunted blood, is associated with a very small decrease in arterial P_{O_2}. This effect is shown graphically in Figure 63 and by the calculations in Table 9.

If the breathing of 12% to 14% O_2 *completely* abolished the P_{O_2} difference owing to the "physiologic shunt," the whole alveolar to arterial P_{O_2} difference under these conditions would be the end-capillary gradient, and all the information required for calculation of the diffusing capacity would be available. However, it does not, and a "trial and error" method (described in the Appendix, p. 304) is necessary to determine the end-capillary P_{O_2} gradient. This permits calculation of the diffusing capacity.

It is fortunate indeed that this one maneuver, the inhalation of 12% to 14% O_2 solves two problems. It increases the "membrane component," so that it becomes a measurable value and at the same time practically eliminates the "physiologic shunt" component, so that the "membrane component" is practically equal to the alveolar-arterial P_{O_2} difference. A summary of these effects is given in Table 10.

This method depends upon the assumptions that the diffusing capacity, cardiac output, and venous admixture are all the same during the breathing of 21% and 12% to 14% O_2, although at least for cardiac output this is unlikely to be the case.

C. NORMAL VALUES FOR PULMONARY DIFFUSING CAPACITY

Approximate values are given in Table 11. Factors that have been found to influence $\dot{D}_L$ are as follows:

---

and of alveolar gas are almost identical. When the patient breathes a low O_2 mixture (12% to 14% O_2), the initial gradient is low, O_2 is transferred at a slower rate, and a measurable end-capillary gradient is present. The curves are plotted from data obtained by the procedure outlined on page 301. Once the curve of increase in P_{O_2} vs. time is plotted, the *mean* capillary pressure is determined graphically by drawing a horizontal line *(dotted)* so that the shaded area above the line *(right)* equals the shaded area below the line *(left)*. The mean gradient (mean alveolar P_{O_2}—mean pulmonary capillary P_{O_2}) must be the same breathing the low O_2 mixture as breathing air if the diffusing capacity and amount of O_2 transferred are the same in the two cases.

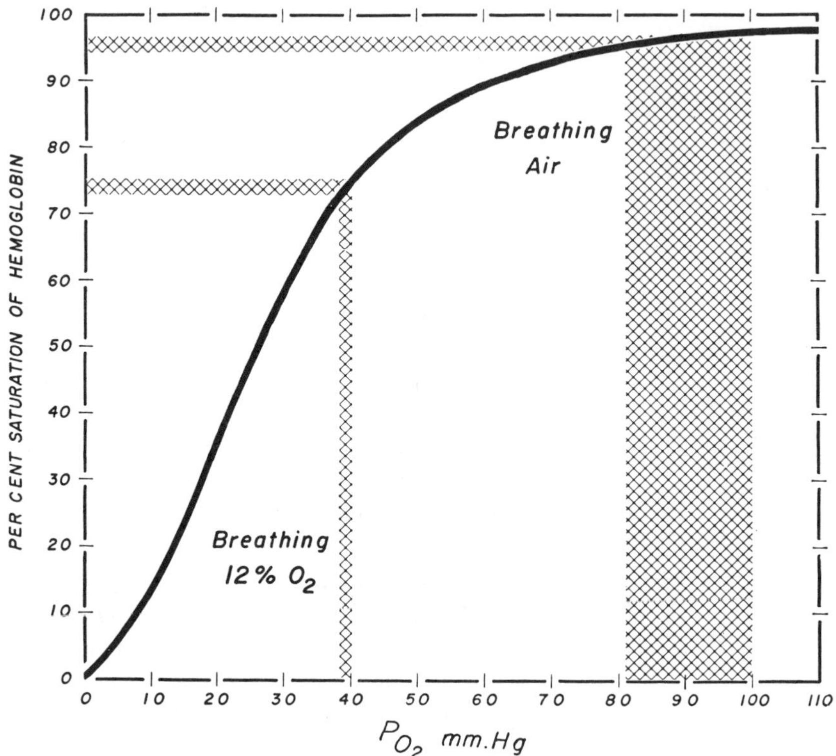

Fig 63.—Effect of Venous to Arterial Shunt on Arterial P_{O_2}. If 10% of the mixed venous blood bypasses the lungs, arterial P_{O_2} is reduced by 19 mm Hg when the patient breathes room air, but only by 1.2 mm Hg when the patients breathes 12% O_2. This is a graphic representation of the calculations in Table 9. In each case, the arteriovenous O_2 saturation difference is 22% and a 10% shunt results in a 2.2% reduction in arterial O_2 saturation.

Body Size

The $D_{L}CO$ has been found to increase with increasing body size, as measured with a variety of parameters such as weight, height, and surface area.

TABLE 9.—EFFECT OF VENOUS-TO-ARTERIAL SHUNT UPON ARTERIAL O_2 SATURATION AND TENSION IN SUBJECT BREATHING *(A)* 20.93% AND *(B)* 12% O_2

	(A) BREATHING AIR	(B) BREATHING 12% O_2
Assume:		
Cardiac output =	5.0 L	5.0 L
Shunted blood =	0.5 L	0.5 L
Nonshunted blood =	4.5 L	4.5 L
Blood O_2 capacity =	20 vol% or 200 ml O_2/L of blood	20 vol% or 200 ml O_2/L of blood
O_2 tension of mixed venous blood =	40 mm Hg	27.5 mm Hg
HbO_2 saturation of mixed venous blood =	75%	53%
Alveolar oxygen tension =	101 mm Hg	44 mm Hg
O_2 tension of end-pul. capillary blood =	100+ mm Hg	40 mm Hg
HbO_2 saturation of end-pul. capillary blood =	97%	75%
Then:		
4.5 L nonshunted blood contains	4.5(0.97 × 200 ml) = 873 ml O_2	4.5(0.75 × 200 ml) = 675 ml O_2
0.5 L shunted blood contains	0.5(0.75 × 200 ml) = 75 ml O_2	0.5(0.53 × 200 ml) = 53 ml O_2
5.0 L arterial blood contains	948 ml O_2	728 ml O_2
100 ml arterial blood contains	948/50 = 18.96 ml O_2	728/50 = 14.56 ml O_2
HbO_2 saturation of arterial blood =	$\frac{18.96}{20} = 94.8\%$	$\frac{14.56}{20} = 72.8\%$
O_2 tension of arterial blood =	81 mm Hg	38.8 mm Hg
Difference between end-pul. capillary and arterial O_2 tension =	100 − 81 = 19 mm Hg	40 − 38.8 = 1.2 mm Hg

Age

D_LCO increases with age from infancy to adulthood, reaching a maximum value in about 20 years. Body size is also increasing during this period and is probably at the dominant factor. From 20 years on D_LCO decreases at the rate of approximately 2% a year. This appears to be an effect of age (or living) itself. At the same age and body size, women have a lower single-breath D_LCO than men by about 10%.

Lung Volume

If D_LCO (single-breath) is measured at two different lung volumes, D_LCO is increased 10% to 25% when lung volume is increased approx-

TABLE 10.—ANALYSIS OF ALVEOLAR – ARTERIAL PO_2

	WHEN PATIENT IS BREATHING		
	12% to 14% O_2	AIR	50% to 100% O_2
Total difference between PO_2 in alveolar gas and arterial blood is*	10 mm Hg	9 mm Hg	35–50 mm Hg
"Venous admixture component" is	1	8	35–50
"Membrane component" is	9	1	0

*The calculations of alveolar PO_2 – arterial PO_2 and of the "venous admixture" component are made on the assumption that this is the result of a shunt. If the "venous admixture" component is produced by nonuniform alveolar ventilation/capillary blood flow, the alveolar PO_2 – arterial PO_2 will decrease at higher inspired O_2 concentrations as shown in Figure 54.

TABLE 11.—NORMAL VALUES FOR PULMONARY DIFFUSING CAPACITY*

	D_LO_2 ML/MIN/MM HG	D_LCO ML/MIN/MM HG	REFERENCE
Carbon monoxide methods			
Steady-state technique (mean alveolar CO tension calculated)	(21)†	17	*J. Clin. Invest.* 33:530, 1954
Steady-state technique (expired alveolar CO tension measured)	(22)	18	*J. Physiol.* 129:237, 1955
Single-breath test (10 sec breath-holding)	(39)	31	Cotes: *Lung Function Assessment.* 1973, p. 373
Rebreathing technique	(33)	27	*J. Appl. Physiol.* 29:896, 1970
Oxygen method			
Steady state	21	(17)†	*Am. J. Physiol.* 147:199, 1946

*Data are average values for resting subjects.
†Numbers in parentheses were computed from the equation $DO_2 = 1.23\ DCO$.

imately 50%. The single-breath test is performed at a large lung volume, and this may be a partial explanation of higher "normal" values obtained when it is used. D_LCO apparently does not increase with increased end expiratory volume in steady-state measurements. The increase may represent an increase in pulmonary capillary blood volume (V_C), an increase in the diffusing capacity of the pulmonary membrane (D_M), a reduction in the nonuniformity of D_LCO/alveolar volume, or all three. If D_LCO increases proportionately* to the increases in alveolar volume, the effect of changes in alveolar volume in a given patient can

*Generally the proportional increase in D_LCO is not as great as the proportional increase in alveolar volume so that D_LCO/alveolar volume is not constant.

be eliminated by measuring D_LCO/alveolar volume (K_{CO} or Krogh's constant). This is useful in patients such as those with emphysema who have a large lung volume, which may of itself increase the measured D_LCO and obscure a real functional decrease in the pulmonary capillary bed. D_LCO/alveolar volume can be obtained by the single-breath technique, eliminating the need for an independent measure of alveolar volume, which is generally obtained by the He equilibration method or the body plethysmograph (see Appendix).

Exercise

D_LCO increases immediately with the onset of exercise and decreases rapidly with its cessation. The changes with cardiac output can double the value of the pulmonary diffusing capacity. Presumably, the increase is not caused by an increase in pulmonary blood flow or its velocity through the pulmonary capillaries per se, but by an increase in the surface contact area of functioning pulmonary capillaries or by an increase in the volume of red blood cells exposed to alveolar gas (V_C). These increases may be produced by the opening of previously closed capillaries and/or the dilation of those already opened. It has so far been difficult to distinguish between these two mechanisms.

In view of the enormous reserves of the pulmonary capillary bed, which could conceal destruction of the pulmonary vasculature by disease, it has been proposed to measure the *maximal* diffusing capacity at high levels of exercise. However, in healthy patients D_LCO continues to increase as long as cardiac output increases; there is no clear maximal value independent of pulmonary blood flow.

Body Position

The D_LCO is 15% to 20% greater in the supine than in the sitting position and about 10% to 15% greater sitting than standing, possibly because of changes in pulmonary capillary blood volume associated with changes in posture. D_LCO/alveolar volume is greater in the bases than the apices of the lung because of the larger capillary bed in the lower alveoli secondary to the higher hydrostatic blood pressure (see Fig 46) and the smaller relative alveolar volume (see Fig 27).

Alveolar PO_2

Because of its influence on the rate of chemical combination of CO with Hb (θCO) increases in alveolar oxygen partial pressure reduce

D_LCO. For example, the diffusing capacities measured at alveolar oxygen tensions of 40 and 600 mm of Hg were 45 and 18 ml × min^{-1} × mm Hg^{-1}, respectively. The changes in D_LCO that are caused by variations in alveolar PO_2 in the physiologic range are much smaller. In patients with severe hypoxia, increases in pulmonary blood flow and dilatation of the pulmonary capillary bed may occur; D_LCO may change on this account, as well as because of change in the reaction rate of CO with Hb.

Alveolar PCO_2

The addition of 6% to 7.5% CO_2 to the inspired gas for some minutes before measuring D_LCO increases it by 5% to 25%. When 6% CO_2 is added just for the 10-second breath-holding period that is required by the single-breath test, only a 5% increase occurs.

D. MEASUREMENTS OF THE DIFFUSING CAPACITY OF THE ALVEOLAR-CAPILLARY MEMBRANE (D_M) AND OF THE PULMONARY CAPILLARY BLOOD VOLUME (V_C)

The reciprocal of D_LCO, can be considered a resistance, pressure difference for CO/flow, where flow is the CO uptake. This resistance can be broken up into the sum of two resistances: (1) resistance to CO diffusion through the pulmonary membrane ($1/D_M$), and (2) the resistance to CO uptake of the total volume of red blood cells in the capillary bed ($1/\theta\ V_C$). Adding resistances (1) and (2), we obtain the following relationship:

$$\frac{1}{D_LCO} = \frac{1}{D_M} + \frac{1}{\theta\ V_C}$$

If we measure D_LCO at increasing values of alveolar PO_2, D_LCO decreases because increased PO_2 causes θCO to decrease. θCO has been measured at different PO_2 for normal human red blood cells in rapid-mixing experiments in vitro and decreases approximately reciprocally with increasing PO_2 (Appendix), so we know the θCO corresponding to each D_LCO. We can solve graphically for the diffusing capacity of the pulmonary membrane, D_M, and the pulmonary capillary blood volume V_C, by plotting the reciprocal of D_LCO against the reciprocal for θCO as shown in Figure 64. The intercept on the ordinate is .018, so that D_M is 53 ml × min^{-1} × mm Hg.$^{-1}$ The slope is 0.0126, so V_C is 79 ml.

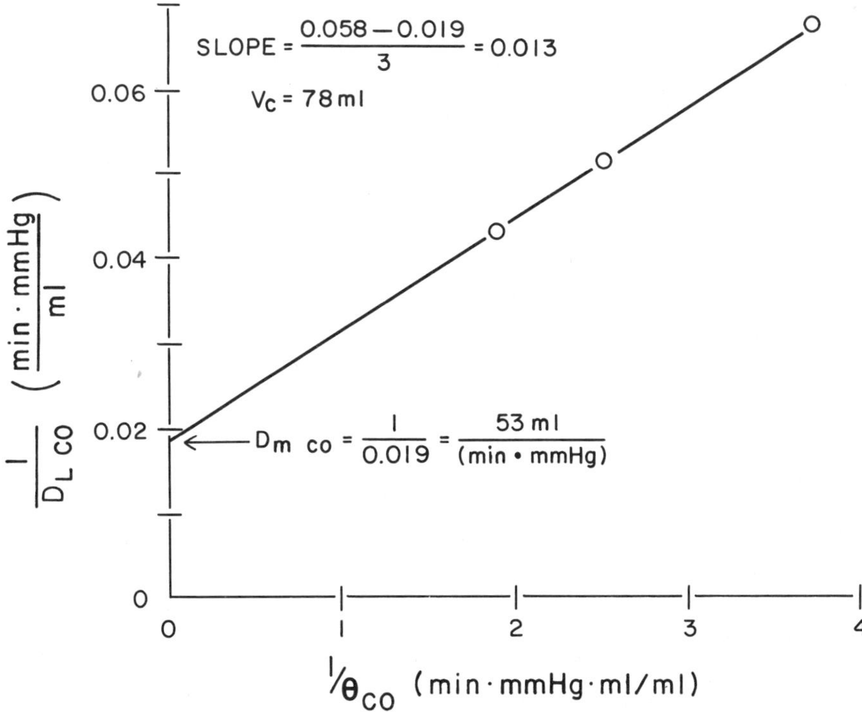

Fig 64.—A calculation of pulmonary capillary blood volume (V_C) and the diffusion capacity of the pulmonary membrane (D_M) from measurements of the diffusing capacity of the lung for D_LCO at different alveolar Po_2. This is a graphical solution of equation:

$$\frac{1}{D_LCO} = \frac{1}{D_M} + \frac{1}{\theta_{CO}V_C}$$

The general equation for a straight line is:

$$Y = A + BX;\ \text{in this case}\ Y = \frac{1}{D_LCO},\ A = \frac{1}{D_M}$$

and B = $1/V_C$. Thus the intercept on the ordinate is $1/D_M$, 53.7 ml/(min x mm Hg). V_C = 1/slope, or 78 ml.

These measurements are made using CO, as no method for changing θO_2 is available. The breath-holding D_LCO method is preferred here because the alveolar Po_2 can be changed rapidly (within 1 second) by altering the O_2 content of the inspired CO mixture and the whole procedure is complete within ten seconds. This means there is little time for possible hemodynamic changes in the pulmonary capillary bed.

It is the capillary Po_2, not the alveolar Po_2, that determines the value of θCO. Therefore, it is necessary to have a high alveolar PO_2 (over 150 mm Hg) in order to equilibrate capillary PO_2 early in transit because it enters the alveolus at the PO_2 of mixed venous blood (about 46 mm Hg).

E. LABORATORY DIAGNOSIS OF IMPAIRMENT OF DIFFUSION

At the beginning of this chapter we indicated that measurements of diffusing capacity have become helpful in the diagnosis of certain types of pulmonary disease, but we did not state why the estimation of diffusing capacity is of more diagnostic help than other laboratory methods, such as the measurement of arterial blood O_2 or PO_2 at rest, during exercise or during inhalation of O_2.

Arterial O_2 saturation may be reduced for many reasons; an impairment of diffusion is only one of these. Arterial O_2 saturation may be normal even though there is definite impairment of the diffusion process. The reason for this may be found in Figure 61 and Table 8. In *A,* the diffusing capacity is normal (27.7) and the end-capillary PO_2 is more than 99.9 mm Hg; in *B,* it is reduced (16.6), but the end-capillary PO_2 is still approximately 99.9; in *C,* it is further reduced (9.1), but the end-capillary PO_2 is reduced to only 96 mm Hg. The arterial O_2 saturation will be "normal" in all three cases; only in *D,* in which the end-capillary PO_2 is 81.4 mm Hg, will the arterial O_2 saturation be decreased sufficiently to be detected by ordinary laboratory methods.

During exercise, the arterial O_2 saturation may decrease below normal in *B* and *C,* because a further increase in pulmonary blood flow shortens the time that the blood spends in the pulmonary capillaries and may exaggerate the lack of equilibrium of capillary blood and alveolar gas. However, the decrease in arterial O_2 saturation during exercise is not diagnostic because such a decrease may occur during exercise in patients with many types of pulmonary disease (venous-to-arterial shunt, uneven distribution, and hypoventilation) and impairment of diffusion is only one of these.

A measurement of arterial PO_2 means little as far as the process of diffusion is concerned unless related to the simultaneously measured alveolar PO_2 (alveolar-arterial PO_2 difference). However, even then the difference between the PO_2 of alveolar gas and that of arterial blood may be due to many causes, of which impairment of diffusion is only one. The test of diffusing capacity specifically measures the diffusing properties of the alveolar-capillary bed.

When O_2 is breathed, arterial O_2 saturation and tension rise to maximal values even in patients suffering from impairment of diffusion. When the alveolar PO_2 rises from 100 to 673 mm Hg, the initial alveolar to blood O_2 gradient (at the beginning of the capillary) is increased tremendously and end-capillary blood is near equilibrium with alveolar gas despite severe impairment of diffusion. However, anoxemia caused by all types of pulmonary disease except a venous-to-arterial shunt is also corrected by O_2 therapy, so that the correction of anoxemia affords no sure diagnostic clue. On the other hand, if impairment of diffusion is associated with a venous-to-arterial shunt, inhalation of O_2 will correct the anoxemia only partially.

Carbon dioxide retention rarely, if ever, results from an impairment of diffusion unless it be in a patient kept alive by O_2 therapy. This is because CO_2 diffuses more readily than O_2 through the pulmonary membranes and particularly because the maximal PCO_2 difference between alveolar gas and mixed venous blood is small (4 to 6 mm Hg) so that a failure of CO_2 to equilibrate between alveolar gas and capillary blood can only represent an end-capillary difference of several millimeters of mercury of PCO_2. This cannot produce much CO_2 retention. Therefore, arterial CO_2 may be (1) normal, (2) low (if there is hyperventilation), or (3) high, if the impairment of diffusion is associated with emphysema or other diseases in which there is hypoventilation or marked nonuniformity of ventilation and blood flow.

Method of Choice for Measuring Diffusing Capacity.—Today the CO methods have displaced the O_2 method, because of the many advantages of the former for clinical studies. The single-breath CO is probably the most widely used at the present time. It does require expensive equipment and patient cooperation. All diffusing capacity tests demonstrate a reduction in diffusing capacity when a diffusion defect is known to be present by other criteria. The steady-state methods are more apt to yield lower values in diseases in which there is both impairment of diffusion and marked unevenness of gas distribution; for this reason they appear to be more sensitive tests than the single-breath (breath-holding) test in patients with emphysema. On the other hand, the single-breath test is more likely to represent a true measure of the characteristics of the membranes and pulmonary capillary bed of the ventilated parts of the patient's lungs. None of the methods can differentiate between impairment of diffusion due to a longer pathway for diffusion of CO and that due to a reduced surface area for diffusion; these can be distinguished only by histologic studies of tissues.

F. DIFFUSING CAPACITY IN PATIENTS WITH CARDIOPULMONARY DISEASE

Some of the diseases in which the diffusing capacity is reduced are discussed here.

Diffuse Interstitial Lung Disease

These disorders involve pathologic changes in the capillary and alveolar walls with thickening, separation by interstitial edema, fibrosis, and destruction of the capillaries themselves. The D_LCO may be markedly decreased; it is not clear whether this results entirely from changes in the permeability characteristics of the alveolar-capillary walls, from an increase their thickness, from a loss of patent capillaries, or from nonuniformity of distribution of capillary diffusing surface in the lung. The interstitial or alveolar pulmonary fibrosis seen in patients with sarcoidosis, berylliosis, asbestosis, and scleroderma falls in this category.

Chronic Obstructive Pulmonary Disease

The diffusing capacity is generally decreased, although the magnitude of the reduction is less than in many types of pulmonary fibrosis. The decreased diffusing capacity results from a destruction of pulmonary capillaries and a reduction in the total surface area and in the pulmonary capillary blood volume. The diffusing capacity is relatively normal in uncomplicated bronchial asthma. Diffusing capacity thus can serve on occasion to differentiate asthma from chronic obstructive lung disease.

Pulmonary Edema

Interstitial edema of the pulmonary membrane is probably not a significant cause of acute decrease in the diffusing capacity of the lung. However, in generalized pulmonary edema some alveoli may fill with fluid, which increases the diffusing distance from alveolar gas to the red blood cells in the capillary by several orders of magnitude. This could be considered "alveolar-capillary block." These alveoli are effectively unventilated. Other alveoli may remain completely airfilled and exchange gas relatively normally. The diffusing capacity of these alveoli (certainly the Krogh constant) will be normal, so that these air-filled alveoli may compensate for the fluid filled alveoli and lung diffusing capacity may be relatively normal.

Loss of Pulmonary Tissue

The pulmonary diffusing capacity is decreased when the total surface area of the capillaries is decreased, as in pneumonectomy or a space-taking lesion of the lung; however, the decrease actually found is generally less than might be expected, because of the great reserve of the pulmonary capillary bed and possibly because of growth of new capillaries.

Vascular Disorders

Any abnormality that occludes the arterial flow to part of the lung tends to decrease the diffusing capacity in that region. For example, congenital absence of, or embolic occlusion of, a pulmonary artery is accompanied by a decreased diffusing capacity in the region supplied. Pulmonary hypertension need not be accompanied by a reduction in diffusing capacity unless there is obliteration of part of the pulmonary *capillary* bed. Pulmonary congestion, such as that associated with mitral stenosis, may cause an increase in diffusing capacity in early stages of the disease because the pulmonary capillary bed may be enlarged; however, when deposition of fibrous tissue occurs, the diffusing capacity decreases. In conditions associated with increase in blood volume, the pulmonary capillary blood volume may also be increased, with a consequent increase in diffusing capacity.

Anemia and Polycythemia

The diffusing capacity (at least for CO) is decreased in anemia. This is most likely to result from a decrease in the hematocrit of the pulmonary capillary blood (which decreases θ_{CO}), at least in simple, uncomplicated anemia. Since the rate of CO uptake (and to a lesser extent of O_2 uptake) in the lung is dependent on the number of red cells in the capillary bed available to react with the gases, a decrease in the number of these cells will decrease D_L. There may of course be other changes in the pulmonary capillary bed; an increased cardiac output in anemia will tend to increase pulmonary capillary blood volume (V_C) and increase the number of red cells present. Polycythemia has the opposite effect.

"Stagnant blood," such as occurs in hemorrhage, may take up CO during a single breath test and give a falsely high value of D_LCO. Either of the steady-state methods, D_LO_2 or D_LCO, on the other hand, measure only the gas uptake of blood in motion.

G. SUMMARY

The exchange of gases between alveolar air and pulmonary capillary blood occurs by the passive physical process of diffusion and not by active processes of gas secretion; the work is done by the respiratory muscles (ventilation of the alveoli) and by the right ventricle (pulmonary blood flow). The process of diffusion can be measured quantitatively in man by determining the pulmonary diffusing capacity (D_L) for oxygen (O_2) or carbon monoxide (CO). The units of D_LO_2 or D_LCO are milliliters of O_2 or CO per minute for a pressure difference (mm Hg) between the O_2 or CO in alveolar gas and the interior of the red cells in the pulmonary capillary blood. The D_LO_2 or D_LCO may be decreased when (1) the alveolar and/or capillary membrane is thickened; these membranes are separated by transudate, exudate, or abnormal tissue; or the total surface area of contact between ventilated alveoli and functioning pulmonary capillaries is reduced; or (2) the total number of red blood cells exposed to alveolar gas in the pulmonary capillary bed is reduced, either by a decrease in the capillary blood volume (V_C) or in the number of red cells per milliliter of capillary blood. By measuring D_LCO at several alveolar PO_2 over 150 mm Hg, it is possible to calculate V_C and the diffusing capacity of the membrane alone, D_M.

9

Blood Oxygen, Carbon Dioxide, and pH

So far we have discussed the dynamic processes of ventilation, diffusion, and ventilation-perfusion matching. These have as their function the maintenance of normal pressures of O_2 and CO_2 in the alveolar gas and pulmonary capillary blood, i.e., the arterialization of the venous blood. For this reason it is logical to examine the *arterial* blood for its O_2 and CO_2 pressure and content to determine how adequately the lung has accomplished its primary purpose. The O_2 and CO_2 in the venous blood from any part of the body (such as the arm, leg, kidney, brain, or heart muscle) depend not only on the O_2 and CO_2 in the arterial blood, but also on the metabolism and rate of blood flow through the tissues. Consequently, venous blood O_2 depends on the adequacy of oxygen delivery in relation to tissue metabolism.

I. ARTERIAL BLOOD OXYGEN

A. THE OXYGEN-HEMOGLOBIN DISSOCIATION CURVES

Blood combines with O_2 in two ways: (1) in physical solution in the watery parts of the blood as dissolved O_2, and (2) in chemical combination with hemoglobin as HbO_2. In each case, the amount of O_2 taken up depends on the PO_2 to which the plasma or blood is exposed (see Table in Fig 65). If plasma is exposed to 10, 20, 30, 40, 50, 60, 70, 80,

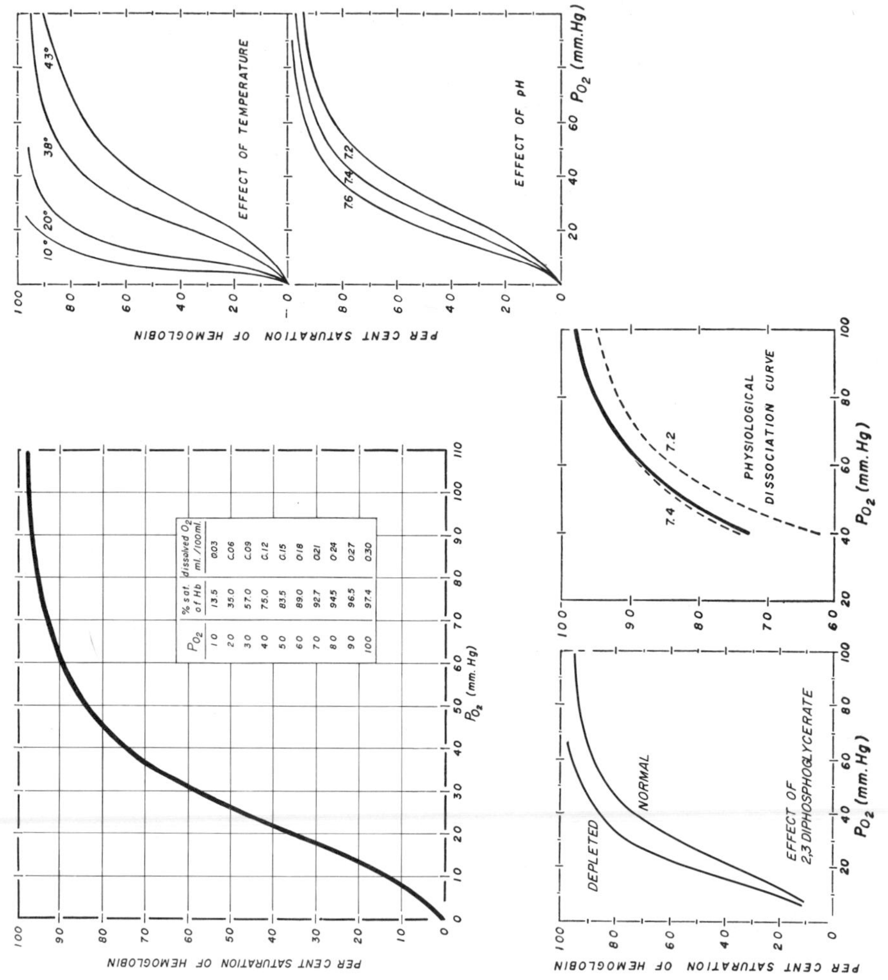

P_{O_2}	% sat. of Hb	dissolved O_2 ml. /100ml.
10	13.5	0.03
20	35.0	0.06
30	57.0	0.09
40	75.0	0.12
50	83.5	0.15
60	89.0	0.18
70	92.7	0.21
80	94.5	0.24
90	96.5	0.27
100	97.4	0.30

Fig 65.—The large graph shows a single dissociation curve, applicable when the pH of the blood is 7.4 and the temperature 37° C. The blood O_2 tension and saturation in patients with CO_2 retention, acidosis, alkalosis, fever, or hypothermia, or 2, 3-diphosphoglycerate (2, 3-DPG) will not fit this curve because the curve "shifts" to the right or left when temperature, pH, P_{CO_2}, or 2,3-DPG concentration is changed.

Effects on the O_2-hemoglobin dissociation curve of change in temperature *(upper right),* pH *(lower right),* and 2,3-DPG concentration *(bottom left)* are shown in the smaller graphs. A small change in blood pH occurs regularly in the body; e.g., when mixed venous blood passes through the pulmonary capillaries, P_{CO_2} decreases from 46 to 40 mm Hg, and pH rises from 7.37 to 7.40. During this time, blood changes from a pH 7.37 dissociation curve to a pH 7.40 curve; an approximate "physiologic" dissociation curve *(bottom center)* has been drawn to describe this change.

Practically all the 2,3-DPG in normal whole blood is removed by incubating for 12 hours at 37° C under sterile conditions.

90, and 100 mm Hg PO_2 in ten different flasks at body temperature, and the amount of O_2 in the plasma is measured in each flask after the plasma has dissolved as much O_2 as it will at each PO_2, it is found that at 10 mm Hg PO_2, 0.03 ml of O_2 is dissolved in 100 ml of plasma, at 20 mm Hg PO_2, twice this amount, and at 100 mm Hg, ten times this amount. Therefore, the amount of dissolved O_2 is directly proportional to the partial pressure (i.e., 0.003 ml O_2/100 ml blood/mm Hg PO_2 at 37° C); this is true no matter how high the O_2 pressure rises. For example, if the arterial PO_2 rose to 600 (because the patient breathed a high O_2 mixture), the dissolved O_2 would be 1.8 ml; if a subject breathed O_2 at an ambient pressure of 3 atmospheres and the arterial PO_2 was 2,000 mm Hg, the dissolved O_2 would be 6 ml O_2/100 ml blood. Only in the latter case would the *dissolved* O_2 be sufficient to supply the O_2 needed by man, and even then only for a man at rest.

Fortunately, a special protein, hemoglobin, is present in red blood cells. One gram of this substance is capable of combining chemically with 1.34 ml of O_2*; thus, if 100 ml of blood contains 15 gm of Hb, it can combine chemically with 15 × 1.34 = 20.1 ml O_2. However, the *actual* amount of O_2 combined depends on the partial pressure of O_2 in the blood.

In the case of Hb, the amount of O_2 associated is *not* linearly related to the PO_2, as it is in the case of dissolved O_2. If *whole blood* is exposed in ten different flasks to ten different O_2 pressures ranging from 10 to 100 mm Hg and the amount of O_2 combined with Hb (total O_2 minus dissolved O_2) is measured in each when equilibrium is reached, the values in Figure 65 will be found. A graph of O_2 content (or % saturation) against PO_2 is not a straight line but an S-shaped curve that has a very steep slope (between 10 and 50 mm Hg PO_2) and a very flat portion (between 70 and 100 mm Hg PO_2). The affinity of Hb for O_2 can be expressed by the P_{50} defined as the PO_2 at which Hb is 50% saturated with O_2. The P_{50} is decreased (indicating higher O_2 affinity) by lower temperature, lower $[H^+]$ (i.e., alkaline pH), and lower concentration of some organic phosphates such as 2,3-diphosphoglycerate (2,3-DPG).

*The molecular weight of hemoglobin is approximately 67,000 gm; therefore 1 mole of Hb = 67,000 gm. One mole of Hb can combine with 4 moles of O_2 because each molecule of Hb contains 4 F_E^{2+} atoms.

Four moles of O_2 occupy 4 × 22.4 L = 89.6 L STPD. Therefore, 1 gm of Hb combines with:

$$\frac{1}{67{,}000} \times 89.6 \text{ L } O_2 = 0.00134 \text{ L } O_2 = 1.34 \text{ ml } O_2.$$

The unusual shape of this HbO_2 dissociation curve† is a distinct advantage to the patient for several reasons: (1) If arterial PO_2 decreases from 100 to 80 mm Hg as the result of cardiopulmonary disease, the Hb of arterial blood will still be almost maximally saturated (94.5%) and the tissues will not suffer from hypoxia. (2) When the arterial blood passes into tissue capillaries and is exposed to the tissue tension of O_2 (about 40 mm Hg), Hb gives up large quantities of O_2 for utilization by the tissues. The shape of the dissociation curve is also of advantage for physiologic diagnosis because, by deliberately varying the position of the patient's arterial blood on this curve (by administration to the patient of low O_2, air, or high O_2 to breathe), it is possible to distinguish among hypoxia caused by impairment of diffusion, ventilation-perfusion imbalance, and "physiologic shunts."

The question is often asked, "Which is more important to normal body function—normal arterial blood PO_2 or O_2 content?" *Both* are important. The body tissues extract 4 to 5 ml of O_2 from each 100 ml of capillary blood in man at rest and much larger amounts during exercise; this can be supplied only from stores of O_2 associated with Hb. On the other hand, it is the difference in PO_2 that causes oxygen to move from alveolar gas into the pulmonary capillary blood. Similarly, in the tissues it is the difference between the PO_2 in the blood and that in the tissue cells, not the blood O_2 content, that causes oxygen to diffuse out of the capillary and into and through the tissue cells to reach the mitochondria. An adequate PO_2 is necessary for the loading of O_2 from the tissue capillaries to the cells. In vitro cellular respiration continues at very low O_2 tensions (less than 1 mm Hg intracellular PO_2), but intact man has symptoms of cerebral anoxia when the inspired PO_2 is lowered abruptly to 60 to 70 mm Hg, and an arterial PO_2 of less than 20 mm Hg is incompatible with survival.

B. METHODS OF MEASURING BLOOD O_2

Arterial O_2 Tension (Arterial PO_2)

In a blood sample, PO_2 is measured most frequently by an oxygen "electrode" immersed in it. This "electrode" consists of an electrical cell made of a thin layer of electrolyte solution bathing a platinum cathode

†The relation between oxygen bound to hemoglobin and PO_2 at equilibrium is called the oxygen-hemoglobin dissociation curve, but is also called the oxygen-hemoglobin equilibrium curve, the hemoglobin dissociation curve, or oxyhemoglobin saturation curve; the terms all mean the same thing.

(negative) and a silver anode (positive) covered by a thin water-impermeable gas-permeable plastic membrane. The electric current required to supply electrons to the cathode to reduce the molecular oxygen in the electrolyte is a measure of the rate of oxygen diffusion from the blood sample across the membrane into the electrolyte, and this in turn is proportional to the PO_2 in the blood. The PO_2 at the cathode remains close to zero. The membrane prevents cells and other blood constituents from interfering with the electrode reactions.

The measurement of O_2 tension has significant advantages over the measurement of O_2-hemoglobin saturation or O_2 content of blood in evaluating pulmonary function: (1) It is a more sensitive test when the arterial blood saturation is near-normal: Because of the shape of the hemoglobin-oxygen equilibrium curve there may be significant changes in arterial PO_2 when there are minimal or undetectable changes in arterial HbO_2 saturation. For example, when *saturation* has decreased from 97.4% to 96.5% (a barely detectable change in saturation), PO_2 has decreased from 100 to 90 mm Hg (an easily measurable change). (2) During the change from breathing air to inhalation of O_2, the saturation increases only 2.6%, whereas O_2 tension increases by 573 mm Hg.

Arterial Blood O_2 Saturation

The actual amount of O_2 in arterial blood combined with hemoglobin is usually related to the capacity of the blood hemoglobin to bind O_2. This ratio, the *% saturation* is defined by

$$\frac{\text{ml of } O_2 \text{ actually combined with Hb} \times 100}{\text{maximum ml of } O_2 \text{ capable of combining with Hb}}$$

The numerator equals the total O_2 content of the blood minus the dissolved O_2; the dissolved O_2 is normally 0.3 ml/100 ml and is often neglected. The denominator is known as the *capacity* of blood for oxygen. The arterial blood O_2 saturation expresses the ability of the lungs to raise alveolar, and thus pulmonary capillary, PO_2 and so oxygenate the mixed venous blood; O_2 content, on the other hand, varies with the amount of Hb per 100 ml of blood (is less in anemia and greater in polycythemia) as well as with the oxygenating function of the lung. Arterial blood O_2 content is generally estimated from measurement of PO_2, blood hemoglobin concentration and reference to a standard O_2 Hb dissociation curve with corrections for temperature and pH. This estimate may be in error if the affinity of Hb for O_2 is abnormal.

There are several ways of actually measuring, as contrasted with calculating, the saturation of arterial blood with O_2. In the manometric method of Van Slyke and Neil, O_2 content (O_2 combined with Hb plus dissolved O_2) of arterial blood is measured; part of the blood is then exposed to atmospheric O_2 (air) so that its hemoglobin combines fully with O_2 and the capacity is measured. Saturation is calculated after corrections are made for dissolved O_2. The method can be very accurate but is too laborious for general use.

The spectrophotometric method measures the ratio of reduced† or oxyhemoglobin to total hemoglobin. Changes in absorption coefficients due to the presence of other pigments in blood limit the accuracy of this approach.

The ear oximetric method uses a filter photometer that passes white light through the ear and compares transmission at two colors that are determined by two filters. Arterial O_2 saturation can be estimated continuously and without withdrawing arterial blood. Although less accurate than other methods for measuring absolute values, it has usefulness in measuring changes in saturation (e.g., rate of increase during inhalation of O_2, or change during exercise or hyperventilation) and in comparing the effectiveness of measures designed to increase arterial O_2 saturation.

C. ALVEOLAR-ARTERIAL Po_2 GRADIENT

The Po_2 and saturation of arterial blood may be normal even though there is definite pulmonary disease (uneven distribution or impaired diffusion). This is because hyperventilation can raise alveolar Po_2 well above usual values and bring arterial Po_2 to normal. However, in this situation there will be a large alveolar-arterial Po_2 difference. The method for estimating alveolar Po_2 is presented in chapter 3. The required measurements are inspired Po_2, arterial Pco_2, and respiratory exchange ratio. The alveolar-arterial O_2 gradient in normal young subjects breathing air is 5 to 10 mm Hg, is higher in normal older people, and normally widens with an increase in inspired O_2 because of the normal degree of unevenness of ventilation/blood flow (see Fig 54). Conversely, arterial Po_2 can be decreased in the absence of lung disease if the alveolar Po_2 is low (see Fig 62) (e.g., breathing air at altitude or breathing gases with a low percentage of O_2). In this situation, the al-

†It is better to say "unoxygenated" since the iron in both unoxygenated and oxygen hemoglobin is reduced, that is, has a charge of $2.^+$ When the iron is oxidized to $3,^+$ hemoglobin becomes methemoglobin.

veolar-arterial O_2 difference is normal. Therefore, the alveolar-arterial O_2 gradient is useful to diagnose the presence of abnormal gas exchange in the lung. Clinically, the measurement is useful to indicate changes in lung gas exchange function in seriously ill patients maintained on enriched O_2 mixtures. In these patients, changes in the arterial blood O_2 can be misleading.

D. CAUSES OF HYPOXEMIA

Hypoxia is a general term referring to a decrease in O_2 content or tension. *Hypoxemia* refers specifically to a decrease in the amount of O_2 in blood. There are many causes of hypoxemia, and some of these occur even though pulmonary function is completely normal.

1. A decrease in inspired P_{O_2}, either because of decreased barometric pressure breathing air (as at altitude) or decreased concentration of oxygen in inspired gas at sea level pressure, will produce hypoxemia.

2. Any type of alveolar hypoventilation, whether due to central respiratory depression or neuromuscular disorder in a patient with normal lungs or due to airway obstruction or rigid lungs or pleura, must decrease alveolar P_{O_2}, decrease arterial P_{O_2}, and decrease arterial O_2 saturation.

3. When there is *uneven distribution* of alveolar ventilation and blood flow there must be a decrease in arterial blood P_{O_2} relative to mean alveolar P_{O_2}. Unless total alveolar ventilation is increased, this must result in arterial hypoxemia (p. 178). However, the patient may increase his total alveolar ventilation enough so that even previously poorly ventilated regions of his lungs receive enough O_2 to arterialize the blood flowing through alveolar capillaries there. It is not proper to say that such lungs are functioning normally simply because the patient's arterial O_2 saturation is normal; in order to maintain a normal P_{O_2} in some alveoli, he must be hyperventilating others and forcing his respiratory muscles to expend more than the usual amount of energy.

Intrapulmonary arterial-to-venous shunts or intracardiac right-to-left shunts represent special types of uneven ventilation in relation to blood flow in which ventilation/blood flow is zero. Because some mixed venous blood bypasses ventilated alveoli, both the P_{O_2} and the saturation of arterial blood must be reduced below normal.

4. When there is *impairment of diffusion,* arterial Po_2 must be lower relative to alveolar Po_2; but, as emphasized earlier (p. 209), the difference may be insignificant in a resting patient. Many patients who have a significant decrease in pulmonary diffusing capacity for CO still have normal arterial O_2 saturation; in many cases, this may be achieved by the hyperventilation characteristic of this dysfunction, and arterial O_2 saturation may fall during exercise.

E. DIFFERENTIAL DIAGNOSIS OF HYPOXEMIA CAUSED BY RESPIRATORY OR CARDIOPULMONARY DISEASE

Hypoventilation

This is defined as a decrease in alveolar ventilation per minute in relation to the O_2 consumption of the patient (see Fig 14 and p. 44). It must be associated with a decrease in calculated alveolar ventilation (Figs 7, p. 28; 8, p. 30; and 13, p. 40) or an increase in O_2 consumption. Alveolar gas and arterial blood Po_2 must be decreased and arterial Pco_2 must be increased, but the alveolar-arterial O_2 gradient is normal. All of the effects of hypoventilation are corrected by providing a normal volume of ventilation with air. Inhalation of O_2, with continued hypoventilation, will correct the hypoxemia but not the CO_2 retention (hypercapnea).

Uneven Ventilation in Relation to Blood Flow

This always results in an arterial blood Po_2 that is less than mean alveolar Po_2. When alveolar ventilation is normal, arterial blood Po_2 and saturation must be decreased and Pco_2 must rise. When total ventilation increases, arterial blood Po_2 and saturation may be maintained at normal levels; if the disease is severe, hyperventilation cannot prevent arterial Po_2 and HbO_2 saturation from falling and Pco_2 from rising. Inhalation of O_2 will wash out N_2 even from poorly ventilated alveoli and establish a high alveolar gas Po_2, which results in high arterial blood Po_2 and full saturation of Hb; it will also abolish the alveolar-arterial Po_2 difference due to uneven ventilation/blood flow ratios (see Fig 54), thus differentiating that from a shunt of venous-to-arterial blood. Inhalation of O_2 and relief of hypoxemia may, however, remove peripheral chemoreceptor stimulation to respiration and cause hypoventilation, CO_2 retention, and respiratory acidosis (see p. 128).

Impairment of Diffusion

This may not necessarily result in arterial hypoxemia (see Fig 61), either because of the reserve in the oxygenating mechanism or because of hyperventilation from other causes than decreased arterial P_{O_2}. Hypoxemia may be produced or be worsened when the patient exercises, because the velocity of pulmonary capillary blood flow increases and shortens the time that the blood remains in contact with the diffusing surface. The alveolar-arterial P_{O_2} difference increases when the patient breathes 12% to 14% O_2 (see Fig 62). Hypoxemia, if present, is corrected by inhalation of O_2, which also abolishes any alveolar-arterial P_{O_2} difference due to impairment of diffusion. The very high initial gradient for P_{O_2} diffusion (alveolar gas > 600 mm Hg; mixed venous blood = 40 mm Hg) rapidly saturates Hb, and the capillary blood then comes into tension equilibrium rapidly with alveolar gas. (Oxygen behaves like an inert gas once Hb is fully saturated.)

Since CO_2 diffuses more rapidly than O_2 through the alveolar capillary membranes, hypercapnea does not occur, with the possible exception of a patient with very serious impairment of diffusion kept alive only by breathing 100% O_2. As a rule, blood P_{CO_2} is low, because either the anoxemia or a reflex owing to the disease process in the lungs causes hyperventilation.

Shunts

With shunting of mixed venous blood into the systemic circulation, the systemic arterial blood P_{O_2} and saturation must be low even if the patient is hyperventilating. Inhalation of O_2 cannot oxygenate the blood fully (p. 178). If the shunt is large, inhalation of O_2 may increase systemic arterial O_2 saturation 8% to 10% (e.g., from 70% to 80%). If the shunt is small, inhalation of O_2 may result in 100% saturation of arterial blood (e.g., from 93% to 100%) but the alveolar-arterial P_{O_2} difference increases and the arterial dissolved O_2 or arterial P_{O_2} will not reach maximal values (2.0 ml/100 ml blood and 600 mm Hg, respectively). This is the only type of hypoxemia in which inhalation of O_2 will not eventually increase arterial blood P_{O_2} to 600 mm Hg.

Exercise usually results in a further decrease in arterial blood P_{O_2} and saturation because the shunted venous blood contains less O_2. Inhalation of 12% to 14% O_2 almost eliminates the alveolar-arterial P_{O_2} difference, because of the shape of the O_2 dissociation curve (see Fig 65).

Carbon dioxide tension in the arterial blood may be elevated if the shunt is very large. However, if the lungs are normal and capable of increased ventilation, arterial P_{CO_2} may remain normal. If hypoxemia is severe and results in hyperventilation, arterial P_{CO_2} may be below normal. Severe hypoxemia often causes metabolic acidosis, hyperventilation, and decreased arterial P_{CO_2} on that account.

Combinations of the four types of hypoxemia may occur in the same individual. A patient under anesthesia may have both hypoventilation and uneven ventilation in relation to blood flow. A patient with an open hemithorax may have hypoventilation, uneven ventilation in relation to blood flow, and venous-to-arterial shunts. The physiologic effect of an intracardiac right-to-left shunt is the same as an intrapulmonary shunt.

It must be emphasized that hypoxemia is not always present, even in serious pulmonary disease. When diseased areas of the lungs receive no blood supply (as in some patients with carcinoma, cysts, or tuberculous lesions), arterial O_2 saturation remains normal as long as there is sufficient normal pulmonary tissue; even after pneumonectomy, arterial O_2 saturation can be normal, at least in a resting patient, if the remaining lung is healthy.

F. OXYGEN DELIVERY TO TISSUES

The arterial blood provides O_2 to the tissues to meet their metabolic requirements. However, the arterial P_{O_2} (or saturation) is not the only factor in determining adequacy of tissue oxygenation. The O_2 provided by the arterial blood to each organ (i.e., the O_2 delivery) is the product of the O_2 content of the arterial blood and the organ blood flow. The oxygen extraction by the tissue is the product of the difference in O_2 content between arterial and venous blood perfusing the organ and the organ blood flow. Thus, tissue hypoxia can be caused by either a decrease in the arterial O_2 content or a decrease in blood flow and is made more severe if tissue metabolic rate is high, as in fever. Conversely, an increase in blood flow can compensate for decreased arterial O_2 content and maintain normal O_2 delivery. Consequently, the measurement of arterial P_{O_2} or of O_2 saturation alone does not provide information regarding the P_{O_2} of any particular tissue.

The adequacy of O_2 delivery is reflected in the tissue P_{O_2}, which is determined by the balance between O_2 delivery and O_2 utilization. Tissue P_{O_2} may be estimated by the use of special tissue oxygen electrodes. However, there is no *one* normal value for tissue P_{O_2} since this may vary considerably with different organs as well as within a single organ, reflecting the varying metabolic activity of different cells and differences in diffusion distance from the O_2 source, that is, the blood in the nearest capillary. With measurements of tissue PO_2 at multiple sites using electrodes, a composite picture of PO_2 distribution can be obtained. This approach is not feasible at present for routine clinical use.

Alternatively, organ PO_2 can be estimated from measurements of the PO_2 of venous blood coming from an organ. This measurement indicates a mean value for the organ but cannot indicate whether all cells of the tissue are exposed to this PO_2 or are utilizing O_2.

The normal value for mixed venous blood (i.e., pulmonary artery, reflecting the entire venous return) is about 40 mm Hg. The PO_2 of coronary sinus blood is normally about 20 mm Hg, reflecting a high metabolic rate relative to blood flow in the normal myocardium. PO_2 in the renal vein is about 70 mm Hg, reflecting the high blood flow relative to metabolic rate. Decreased O_2 delivery to tissue with tissue hypoxia can occur with any of the causes of O_2 desaturation of arterial blood. However, there are many important causes of tissue hypoxia that are not reflected in the arterial PO_2.

Hypoxemia could also occur because of a shift in the dissociation curve of Hb, so that less O_2 combines with Hb at a given PO_2 ("shift of the curve to the right"). This occurs when the blood PCO_2 is high, the pH is low, or the blood temperature is increased (see Fig 65). Similar "shifts to the right" have been reported in natives living at high altitudes and in children 2 to 20 years of age. 2,3-Diphosphoglycerate, which is found in high concentration in the erythrocyte, also causes a shift to the right. An increase in this compound is found in many clinical conditions associated with hypoxia. A "shift to the left" (greater affinity of O_2 for Hb) occurs in the fetus because of the existence of a special fetal hemoglobin.

Tissue hypoxia may also occur despite normal rates of O_2 delivery. Tissue edema (by causing impaired capillary-tissue diffusion), or abnormally high O_2 requirements, or poisoning of cellular enzymes can lead to tissue anoxia in the absence of anoxemia. These manifestations can be detected through measurements of cell metabolic parameters such as nicotinamide adenine dinucleotide (NADH) redox state, adenosine triphosphate (ATP) concentration, or altered metabolic pathways. For example, cell hypoxia results in a shift in the normal ratio between production of lactate and of pyruvate. The increased lactate production with hypoxia represents a decreased rate of NADH oxidation by the mitochondria. Because lactate and pyruvate are transported out of the cells, their ratio in the extracellular fluid or blood has been used to estimate tissue oxygenation. Unfortunately, many alterations of tissue metabolism (e.g., increase in glycolysis) also alter the lactate-to-pyruvate ratio so that this test is not specific for hypoxia. While measurements of cellular metabolism may in the future be useful for measuring tissue oxygenation in clinical situations, they presently have limited applicability.

II. ARTERIAL CARBON DIOXIDE AND pH

Inspired air contains insignificant amounts (0.04%) of CO_2. Unless CO_2 has been added to inspired gas, the CO_2 of venous blood, alveolar gas, and arterial blood originates in tissue metabolism. Carbon dioxide diffuses from tissue cells into the capillary blood and is carried in chemical combination and in physical solution in the venous blood to the lungs, where a part of it diffuses into alveolar gas and is eliminated in the expired gas.

A. CO_2 TRANSPORT

The loading, transport, and unloading of CO_2 are described in detail in several books and articles listed in the references. Stated briefly, the processes involved in loading and transport are as follows:

1. *Diffusion of CO_2 from tissue cells into capillary blood.*—In actively metabolizing cells, tissue P_{CO_2} is greater than the P_{CO_2} of arterial blood flowing through systemic capillaries. Carbon dioxide therefore diffuses from the cells into the plasma.

2. *Chemical reactions in the plasma.*—*(a)* Some CO_2 dissolves in the plasma. A very small amount of this reacts slowly with water to form carbonic acid ($H_2O + CO_2 \rightleftharpoons H_2CO_3$). This H_2CO_3 dissociates into $H^+ + HCO_3^-$ and the H^+ is buffered by plasma buffering systems.

(b) Dissolved CO_2 in plasma reacts with amino groups of plasma proteins to form carbamino compounds.

3. *Chemical reactions within the erythrocyte.*—Most of the CO_2 that diffuses from tissue cells into the plasma passes into the erythrocytes. Intra-erythrocytic CO_2 reacts in three ways:

(a) Some remains within the red blood cell as dissolved CO_2.

(b) Some combines with the NH_2 groups of Hb to form carbamino compounds.

$$R - NH_2 + CO_2 \rightleftharpoons R - NHCOO^- + H^+$$

This is a very rapid chemical reaction that requires no special catalyst. The H^+ is buffered by portions of the Hb molecule (isohydric reaction). This process is facilitated by the simultaneous loss of O_2 from capillary blood to the tissues ($HbO_2 \rightleftharpoons Hb + O_2$) because the conversion of oxyhemoglobin to reduced Hb causes Hb to become a weaker acid and to take up additional H^+ with little change in pH.

(c) Some CO_2 combines with water to form H_2CO_3, which then dissociates to form H^+ and HCO_3^- ions. The conversion of CO_2 and H_2O into H_2CO_3 is a very rapid reaction only because of the presence of an enzyme, carbonic anhydrase. Carbonic anhydrase is concentrated within the erythrocyte, and this reaction (the hydration of CO_2) is an important and rapid one within red blood cells.

This reaction results in the formation of H^+ ions which are also buffered by chemical groups of the Hb molecule with minimal change in pH (isohydric reaction); like the reaction in 3*(b)*, this is aided by simultaneous conversion of some HbO_2 to Hb as O_2 passes into the tissues.

This reaction also results in the accumulation of a high level of HCO_3^- ions within the red blood cell. Bicarbonate ions then diffuse into the plasma to reestablish equilibrium of HCO_3^- between cells and plasma. If this diffusion of anions were accompanied by diffusion of an equal number of cations, electrical neutrality of the erythrocyte would be maintained. However, the red cell membrane is not freely permeable to cations and so anions from the plasma (Cl^-) diffuse into the erythrocyte (chloride shift) to achieve electrical neutrality. Some movement of water inward occurs simultaneously to maintain osmotic equilibrium; this results in a slight swelling of erythrocytes in venous blood, relative to those in arterial blood.

The reverse of the foregoing reactions occurs in the pulmonary capillaries when O_2 is added and CO_2 is unloaded.

Several points are of especial interest:

1. Although plasma contains much more CO_2 (in all forms) than do the red blood cells (in all forms), and although the plasma *transports* more than 60% of CO_2 added to capillary blood, the chemical reactions within the red blood cell provide practically all of the additional bicarbonate ions transported in the plasma. If the enzyme carbonic anhydrase is completely inhibited, the reaction $CO_2 + H_2O \rightleftharpoons H_2CO_3$ proceeds slowly and is not complete in the systemic capillary or even in the

time that the blood flows through the veins en route to the heart. The reverse reaction, $H_2CO_2 \rightleftharpoons CO_2 + H_2O$, which normally occurs during the time that venous blood is in the pulmonary capillaries, is also slow in the absence of carbonic anhydrase and continues long after the blood has left the pulmonary capillaries and entered the systemic circulation. Therefore, after inhibition of carbonic anhydrase (as by administration of large doses of acetazolamide), the CO_2 that enters the blood in the tissue does not react with the buffer systems immediately. It continues to form HCO_3^- after the blood has left the capillary bed so that the P_{CO_2} decreases in venous blood until it reaches the pulmonary capillaries. Here the dissolved CO_2 can diffuse into alveolar gas, but blood HCO_3 cannot dehydrate fast enough to maintain the P_{CO_2}. Thus, P_{CO_2} rises as blood flows through the systemic arteries, and the *unloading* reaction goes slowly to completion. The overall result is a rise in tissue P_{CO_2}.

2. Carbon dioxide loading and O_2 unloading in body tissue capillaries are mutually helpful; an increase in capillary blood P_{CO_2} (and decrease in pH) facilitates the unloading of O_2 (the Bohr effect), and the unloading of O_2 (change from HbO_2 to Hb) facilitates the loading of CO_2 (the Haldane effect). This is pictured in Figures 65 and 66.

3. Just as the amount of O_2 carried by the blood is related to the P_{O_2} to which blood is exposed, so the amount of CO_2 in blood is related to the P_{CO_2} of the blood. The CO_2 dissociation curve is pictured in Figure 66. Note that in the physiologic range of CO_2, say between 30 and 50 mm Hg tension, the relationship between the two is almost linear, whereas the O_2 dissociation curve is S-shaped.

B. METHODS FOR MEASURING CO_2 AND pH

Carbon Dioxide Partial Pressure (P_{CO_2})

This is the most useful blood CO_2 measurement for the pulmonary physiologist. The methods used to measure P_{CO_2} have varied with the instruments and techniques available and with practical considerations, but all are based on the relationships among pH, HCO_3^-, and CO_2 expressed in the Henderson-Hasselbalch equation below.

$$pH = pK + \log \frac{[HCO_3^-]}{[CO_2]}$$

P_{CO_2} can be calculated from independent measurements of plasma pH and HCO_3^-. However, this is easier said than done. It is obvious

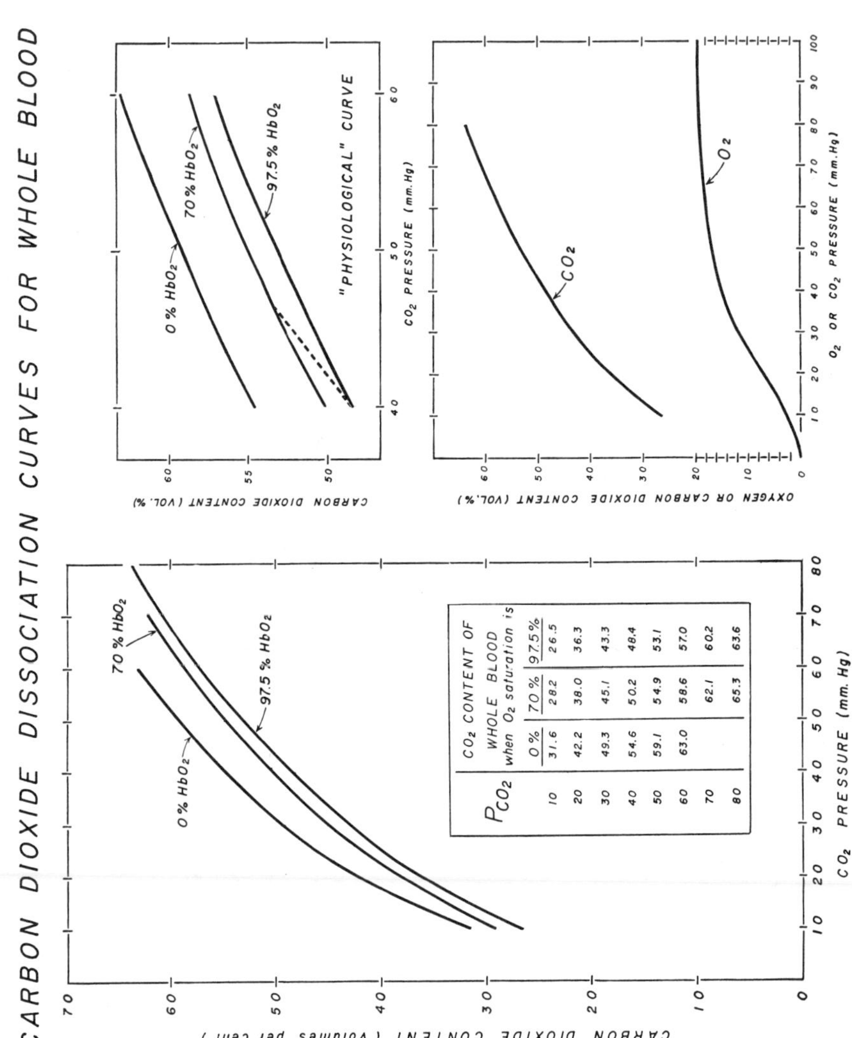

P_{CO_2}	CO_2 CONTENT OF WHOLE BLOOD when O_2 saturation is		
	0 %	70 %	97.5%
10	31.6	28.2	26.5
20	42.2	38.0	36.3
30	49.3	45.1	43.3
40	54.6	50.2	48.4
50	59.1	54.9	53.1
60	63.0	58.6	57.0
70		62.1	60.2
80		65.3	63.6

Fig 66.—The large graph shows relationship between P_{CO_2} and CO_2 content of whole blood; this varies with changes in saturation of hemoglobin with O_2. Thus, CO_2 tension of the blood influences oxygen saturation ("Bohr effect"), and oxygen saturation of the blood influences CO_2 content ("Haldane effect"). The O_2-CO_2 diagram (Fig 71), by combining much of Figures 65 and 66 into one, gives the correct figure for both CO_2 and O_2 at every P_{O_2} and P_{CO_2}.

Above right, greatly magnified portion of the large graph to show the change that occurs as mixed venous blood (70% HbO_2, P_{CO_2} 46 mm Hg) passes through the pulmonary capillaries and becomes arterial blood (97.5% HbO_2, P_{CO_2} 40 mm Hg). Dashed line is a hypothetical transition between the two curves. *Below right,* O_2 and CO_2 dissociation curves plotted on same scale to show the important point that the O_2 curve has a very steep and a very flat portion and the CO_2 curve does not.

from the previous section that the CO_2 content of whole blood, of plasma, and of red blood cells will be different (Table 12). Red blood cells can be separated from plasma by centrifugation, but this must be done in the cold (to slow down chemical reactions that continue in the blood sample) and anaerobically (so that CO_2 and oxygen are not exchanged with the air). This is a tedious, complicated technique that is little used.

Arterial CO_2 content can be measured in whole blood (handled under anaerobic conditions), as part of the determination of arterial blood O_2 content using a gas analysis apparatus (Van Slyke manometric) and plasma $[HCO_3^-]$ calculated from published data. Knowing the proportion of cells to plasma (hematocrit), one can determine the *plasma CO_2 content* from a nomogram. Then, if the pH of whole blood, which is the same as that of plasma, is measured with a glass electrode, P_{CO_2} can be calculated by application of the Henderson-Hasselbalch equation, which requires knowledge of plasma pH, $[HCO_3^-]$, and $[CO_2]$ separately. The laboratory measurement provides a value for *total* CO_2 (or $[HCO_3^-] + [CO_2] + [H_2CO_3]$).The problem is resolved by substituting in the numerator "[total CO_2] − $[CO_2]$" (which = $[HCO_3^-]$). Then

$$pH = pK + \log \frac{[\text{total } CO_2] - [CO_2]}{[CO_2]}$$

TABLE 12.—MEAN VALUES FOR BLOOD O_2, CO_2, AND PH IN HEALTHY YOUNG MEN

	ARTERIAL BLOOD	MIXED VENOUS BLOOD
O_2 pressure (mm Hg)	95	40
Dissolved O_2 (ml O_2/100 ml W.B.*)	0.29	0.12
O_2 content (ml O_2/100 ml W.B.)	20.3	15.5
O_2 combined with Hb (ml O_2/100 ml W.B.)	20.0	15.4
O_2 capacity of Hb (ml O_2/100 ml W.B.)	20.6	20.6
% Saturation of Hb with O_2	97.1	75.0
Total CO_2 (ml CO_2/100 ml W.B.)	49.0	53.1
Plasma CO_2 content (ml CO_2/100 ml plasma)	59.6	63.8
Dissolved CO_2 (ml CO_2/100 ml)	2.84	3.2
Combined CO_2 (ml CO_2/100 ml)	56.8	60.5
(mm)	25.4	27.0
Combined CO_2/dissolved CO_2	20/1	18.9/1
CO_2 pressure (mm Hg)	41	46.5
Plasma pH	7.40	7.376

Modified from Albritton E.C. (ed.): *Standard Values in Blood.* Philadelphia, W.B. Saunders Co., 1952.

*W.B. indicates whole blood.

Since $[CO_2]$ = the partial pressure of CO_2 times the solubility coefficient, the equation becomes

$$pH = pK + \log \frac{\text{total } CO_2 - \alpha \, P_{CO_2}}{\alpha \, P_{CO_2}}$$

The pK for the bicarbonate/CO_2 buffer system = 6.1, and α = 0.0301 mM/mm Hg. Knowing pH and total plasma CO_2, plasma P_{CO_2} can be calculated.

However, the most widely used and convenient method to determine blood arterial blood P_{CO_2} is the CO_2 electrode. This consists of a glass pH electrode covered by a very thin layer of bicarbonate solution and then a membrane, freely permeable to CO_2, but impermeable to water and electrolytes. A reference electrode, usually Ag/AgCl, is also immersed in the bicarbonate electrolyte, which is continuous with the fluid layer covering the pH-sensitive glass surface. When this assembly is immersed in a blood sample, carbon dioxide diffuses through the membrane and forms un-ionized carbonic acid, H_2CO_3, in the watery film; the H_2CO_3 dissociates into H^+ and HCO_3^- ions, and the former are measured by the glass electrode. The relation between pH and P_{CO_2} is described by another slightly different form of the Henderson-Hasselbalch equation.

$$pH = pK + \log \frac{[HCO_3^-]}{\alpha[P_{CO_2}]}$$

The concentration of cation, sodium, and potassium, that balances the HCO_3^- is constant as none can enter or leave the layer of electrolyte. Thus, log P_{CO_2} is linearly related to the measured pH. Rather than actually determine the $[HCO_3^-]$, it is more convenient to calibrate the electrode with solutions of known P_{CO_2}.

Alveolar Gas P_{CO_2}

Alveolar gas P_{CO_2} can be measured in spot samples or continuously by infrared or mass spectrometric analysis. Because gas and blood P_{CO_2} are assumed to be equal across the membranes of any single alveolus, end-tidal P_{CO_2} approximates arterial blood P_{CO_2}. This estimate is probably accurate in individuals with normal lungs, but may be seriously in error when the patient has a large pulmonary arterial-to-venous shunt, pulmonary vascular occlusion, serious maldistribution of blood and gas, and/or rapid and shallow breathing, or has received large doses of carbonic anhydrase inhibitor (acetazolamide). If end-expired P_{CO_2} exceeds 50 mm Hg, it is reasonably certain that arterial blood P_{CO_2} is greater than normal.

Mixed venous blood P_{CO_2} is about 6 mm Hg greater than arterial blood P_{CO_2} and therefore can be used as an approximate measure of the arterial value. It can be estimated by having the patient rebreathe from a bag containing a CO_2 concentration greater than mixed venous P_{CO_2} and containing oxygen to prevent hypoxia. The expired CO_2 is measured at the mouth with a rapidly recording analyzer until a plateau is reached (Fig 67). At this point the P_{CO_2} of the gas inspired from the bag should equal that of oxygenated mixed venous P_{CO_2}, and the arterial value can be obtained by subtracting 6 mm Hg. This approximate method of measuring mixed venous P_{CO_2} requires no arterial sample or cardial catheterization, but does require patient cooperation and has been largely superseded by measurement of arterial samples.

C. SIGNIFICANCE OF CHANGES IN ARTERIAL BLOOD P_{CO_2}

Increase in Arterial Blood P_{CO_2}

This must mean either that the whole lung or a major portion of it is hypoventilated (see Table 3, p. 46). Arterial P_{CO_2} is never increased by pure impairment of diffusion. It may be increased slightly by a venous-

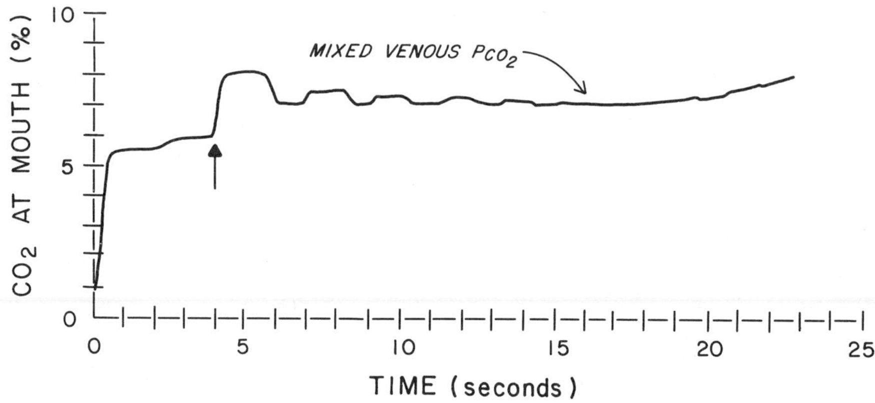

Fig 67.—Rebreathing estimation of mixed venous P_{CO_2}. Continuous record of CO_2 concentration at the mouth as the patient inspires from a rebreathing bag containing 8% CO_2 and 92% O_2. At time 0 the mouthpiece is being attached; the first inspiration from the bag takes place at the first arrow at 4 seconds. The CO_2 concentration of the gas in the bag appears to equilibrate with mixed venous blood at about 7% CO_2 (*second arrow),* corresponding to a P_{CO_2} of 51 mm Hg.

This value for mixed venous P_{CO_2} is higher than the in-vivo value because the blood is oxygenated, while true mixed venous blood is not. Oxygenation will release oxylabile protons and hemoglobin carbamate will dissociate, forming additional CO_2.

to-arterial shunt, though as a rule hyperventilation reduces the P_{CO_2} in the alveolar capillary blood sufficiently to compensate for the higher P_{CO_2} in shunted blood. When there is uneven distribution of gas in relation to blood, arterial P_{CO_2} will rise if alveolar ventilation is decreased or normal; it will also rise when total alveolar ventilation is increased if the major portion of the alveolar ventilation is going to regions with little pulmonary capillary blood flow.

Whenever there is pulmonary insufficiency for CO_2, there must be pulmonary insufficiency for O_2 as well, unless high concentrations of O_2 are breathed.

Decrease in Arterial Blood P_{CO_2}

This occurs whenever all or a major portion of the lungs is being hyperventilated (see p. 46).

Arterial blood P_{CO_2} may be normal or even low in patients with uneven distribution of alveolar ventilation/blood flow ratio. The shapes of O_2 and CO_2 dissociation curves (see Figs 14, p. 45; 65, p. 224; and 66, p. 238) are such that a hyperventilated area can compensate or more than compensate for a poorly ventilated region with respect to CO_2 but not to O_2. For example, in patients with emphysema, a region with a low ventilation/blood flow ratio tends to cause anoxemia and CO_2 retention (Fig 14, *left*), but an area with a high ventilation/blood flow ratio can contribute little additional O_2 to the blood though it can "blow off" enough CO_2 to keep arterial P_{CO_2} normal or low (Fig 14, *right*).

Normal Arterial Blood P_{CO_2}

This does not exclude pulmonary disease. Patients with a major reduction in functioning pulmonary tissue (pneumonectomy, pulmonary embolism) or other types of disease (pulmonary vascular disease, impairment of diffusion) may have normal arterial blood P_{CO_2} if their alveolar ventilation matches the metabolic rate of the body. It is possible to have severe pulmonary disability, because of mechanical difficulties in breathing, without having an elevated P_{CO_2}; in fact, the increased work of breathing which keeps arterial blood P_{CO_2} normal may be responsible for the dyspnea and disability.

D. CARBON DIOXIDE, pH AND ACID-BASE BALANCE

The elimination of CO_2 is of great importance in the regulation of acid base balance because $CO_2 + H_2O \rightleftharpoons H_2CO_3$, or carbonic acid. Since several excellent monographs discuss the subject of acid-base balance in great detail, only a few important points will be discussed here.

1. The lungs are quantitatively the most important organ in the body for acid excretion. In ordinary circumstances, the kidney excretes 40 to 80 mEq/day (of *fixed* acids), whereas the lungs excrete about 13,000 mEq of CO_2, representing an equivalent amount of carbonic acid in a resting subject and two to three times as much with normal rates of activity.*

2. In a strict chemical sense the HCO_3^-/CO_2 system is a poor buffer in blood. It is important physiologically in maintaining the normal pH of the blood, because the CO_2 concentration is maintained constant by the lungs; in order to do this, the lungs vary their instantaneous elimination of CO_2. At the same time, the kidneys regulate the concentration of HCO_3^- (or rather, the cation available to balance the HCO_3^-).

The Henderson-Hasselbalch equation states that it is the *ratio* of HCO_3/CO_2 that determines blood pH, rather than the absolute amounts of each.

$$\mathrm{pH} = \mathrm{pK} + \log \frac{[\mathrm{HCO_3}]}{[\mathrm{CO_2}]\dagger} \qquad (1)$$

The pK for this system is 6.1. Values for HCO_3^- and CO_2 are given in Table 12. Substituting in equation (1):

$$\mathrm{pH} = 6.1 + \log \frac{56.8 \text{ vol\% } \mathrm{CO_2}}{2.84 \text{ vol\% } \mathrm{CO_2}} \text{ or } \frac{25.4\mathrm{mM\ CO_2}}{1.27\mathrm{mM\ CO_2}} \qquad (2)$$

*Concentrations of carbonic acid and bicarbonate are sometimes measured clinically as volumes percent of CO_2. It is important in an analysis of acid-base balance to convert volumes percent of CO_2 into mM or mEq/L, since that is how ions such as sodium and chloride are expressed. Dividing volumes percent of CO_2 by 2.23 converts the concentration to millimolar or milliequivalents per liter. Thus,

$$\frac{59.6 \text{ vol\%}}{2.23} = 26.6\mathrm{mM}$$

The factor 2.23 is obtained as follows:

1 mole (1 gm molecular weight) of CO_2 occupies 22.3 L or 22,300 ml at one atmosphere and 0° C (273° K), standard temperature and pressure dry (STPD);
1 mmole (1/1,000 gm molecular weight) of CO_2 occupies 22.3 ml;
1 mmole of CO_2/L of blood = 22.3 ml of gas/L of blood
= 2.23 ml of gas/100 ml of blood
Therefore, 1 mmole/L (= 1mM) = 2.23 volumes percent

†The denominator $[CO_2]$ is sometimes written as $[H_2CO_3]$. Actually, both dissolved CO_2 and H_2CO_3 are present, since $CO_2 + H_2O \rightleftharpoons H_2CO_3$, but at equilibrium the concentration of dissolved CO_2 in the plasma is almost 1,000 times that of H_2CO_3.

In either case,

$$\begin{aligned} pH &= 6.1 + \log 20 \\ &= 6.1 + 1.30 \\ &= 7.40 \end{aligned}$$

The pH would still be 7.40 if both $[HCO_3^-]$ and $[CO_2]$ doubled (113.6/5.68), or were halved (28.4/1.42), since the ratio remains 20/1

3. Normally, this ratio is maintained by pulmonary ventilation which keeps arterial P_{CO_2} at 41 mm Hg at sea level (equivalent to a dissolved CO_2 of 2.84 vol%).‡ Whenever arterial P_{CO_2} tends to rise, the medullary respiratory center is stimulated, alveolar ventilation is increased and the P_{CO_2} is restored to normal. This delicate mechanism operates only when the sensitivity of the respiratory center is normal, the nervous connections between the center and the respiratory muscles are intact, the respiratory muscles are normal and the lung is not seriously diseased. Whenever hypoventilation occurs (see Table 3, p. 46), either because of depression of the neuromuscular mechanisms or because of mechanical limitations, CO_2 must accumulate in the blood. The very first change is in the dissolved CO_2 or $[CO_2]$. If arterial P_{CO_2} rises to 51 mm Hg, the $[CO_2]$ increases to 1.6mM and equation (1) becomes:

$$\begin{aligned} pH &= 6.1 + \log \frac{25.4\text{mM } CO_2}{1.6\text{mM } CO_2} \\ &= 6.1 + \log 16 \qquad (3) \\ &= 6.1 + 1.20 = 7.30 \end{aligned}$$

According to equation (3), the total increase in CO_2 is 0.3 mM, all of which is due to the increase in $[CO_2]$. However, Figure 66 shows that an increase of 10 mm Hg P_{CO_2} leads to a much greater increase in total blood CO_2 than 0.3 mM. The additional CO_2 represents an increment in $[HCO_3^-]$. What is the origin if this increase in $[HCO_3^-]$? When hypoventilation occurs and blood P_{CO_2} rises, the increase in $[CO_2]$ drives the reaction to the right:

$$CO_2 + H_2O \rightleftharpoons H_2CO_3 \rightleftharpoons H^+ + HCO_3^-$$

Some of the increment of H^+ ion is neutralized by blood buffers (especially by Hb protein) with an increase in $[HCO_3^-]$. The H^+ ions not neutralized cause a decrease in blood pH. In the case mentioned, the increase in the $[HCO_3^-]$ of the *numerator* occurs almost simulta-

‡"Normal" values for arterial P_{CO_2} have been reported as 39, 40, or 41 mm Hg.

neously with the increase in the *denominator* and results in a ratio of about 17:1 instead of 16:1 and a pH of 7.34 instead of 7.30

When CO_2 is retained more gradually, renal compensation has time to occur. The renal tubular cells secrete a more acid urine by exchanging H^+ for Na^+; the H^+ is excreted as HCl or NH_4Cl (the tubular cells can form NH_3^+) and HCO_3^- is reabsorbed. (The bicarbonate ion eventually returned to the extracellular fluid and plasma in combination with sodium is not the filtered anion but rather the intracellular anion derived from $CO_2 + H_2O \rightleftharpoons H_2CO_3 \rightleftharpoons H^+ + HCO_3^-$, but the end result is the same as if $NaHCO_3$ per se had been reabsorbed.)

If renal compensation were complete, equation (2) would become

$$\begin{aligned} pH &= 6.1 + \log \frac{32mM\ CO_2}{1.6mM\ CO_2} \\ &= 6.1 + \log 20 = 6.1 + 1.30 = 7.40 \end{aligned} \tag{4}$$

However, it is important to note three points:

1. Renal compensation is rarely perfect during respiratory acidosis, and the arterial pH is usually less than normal.

2. Total blood CO_2 and plasma P_{CO_2} will be *high* in *respiratory acidosis* and *metabolic alkalosis.*

3. Total blood CO_2 and plasma P_{CO_2} will be *low* in *respiratory alkalosis* and *metabolic acidosis.*

Therefore, to interpret data on total blood CO_2, HCO_3, and CO_2, a measurement of plasma pH is required. If the arterial pH is low and the P_{CO_2} is high, respiratory acidosis is present. If the arterial pH is high and the P_{CO_2} is low, respiratory alkalosis is present.

Generally pH and P_{CO_2} are measured on whole blood with respective electrodes. These data apply to plasma, so that plasma $[HCO_3^-]$ can be calculated using the Henderson-Hasselbalch equation. This permits interpretation of the acid-base data.

III. SUMMARY

Hypoxemia may be due to pulmonary disease that causes inadequate alveolar ventilation, uneven alveolar ventilation in relation to pulmonary capillary blood flow, impaired diffusion, or venous-to-arterial shunts. Measurement of O_2 content, capacity, and tension of arterial blood sampled while the patient breathes air and again while he breathes O_2 often provides data for differential diagnosis. The CO_2 tension of arterial blood or alveolar gas rises when the patient has pulmonary insufficiency; if there is incomplete renal compensation, this leads to respiratory acidosis.

PART TWO

Appendix

USEFUL DATA

1. Typical Values for Pulmonary Function Tests

These are values for a healthy, resting, recumbent young male (1.7 M^2 surface area) breathing air at sea level, unless other conditions are specified. They are presented merely to give approximate figures. These values may change with position, age, size, and sex; there is variability among members of a homogeneous group under standard conditions. For predicted values, see the next section.

TABLE 13.—PULMONARY FUNCTION TEST VALUES

Lung volumes (BTPS)		
Inspiratory capacity, ml (% TLC)	3,000	(50)
Expiratory reserve volume, ml (% TLC)	1,500	(50)
Vital capacity, ml (% TLC)	4,500	(75)
Residual volume (RV), ml (%TLC)	1,500	(25)
Functional residual capacity, ml (% TLC)	3,000	(50)
Thoracic gas volume, ml (% TLC)	3,000	(50)
Total lung capacity (TLC), ml (% TLC)	6,000	(100)
Ventilation (BTPS)		
Tidal volume, ml		500
Frequency, respirations/min		12
Minute volume, ml/min		6,000
Respiratory dead space, ml		150
Alveolar ventilation, ml/min		4,200
Distribution of inspired gas		
Single-breath test (% increase N_2 for 500 ml expired alveolar gas), % N_2		<1.5
Pulmonary nitrogen emptying rate (7 min test), % N_2		<2.5
Helium closed-circuit (mixing efficiency related to perfect mixing), %		76
Alveolar ventilation/pulmonary capillary blood flow		
Alveolar ventilation (L/min)/blood flow (L/min)		0.8
Physiologic shunt/cardiac output × 100, %		<7
Physiologic dead space/tidal volume × 100, %		<30

(continued)

TABLE 13.—*(continued)*

Pulmonary circulation	
Pulmonary capillary blood flow, ml/min	5,400
Pulmonary artery pressure, mm Hg	25/8
Pulmonary capillary blood volume, ml	90
Pulmonary "capillary" blood pressure (wedge), mm Hg	8
Alveolar gas	
Oxygen partial pressure, mm Hg	104
CO_2 partial pressure, mm Hg	40
Diffusion and gas exchange	
O_2 consumption (STPD), ml/min	250
CO_2 output (STPD), ml/min	200
Respiratory exchange ratio, R (CO_2 output/O_2 uptake)	0.8
Diffusing capacity, O_2 (STPD) resting, ml O_2/min/mm Hg	>15
Diffusing capacity, CO (steady state (STPD) resting, ml CO/min/mm Hg	18
Diffusing capacity, CO (single-breath) (STPD) resting, ml CO/min/mm Hg	31
Diffusing capacity, CO (rebreathing) (STPD) resting, ml CO/min/mm Hg	27
Fractional CO uptake, resting, %	53
Maximal diffusing capacity, O_2 (exercise) (STPD), ml O_2/min/mm Hg	60
Arterial blood	
O_2 saturation (saturation of Hb with O_2), %	97.1
O_2 tension, mm Hg	95
CO_2 tension, mm Hg	40
Alveolar-arterial Po_2 difference, mm Hg	9
Alveolar-arterial Po_2 difference (12% to 14% O_2), mm Hg	10
Alveolar-arterial Po_2 difference (100% O_2), mm Hg	35
O_2 saturation (100% O_2), % (+1.9 ml dissolved O_2/100 ml blood)	100
O_2 tension (100% O_2), mm Hg	640
pH	7.4
Mechanics of breathing	
Maximal voluntary ventilation (BTPS), L/min	170
Forced expiratory volume, % in 1 sec	83
% in 3 sec	97
Maximal expiratory flow rate (for 1 L) (ATPS), L/min	>400
Maximal inspiratory flow rate (for 1 L) (ATPS), L/min	>300
Compliance of lungs and thoracic cage, L/cm H_2O	0.1
Compliance of lungs, L/cm H_2O	0.2
Airway resistance, cm H_2O/L/sec	1.6
Pulmonary resistance, cm H_2O/L/sec	1.9
Work of quiet breathing, kgM/min	0.5
Maximal work of breathing, kgM/breath	10
Maximal inspiratory and expiratory pressures, mm Hg	60–100

2. Predicted Normal Values for Pulmonary Function Tests

TABLE 14.—Prediction of Lung Volumes in Liters From Age (A) in Years, Height (H) in Centimeters, and Sex*

LUNG VOLUME	SUBJECT	FORMULA			95% CONFIDENCE INTERVAL
VC (L)	Men	0.0600H	−0.0214A	−4.650	±1.12
	Women	0.0491H	−0.0216A	−3.590	±0.68
TLC (L)	Men	0.0795H	+0.0032A	−7.333	±1.61
	Women	0.0590H		−4.537	±1.08
FRC (L)	Men	0.0472H	+0.0090A	−5.290	±1.46
	Women	0.0360H	+0.00310A	−3.182	±1.06
RV (L)	Men	0.0216H	+0.0207A	−2.840	±0.76
	Women	0.0197H	+0.0201A	−2.421	±0.78
RV/TLC%	Men		+0.3090	+14.06	±8.8
	Women		+0.416A	+14.35	±11.0

*From Morris A.M., et al.: *Clinical Pulmonary Function Testing: A manual of Uniform Laboratory Procedures,* ed. 2. Salt Lake City, Intermountain Thoracic Society, 1984.

TABLE 15.—Effect of Postural Change on Lung Volumes*

DIVISION OF LUNG VOLUMES	MEAN VALUES (L) SITTING	LYING	MEAN DIFF., SITTING MINUS LYING (L)
40 male subjects			
Total lung capacity	5.788	5.483	+0.305
Vital capacity	4.098	4.018	+0.080
Inspiratory capacity	2.708	3.027	−0.319
Expiratory reserve volume	1.389	0.991	+0.398
Functional residual capacity	3.080	2.456	+0.624
Residual volume	1.691	1.465	+0.226
16 female subjects			
Total lung capacity	4.659	4.320	+0.339
Vital capacity	3.107	3.109	−0.002
Inspiratory capacity	2.094	2.451	−0.357
Expiratory reserve volume	1.013	0.659	+0.354
Functional residual capacity	2.565	1.869	+0.696
Residual volume	1.553	1.211	+0.342

*From Whitfield A.G.W., et al.: *Br. J. Soc. Med.* 4:90, 1950.

TABLE 16.—NORMAL VALUES FOR SPIROMETRY IN CHILDREN*

	FORMULA	SD %
Vital capacity, ml		
Boys	$3.58 \times 10^{-4} \times H^{3.18}$	13 (64)
Girls	$2.57 \times 10^{-3} \times H^{2.78}$	14 (60)
FEV_1, ml		
Boys	$7.74 \times 10^{-4} \times H^{3.00}$	13 (65)
Girls	$3.79 \times 10^{-3} \times H^{2.68}$	14 (61)
$FEV_{25-75\%}$, L/min		
Boys	$7.98 \times 10^{-4} \times H^{2.46}$	26 (67)
Girls	$3.79 \times 10^{-3} \times H^{2.16}$	28 (63)

H = height in centimeters.
*From Morris A.M., et al.: *Clinical Pulmonary Function Testing: A Manual of Uniform Laboratory Procedures,* ed. 2. Salt Lake City, Intermountain Thoracic Society, 1984.

TABLE 17.—PREDICTION OF MINUTE VOLUME OF VENTILATION, BASAL CONDITIONS*

AGE RANGE (YR)	MINUTE VOLUME (L/MIN, BTPS)	
	MALES	FEMALES
16–34	3.6 × SA (SD 0.3 × SA)	3.2 × SA (SD 0.4 × SA)
35–49	3.1 × SA (SD 0.5 × SA)	3.2 × SA (SD 0.4 × SA)
50–69	3.9 × SA (SD 0.45 × SA)	3.4 × SA (SD 0.4 × SA)

SA = surface area in liters.
*From Baldwin E. de F., et al.: *Medicine* 27:243, 1948.

A method of predicting standard (basal) ventilation from breathing frequency by weight and sex is shown in Figure 68 on page 256.

TABLE 18.—NORMAL VALUES FOR DYNAMIC MEASUREMENTS OF VOLUMES*

FEV_1 (L)	Men	0.0414H	−0.0244A	−2.190	±0.84
	Women	0.0342H	−0.0255A	−1.578	±0.56
FEV_1/VC%	Men	−0.1300H	−0.152A	+110.49	±8.3
	Women	−0.2020H	−0.252A	+126.58	±9.1
$FEV_{25-75\%}$ (L/sec)	Men	0.0204H	−0.0380A	+2.133	±1.67
	Women	0.0154H	−0.0460A	+2.683	±1.36
MVV (L/min)	Men	1.34H	−1.26A	−21.4	±56.8
	Women	0.807H	−0.57A	−5.50	±21.0

H = height in centimeters. A = surface area in liters.
*From Morris A.M., et al.: *Clinical Pulmonary Function Testing: A Manual of Uniform Laboratory Procedures,* ed. 2. Salt Lake City, Intermountain Thoracic Society, 1984.

TABLE 19.—NORMAL VALUES FOR LUNG COMPLIANCE (C_L)*

SUBJECTS	FORMULA ($L/CM\ H_2O$)	RANGE OF NORMAL
Young adults	C_L = (0.00343 × height in cm) − 0.425	65–145% of C_L
Adults	C_L = 0.05 × FRC in L	0.070 × FRC to 0.038 × FRC
Age 50–89 yr	C_L = 0.13	0.08 to 0.23

*From Frank N.R., et al.: *J. Appl. Physiol.* 9:38, 1956; Marshall R.: *Clin. Sci.* 16:507, 1957; Frank N.R., et al.: *J. Clin. Invest.* 36:1680, 1957.

TABLE 20.—AIRWAY RESISTANCE*

SUBJECTS	FORMULA ($CM\ H_2O/L/SEC$)	RANGE ($CM\ H_2O/L/SEC$)
Men, women, and children, panting	Airway resistance = $\frac{4.2}{\text{lung volume}}$	$\frac{7.7}{\text{lung volume}}$ to $\frac{2.9}{\text{lung volume}}$
	Airway conductance = 0.24 × lung volume	0.13 × lung volume to 0.34 × lung volume

*Lung volume is that at which the measurement is made in liters BTPS. From Briscoe W.A., et al.: *J. Clin. Invest.* 37:1279, 1958.

USEFUL EQUATIONS AND CALCULATIONS

For Chapter 1, Introduction

Symbols and Abbreviations Used in Pulmonary Function Tests (Based on **Federation Proc.** *9:602–605, 1950 and* **Symbols and Abbreviations for Use in The Handbook of Physiology: The Respiratory System***)*

SPECIAL SYMBOLS

— Dash above any symbol indicates a mean value.

. Dot above any symbol indicates a time derivative.

PRIMARY SYMBOLS		EXAMPLES	
V	= Gas volume	V_A	= Volume of alveolar gas
$\dot{V}$	= Gas volume/unit time	$\dot{V}_{O_2}$	= O_2 consumption/min
P	= Gas pressure	$P_{A_{O_2}}$	= Alveolar O_2 pressure
$\bar{P}$	= Mean gas pressure	$\bar{P}_{C_{O_2}}$	= Mean capillary O_2 pressure
F	= Fractional concentration in dry gas phase	$F_{I_{O_2}}$	= Fractional concentration of O_2 in inspired gas
f	= Respiratory frequency (breaths/unit time)		

t	=	Time	DO_2	=	Diffusing capacity for O_2 (ml O_2/min/mm Hg)
D	=	Diffusing capacity			
R	=	Respiratory exchange ratio	R	=	$\dot{V}CO_2/\dot{V}O_2$

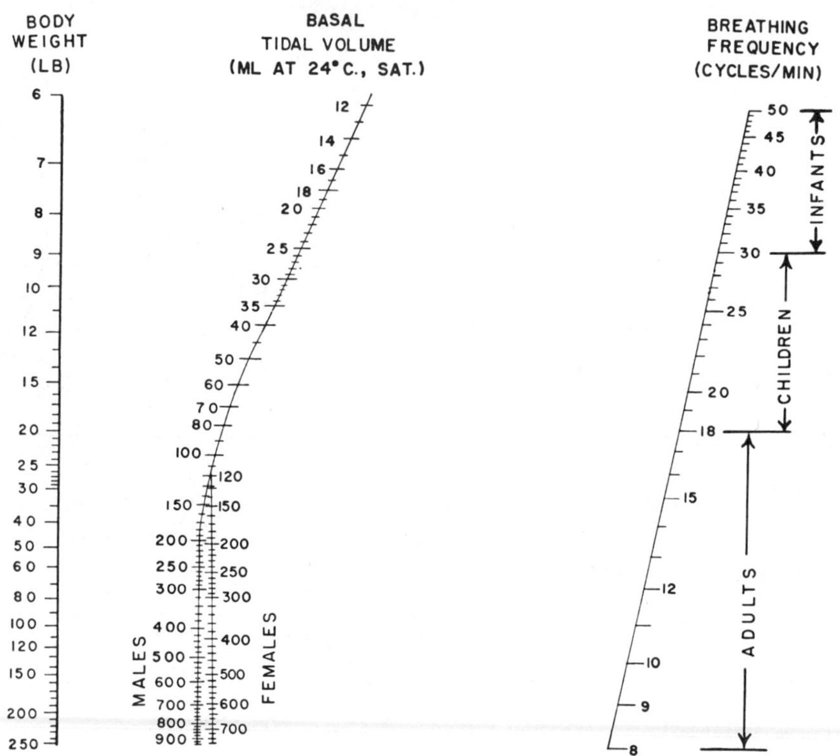

Fig 68.—To determine tidal volume required of mechanical ventilator, connect body weight of patient and cycles/min of the device with a straight line and determine where it crosses the basal tidal volume line. Corrections to be applied as required: *daily activity*, add 10%; *fever*, add 5% for each degree F above 99 (rectal); *altitude*, add 5% for each 2000 ft above sea level; *metabolic acidosis during anesthesia*, add 20%; *tracheotomy and endotracheal intubation*, subtract a volume equal to ½ the body weight; *added dead space with anesthesia apparatus*, add volume of apparatus and mask dead space. Tidal volumes are adequate only in patients with uniform (or matched) alveolar ventilation and capillary blood flow and no impairment of diffusion; in patients with abnormal lungs, measurement of arterial O_2 saturation and end-tidal PCO_2 may be necessary. (From Radford, E.P. Jr.: *N. Engl. J. Med.* 251:877, 1954, and *J. Appl. Physiol.* 7:451, 1955.)

Secondary Symbols		Examples	
I	= Inspired gas	$F_{I_{CO_2}}$	= Fractional concentration of CO_2 in inspired gas
E	= Expired gas	V_E	= Volume of expired gas
A	= Alveolar gas	$\dot{V}_A$	= Alveolar ventilation/min
T	= Tidal gas	V_T	= Tidal volume
D	= Dead space gas	V_D	= Volume of dead space gas
B	= Barometric	P_B	= Barometric pressure
STPD	= 0° C, 760 mm Hg, dry		
BTPS	= Body temperature and pressure saturated with water vapor		
ATPS	= Ambient temperature and pressure saturated with water vapor		

For Blood

Primary Symbols (Large Capital Letters)		Examples	
Q	= Volume of blood	Q_C	= Volume of blood in pulmonary capillaries
$\dot{Q}$	= Volume flow of blood/unit time	$\dot{Q}_C$	= Blood flow through pulmonary capillaries/min
C	= Concentration of gas in blood phase	Ca_{O_2}	= ml O_2 in 100 ml arterial blood
S	= % saturation of Hb with O_2 or CO	$S\bar{v}_{O_2}$	= Saturation of Hb with O_2 in mixed venous blood

Secondary Symbols (Small Letters)		Examples	
a	= Arterial blood	Pa_{CO_2}	= Partial pressure of CO_2 in arterial blood
v	= Venous blood	$P\bar{v}_{O_2}$	= Partial pressure of O_2 in mixed venous blood
c	= Capillary blood	Pc_{CO}	= Partial pressure of CO in pulmonary capillary blood

Subdivision of Lung Volumes

VC	= Vital capacity	= Maximal volume that can be expired after a full inspiration
IC	= Inspiratory capacity	= Maximal volume that can be inspired from resting expiratory level
IRV	= Inspiratory reserve volume	= Maximal volume that can be inspired from end-tidal inspiration
ERV	= Expiratory reserve volume	= Maximal volume that can be expired from resting expiratory level
FRC	= Functional residual capacity	= Volume of gas in lungs at resting expiratory level
RV	= Residual volume	= Volume of gas in lungs at end of maximal expiration
TLC	= Total lung capacity	= Volume of gas in lungs at end of maximal inspiration

For Mechanics

Primary Symbols		Examples	
R	= Resistance, pressure/flow	R_{aw}	= Airway resistance
C	= Compliance	C_{stL}	= Static lung compliance
E	= Elastance	E_L	= Lung elastance
G	= Conductance, flow/pressure	G_{aw}	= Airway conductance
I	= Inertance	I_L	= Lung inertance
Z	= Impedance	Z_{aw}	= Impedance of airways

Secondary Symbols		Examples	
aw	= Airway	G_{aw}	= Airway conductance
w	= Chest wall	C_w	= Compliance chest wall
L	= Lung	D_L	= Diffusing capacity of the lung
m	= Mouth	P_m	= Pressure at the mouth
pl	= Pleural	P_{pl}	= Pleural pressure
st	= Static	P_{st}	= Static pressure
dyn	= Dynamic	C_{dyn}	= Dynamic compliance

FORCED RESPIRATORY MANEUVERS

FVC	= Forced vital capacity
FEV_t	= Forced expiratory volume in time interval *t*
$FEV_t/FVC\%$	= Percent of FVC expired in time interval *t*
MVV	= Maximum voluntary ventilation
MEFV curve	= Maximum expiratory flow-volume curve
MIFV curve	= Maximum inspiratory flow-volume curve
PEFV curve	= Partial expiratory flow-volume curve

For Chapter 2, Lung Volumes

A. The Gas Laws

A gas, or mixture of gases, behaves not as a continuous fluid but rather as an enormous number of tiny particles. These particles (molecules) are separated by distances large in comparison to their own dimensions and are in a continual state of random motion. They exert no forces on one another except when they collide. During collisions with other molecules or with the walls of the containing vessel, energy is conserved, and there is no chemical reaction; therefore the collisions may be regarded as perfectly elastic. The gas laws describe how the gases behave in or out of the lungs, during various conditions of pressure, temperature, flow, and diffusion.

Strictly speaking, these laws apply only to an ideal gas. Real gases deviate from them particularly at high pressure and low temperatures, although deviations are generally small over physiologic ranges. Carbon dioxide is particularly disobedient.

Boyle's Law.—At a constant temperature, the volume of any gas varies inversely as the pressure to which the gas is subjected. For a perfect gas, changing from pressure P_1 and volume V_1 to pressure P_2 and V_2 without change of temperature, $P_1V_1 = P_2V_2$. The basis for this relationship is that gas molecules in a container produce pressure by colliding with the walls of the container; if the volume is compressed, the molecules become more crowded so that collisions are more frequent, and the pressure on the walls is greater. For adiabatic compression (non-isothermal), a different relationship must be used.

Charles' Law.—The volume of a gas at constant pressure increases proportionately to the absolute temperature. If V_1 and V_2 are volumes of the same mass of gas at absolute temperatures, T_1 and T_2,

$$\frac{V_1}{V_2} = \frac{T_1}{T_2}$$

The basis for this is that at absolute zero ($-273°$ C), molecular motion ceases. At warmer temperatures, molecular velocity is proportional to the square root of the absolute temperature. By heating a gas, the molecules rebound more following collisions, so that either the pressure in the container must rise or the space between the molecules of gas must increase (i.e., increased gas volume) if the pressure is kept constant.

Dalton's Law.—The pressure exerted by each component in a gaseous mixture is independent of other gases in the mixture, and the total pressure of the mixture of gases is equal to the sum of the separate pressures which each gas would exert if it alone occupied the whole volume. For example, the gases in the lung are CO_2, O_2, N_2, and H_2O. Each of these behaves in the alveoli as if it were independent of the others present, and yet the partial pressures of all together add up to the atmospheric pressure (P_B) in the lungs:

$$P_{CO_2} + P_{O_2} + P_{N_2} + P_{H_2O} = P_B$$

The independent action can be explained on the basis that CO_2 molecules, on the average, colliding with O_2 molecules behave as they do when they collide with other CO_2 molecules.

Partial Pressure of a Gas in a Liquid.—The O_2, CO_2, N_2, or H_2O molecules which are in physical solution in a liquid, such as plasma, continually escape through the liquid surface into the gas phase and may also return from the gas phase into solution. When the partial pressure of a particular gas tending to come out of solution is equal to the partial pressure of the same gas tending to go back into solution, the system is in equilibrium for that particular gas. Therefore, a liquid may also have a partial pressure of O_2, CO_2, CO, or N_2. The technical problem in determining the partial pressure of a gas in a liquid sample is that the analytical process may consume enough of the gas to lower the partial pressure in the sample and produce an erroneous measurement. The problem has been solved by the development of physical or physicochemical instruments that can detect minute fluxes of gas out of a blood sample through a relatively impermeable membrane. The partial pressure of gas in the blood sample is proportional to this flux. An oxygen electrode measures the electron current needed to reduce this flux of oxygen. A mass spectrometer measures the flux of any gas that is separable by mass/charge. The CO_2 electrode (p. 241) does not consume CO_2, but measures the pH of a thin layer of bicarbonate solution in gaseous equilibrium with the blood sample through a gas permeable membrane. Blood gas partial pressure may be analyzed by equilibrating a small bubble of gas with a large volume of blood sample and then chemically analyzing the composition of the bubble. However, this technique is not accurate for inert gases or high P_{O_2} because of the amount of gas lost from the sample.

Partial Pressure of Water Vapor.—This obeys similar laws. H_2O molecules tend to leave or enter the aqueous medium, and equal exchange occurs when the partial pressure of water vapor equals the "vapor pressure" of the liquid water. The warmer the liquid, the greater the vapor pressure. Water vapor in a gas in contact with a liquid phase maintains a partial pressure of 47 mm Hg (at 37° C) regardless of changes in barometric pressure. Some water vapor pressures covering the range encountered in physiologic conditions are given in Table 21.

Examples of Use of the Gas Laws

1. Calculation of Partial Pressure of CO_2 in Alveolar Gas.—Most chemical gas analyzers yield data in terms of "percent of dry gas." To calculate the partial pressure at body temperature, saturated with water vapor, the fraction of dry gas must be multiplied by (B − 47). For example: Alveolar gas, on analysis, contained 5.6% CO_2. Then $F_{CO_2} = 0.056$. Barometric pressure was 760 mm Hg. $P_{CO_2} = 0.056\ (760 - 47) = 40$ mm Hg.

2. Correction of Volumes of Gases Collected and Measured at Room Temperature.—A subject has just exhaled into a spirometer. Correct the volume to BTPS. After exhalation, the change of volume in the spirometer is 4.0 L. The temperature of the gas under the bell is 25° C. The barometric pressure is 750 mm Hg.

Air inside the spirometer is assumed to be saturated with water vapor at the spirometer temperature (T = 25° C; $P_{H_2O} = 24$ mm Hg), whereas air in the lungs is assumed to be saturated at body temperature (T = 37° C; $P_{H_2O} = 47$ mm Hg). The volume of gas in the spirometer must be increased by a factor $\frac{750 - 24}{750 - 47}$, in order to correct for the effect of a change in temperature on water vapor. Since the temperature of the gas in the body was greater than in the spirometer, the volume must also be increased by another factor $\frac{273° + 37°}{273° + 25°}$ to cor-

TABLE 21.—FACTORS TO CONVERT GAS VOLUMES FROM ROOM TEMPERATURE, SATURATED, TO 37°C, SATURATED

FACTOR TO CONVERT VOL. TO 37°C SAT.	WHEN GAS TEMPERATURE (°C) IS	WITH WATER VAPOR PRESSURE (MM HG)* OF
1.102	20	17.5
1.096	21	18.7
1.091	22	19.8
1.085	23	21.1
1.080	24	22.4
1.075	25	23.8
1.068	26	25.2
1.063	27	26.7
1.057	28	28.3
1.051	29	30.0
1.045	30	31.8
1.039	31	33.7
1.032	32	35.7
1.026	33	37.7
1.020	34	39.9
1.014	35	42.2
1.007	36	44.6
1.000	37	47.0

*H_2O vapor pressures from *Handbook of Chemistry and Physics,* ed. 34. Cleveland, Chemical Rubber Publishing Co., 1952, p. 1981.

NOTE: These factors have been calculated for barometric pressure of 760 mm Hg. Since factors at 22°C, for example, are 1.0904, 1.0910, and 1.0915, respectively, at barometric pressures 770, 760, and 750 mm Hg, it is unnecessary to correct for small deviations from standard barometric pressure.

rect for the temperature change itself. Therefore, combined corrections on the volume in the spirometer are

$$V\ (\text{BTPS}) = (4.0)\left(\frac{273 + 37}{273 + 25}\right)\left(\frac{750 - 24}{750 - 47}\right)$$

$$\text{or } V = 4.3\ \text{L}$$

Table 21 gives correction factors so calculated.

For Chapter 3, Pulmonary Ventilation

Quantitative analysis of the exchange of gas between alveoli and blood requires knowledge of the quantity of alveolar ventilation and pulmonary capillary blood flow and of the gaseous composition of alveolar gas and capillary blood. Representative samples of alveolar gas and pulmonary capillary blood cannot be obtained, but gas entering and leaving the alveoli (inspired and expired gas) and blood entering the pulmonary capillaries (mixed venous) and arterial blood can be obtained and analyzed. By means of a series of equations, the desired relationships can be calculated. These equations permit:

1. Calculation of the respiratory dead space.
2. Calculation of the composition of alveolar gas.
3. Calculation of alveolar ventilation.

A. Bohr's Equation for Respiratory Dead Space

Bohr's equation as it applies to a particular gas x is developed as follows:

$$\text{Total vol. of expired gas } (V_E) = \text{vol. of alv. gas portion } (V_A) + \text{vol. of dead space portion } (V_D) \quad (1)$$

Expired gas is defined as the total volume of gas that leaves the nose and mouth between the onset and end of a single expiration. V_A is used here to denote the volume of alveolar gas contributed to the expired gas and does not refer to the total volume of gas in the alveoli.

The amount of gas x in V_E, V_A, or V_D is its fractional concentration, F_X, times the total gas volume in which gas x is contained. Therefore, as in (1)

$$F_{E_x} V_E = F_{A_x} V_A + F_{D_x} V_D \quad (2)$$

The gas in the dead space at the beginning of expiration is inspired gas; therefore, $F_{D_x} = F_{I_x}$ and

$$F_{E_x} V_E = F_{A_x} V_A + F_{I_x} V_D \quad (3)$$

Since the volume of the alveolar gas portion (V_A) = volume of expired gas (V_E) − volume of dead space gas (V_D), equation (3) becomes

$$F_{E_x} V_E = F_{A_x} (V_E - V_D) + F_{I_x} V_D \quad (4)$$

Rearranging

$$V_D = \frac{[F_{A_x} - F_{E_x}]\, V_E}{[F_{A_x} - F_{I_x}]} \quad (5)$$

When the gas in question is CO_2, equation (5) can be simplified because inspired air normally contains practically no CO_2 and $F_{I_{CO_2}} = 0$

$$V_D = \frac{[F_{A_{CO_2}} - F_{E_{CO_2}}]\, V_E}{F_{A_{CO_2}}} \quad (6)$$

A sample calculation may be made from the data in Figure 13 (p. 40), where the fraction of CO_2 in alveolar gas ($F_{A_{CO_2}}$) is 0.056 (5.6%), the fraction of CO_2 in dead space gas is 0.0, the volume of a single expiration (V_E) is 450 ml, and the fraction of CO_2 in expired gas ($F_{E_{CO_2}}$) is 0.0373 (3.73%). Then

$$V_D = \frac{(0.056 - 0.0373)}{0.056} \times 450 = 150 \text{ ml}$$

The same calculation may be applied to a single breath (as above) or to multiple breaths, in which case the expired gas is collected over a period of several minutes.

B. Single-Breath Measurement of Anatomic Dead Space

This technique for measuring the respiratory dead space requires a continuous analysis of the concentration of a gas in the expired breath plus simultaneous measurement of the expired volume flow rate. A typical record is shown in Figure 69, in which N_2 concentration and flow rate at the mouth are recorded during expiration following a single inspiration of N_2-free gas (O_2) (see Fig 10, p. 34).

If a square front (see Fig 9, p. 31) were maintained during expiration between the dead space gas (0% N_2) and alveolar gas (in this example, about 60% N_2, because of dilution by O_2), the expired N_2 concentration would remain zero until a volume equal to the dead space had been expired, at which point the expired N_2 concentration would suddenly rise (thin vertical line in Fig 69) to the N_2 concentration of alveolar gas. In this hypothetical case, the dead space volume would simply be the volume expired up to the point where the alveolar gas suddenly appeared. However, alveolar gas does mix with dead space gas during expiration (see Fig 9), so that the exact point at which a volume equal to the anatomic dead space has been expired is not immediately apparent. However, it is possible to construct a "square front" on the record by numerical methods. It is only necessary to place a vertical line (the thin vertical line in Fig 69) so that the amount of N_2 in shaded area *A* exactly equals the N_2 that could be contained in the nonshaded area *B*. (The amount of N_2 equals the concentration of N_2 times the total volume of expired gas; in the example in Figure 69, where the expiratory volume flow rate is constant, equal amounts of N_2 are contained in equal areas of the N_2 meter record.) Once the square front is constructed, the dead space volume is simply the volume expired up to that point.

Bohr's equation (5) can also be applied to these data.

$$V_D = \frac{[F_{A_x} - F_{E_x}]\, V_E}{[F_{A_x} - F_{I_x}]}$$

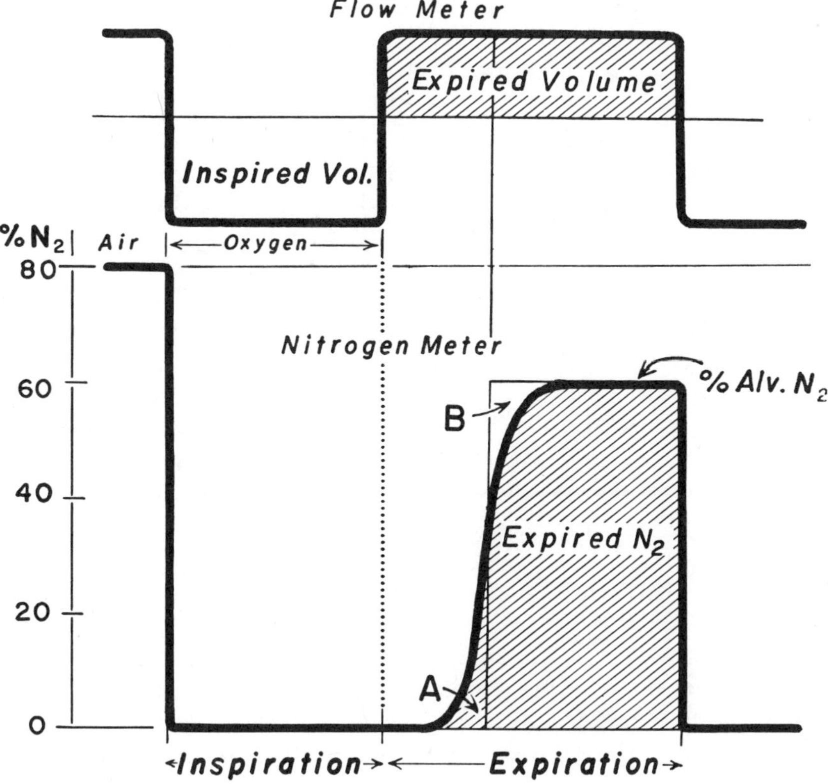

Fig 69.—Single breath analysis for measurement of anatomic dead space. *Above,* volume flow of inspired and expired gas. A constant flow rate is pictured for ease of measurement, though this would not be obtained in actual practice. *Below,* nitrogen concentration of inspired and expired gas following a single breath of O_2. For further explanation, see text.

In this case, N_2 is measured instead of CO_2. At the end of the single breath of O_2 the dead space is filled with O_2, a N_2-free gas. Therefore, $F_{I_{N_2}} = 0$, and the equation is simplified to the following:

$$V_D = \frac{[F_{A_{N_2}} - F_{E_{N_2}}]\, V_E}{F_{A_{N_2}}} \qquad (7)$$

$F_{A_{N_2}}$ is read directly from the nitrogen meter record of expired alveolar gas. V_E is computed from the flow meter record. $F_{E_{N_2}}$ equals the volume of N_2 expired (obtained from measuring the area under the curve of N_2 concentration) divided by the total volume of expired gas (V_E).

C. 'Physiologic' Dead Space

In Bohr's equation (6) for respiratory dead space, $F_{E_{CO_2}}$ and V_E can be measured easily, but the *alveolar* CO_2 concentration ($F_{A_{CO_2}}$) is difficult to obtain (see p. 52), and V_D cannot be calculated without knowing the correct value for $F_{A_{CO_2}}$. The controversy between Krogh and Haldane about the size of V_D centered largely on what constituted representative alveolar gas. This has been resolved by the following reasoning.

There is almost always complete equilibrium between the alveolar P_{CO_2} and end-pulmonary capillary P_{CO_2}. Therefore, in patients who do not have significant venous-to-arterial shunts, the arterial P_{CO_2} represents a mean alveolar P_{CO_2} over several respiratory cycles if the arterial blood is drawn over this period of time. Thus, arterial P_{CO_2} can be used to replace alveolar P_{CO_2}. When this is done and F is changed to P (P = F × 713 mm Hg), equation (6) becomes

$$\underset{\text{(physiologic)}}{V_D} = \frac{[Pa_{CO_2} - P_{E_{CO_2}}]\, V_E}{Pa_{CO_2}} \tag{8}$$

In the "ideal" case (p. 164), the anatomic dead space equals the physiologic dead space. However, in patients with uneven ventilation/blood flow ratios throughout the lung, the "physiologic dead space" is larger than the anatomic dead space (see Fig 12, p. 38). This is because regions with a high alveolar ventilation in relation to blood flow may be considered to be partly respiratory dead space regions.

A calculation of anatomic and physiologic dead spaces in an extreme case will make this point clear:

One pulmonary artery has been ligated but the lung has been left in situ (see Fig 55, p. 184). As a result of hyperventilation, the normal lung, *B*, receives 4 L of alveolar ventilation per minute and so is able to arterialize the entire cardiac output (5 L/min) and maintain an arterial P_{CO_2} of 40 mm Hg (equivalent to 5.6% CO_2 in alveolar gas). Frequency of breathing is 20/min. Total expired volume is 11 L/min, and the expired CO_2 (all of which comes from alveoli *B*) is 224 ml/min, or 2.04% CO_2 [(224/11,000) × 100 = 2.04%]; the P_{CO_2} of expired gas is 2.04% of 713, or 14.5 mm Hg. *Expired alveolar* gas contains not 5.6% CO_2 but only 2.8% CO_2 since the gas from alveoli *B* is diluted equally with CO_2-free gas from alveoli *A*.* Tidal volume (V_E) is 11,000/20 or 550 ml.

According to equation (6),

$$\underset{\text{(anatomic)}}{V_D} = \frac{[0.028 - 0.0204]\ 550}{[0.028]} = 150 \text{ ml}$$

According to equation (8),

$$\underset{\text{(physiologic)}}{V_D} = \frac{[40 - 14.5]\ 550}{40} = 350 \text{ ml}$$

Since expired volume = tidal volume, some express equation (8) as

$$\frac{V_D}{V_T} = \frac{Pa_{CO_2} - P_{E_{CO_2}}}{Pa_{CO_2}}$$

The fraction V_D/V_T is considered to be normal if it does not exceed 0.3.

D. Calculation of Composition of Alveolar Air (Alveolar Air Equation)

It was stated earlier that the determination of alveolar P_{O_2} and P_{CO_2} from analyses of a spot sample of expired alveolar gas is subject to considerable error, but that mean alveolar P_{O_2} can be *calculated* with reasonable accuracy. The basis for the calculation, stated in words, is given on page 43. The precise formula (assuming that inspired P_{CO_2} is zero) is

$$\underset{\text{(unknown)}}{P_{A_{O_2}}} = \underset{\text{(known)}}{P_{I_{O_2}}} - \underset{\text{(measured)}}{P_{A_{CO_2}}} \underset{\text{(correcting factor)}}{\left[F_{I_{O_2}} + \frac{1 - F_{I_{O_2}}}{R}\right]}$$

$P_{I_{O_2}}$ is inspired O_2 tension (moist); at sea level, this is 20.93% of (760 − 47) = 149 mm Hg. $P_{A_{CO_2}}$ is alveolar CO_2 tension. It is assumed to be equal to arterial P_{CO_2}; the latter is measured. The *"correcting" factor* introduces no correction when R, the respiratory exchange ratio $\dot{V}_{CO_2}/\dot{V}_{O_2}$, is 1.0.

If R = 1, the correcting factor is

$$\left[F_{I_{O_2}} + \frac{1 - F_{I_{O_2}}}{R}\right] = 0.2093 + \frac{1 - 0.2093}{1} = 1$$

*This is not strictly true since some end-expiratory dead space gas (2.8% CO_2) does enter alveoli *A* during inspiration. Furthermore, the flow of blood through the bronchial arteries supplying alveoli *A* does contribute some CO_2 to the expired gas. Finally, the assumptions do not allow for bronchiolar constriction on the vascularly occluded side (p. 175).

Usually, R is less than 1.0 (the volume of O_2 absorbed exceeds the CO_2 excreted), so that the volume of expired gas is slightly less than the volume of inspired air. In chapter 3, "Pulmonary Ventilation," this slight difference was ignored; here it cannot be, if great accuracy is desired.

For example, if R = 0.8, the correcting factor is

$$\left[F_{I_{O_2}} + \frac{1 - F_{I_{O_2}}}{R}\right] = 0.2093 + \frac{1 - 0.2093}{0.8} = 1.2$$

If R = 1, $P_{A_{CO_2}}$ = 40 and the correcting factor is 1.0, $P_{A_{O_2}}$ = 109 mm Hg. If R = 0.8, $P_{A_{CO_2}}$ = 40 and the correcting factor is 1.2, $P_{A_{O_2}}$ = 101 mm Hg.

The actual derivation of the alveolar air equation follows:

It is based on the knowledge that N_2 is not metabolized in the body and that, under steady-state conditions, the quantity of N_2 entering the alveoli per minute in inspired gas must equal the quantity of N_2 leaving the alveoli each minute in expired gas.

$$\dot{V}A_I\ (1 - F_{I_{O_2}} - F_{I_{CO_2}}) = \dot{V}A_E\ (1 - F_{A_{O_2}} - F_{A_{CO_2}}) \qquad (1)$$

This equation is based on the fact that when O_2, N_2, and CO_2 are the only gases present in the lungs (the gases here are measured as dry gases), the sum of their fractional concentrations must add up to 1.0. Therefore, $1 - F_{O_2} - F_{CO_2}$ must equal F_{N_2}. Note that the volumes of alveolar ventilation on inspiration and on expiration are given different symbols ($\dot{V}A_I$ and $\dot{V}A_E$, respectively) because these volumes differ when R is less than or greater than 1.0. Since the *number of N_2 molecules* must be the same in inspired and expired gas but the total volume of gas in which they are contained may change on expiration, it is obvious that F_{N_2} may be different in inspired and expired gas.

If we rearrange this equation, considering $F_{I_{CO_2}}$ negligible when the patient breathes air,

$$\frac{\dot{V}A_I}{\dot{V}A_E} = \frac{1 - F_{A_{O_2}} - F_{A_{CO_2}}}{1 - F_{I_{O_2}}} \qquad (2)$$

The correction factor requires knowledge of $\dot{V}_{O_2}$ and $\dot{V}_{CO_2}$. O_2 consumption ($\dot{V}_{O_2}$) equals the quantity of O_2 entering the alveoli in inspired gas less the quantity leaving the alveoli in expired gas.

$$\dot{V}_{O_2} = \dot{V}A_I F_{I_{O_2}} - \dot{V}A_E F_{A_{O_2}} \qquad (3)$$

CO_2 production ($\dot{V}_{CO_2}$) equals the quantity expired, since no appreciable amount of CO_2 is inspired while the patient breathes air.

$$\dot{V}_{CO_2} = \dot{V}A_E F_{A_{CO_2}} \qquad (4)$$

Respiratory exchange ratio (R) =

$$\frac{\dot{V}_{CO_2}}{\dot{V}_{O_2}} \tag{5}$$

Substituting equations (3) and (4) in equation (5)

$$R = \frac{\dot{V}A_E FA_{CO_2}}{\dot{V}A_I FI_{O_2} - \dot{V}A_E FA_{O_2}} = \frac{FA_{CO_2}}{\left[\frac{\dot{V}A_I FI_{O_2}}{\dot{V}A_E}\right] - FA_{O_2}} \tag{6}$$

Substitute equation (2) in equation (6)

$$R = \frac{FA_{CO_2}}{\left[\frac{1 - FA_{O_2} - FA_{CO_2}}{1 - FI_{O_2}}\right] FI_{O_2} - FA_{O_2}} \tag{7}$$

Clearing and solving for FA_{O_2}

$$FA_{O_2} = FI_{O_2} - FA_{CO_2}\left[FI_{O_2} + \frac{1 - FI_{O_2}}{R}\right] \tag{8}$$

If PA_{O_2} is desired, the equation becomes

$$PA_{O_2} = FI_{O_2}\,(713) - PA_{CO_2}\left[FI_{O_2} + \frac{1 - FI_{O_2}}{R}\right] \tag{9}$$

In some circumstances it is more convenient to calculate PA_{O_2} directly from the experimental data and use the form of alveolar air equation given on page 296.

E. Calculation of Alveolar Ventilation

The derivation of the equation in Figure 13 (p. 40) is as follows: The CO_2 in expired gas must all come from alveolar gas. The volume of CO_2 leaving the alveoli and entering the expired gas per unit time ($\dot{V}CO_2$) must equal the volume of alveolar ventilation in that same time ($\dot{V}A$) × the fractional concentration of CO_2 in the alveolar gas (FA_{CO_2}). Thus,

$$\dot{V}CO_2 = \dot{V}A \times FA_{CO_2}$$

or

$$\dot{V}A = \frac{\dot{V}CO_2}{FA_{CO_2}}$$

$$FA_{CO_2} = \frac{\%\ \text{alveolar } CO_2}{100}$$

Therefore

$$\dot{V}_A = \frac{\dot{V}_{CO_2}}{\% \text{ alveolar } CO_2} \times 100$$

This equation is correct only when $\dot{V}_A$ and $\dot{V}_{CO_2}$ are corrected to BTPS. $\dot{V}_A$ is usually corrected to BTPS, but $\dot{V}_{CO_2}$ to STPD. If this is the case, the right-hand side of the above equation must be multiplied by a factor of 1.21, or the left by 0.83.

The equation is often used with alveolar P_{CO_2} instead of % alveolar CO_2. This requires the use of a new factor to include the above correction and to convert % CO_2 into mm Hg pressure. The equation then becomes

$$\dot{V}_A \text{ (ml)} = \frac{\dot{V}_{CO_2} \text{ (ml)} \times 863}{\text{alv. } P_{CO_2}}$$

For Chapter 4, Mechanics of Breathing

A. Viscosity of a Gas

The pressure required to cause gas to flow through small tubes is proportional to the viscosity of the gas, the rate of flow, and the dimensions of the tubes. The property called "viscosity" can be pictured as fluid friction between adjacent layers of gas moving, or slipping, layer upon layer. The molecular basis for this property can be described as follows:

If there are two parallel layers of gas, one slipping across the other, the layer that is slipping can be said to move faster than the other. If gas molecules from the slower layer move sideways and cross over into the faster layer, the latter will be slowed down by the inertia of the molecules. It is this random sideways interchange of gas molecules that accounts for "viscosity," and explains why it takes pressure to make gas flow from one place to another. This type of flow is called "laminar" or "streamline" flow, and is found in the bronchioles of the lung in the absence of turbulence. Under these conditions, the pressure to produce a given rate of air flow depends on the viscosity and not on the density of the flowing gas (see Fig 28, p. 87).

B. Effects of Density of a Gas on the Gas Flow

At rapid rates of air flow, the density of the gas produces certain definite effects that require pressure to maintain the air flow. For example, to maintain flow through a constricted region of the trachea, the gas molecules must accelerate. This requires pressure in proportion to the density of the gas and the square of the velocity. (Calculations are based on equating the potential energy with the kinetic energy of the gas.)

Again, pressure is required to move the gas molecules when they become abruptly stopped by protrusions in the walls of the airways, or when they change their direction and form eddy currents or turbulence. These effects involve acceleration of molecules that have become "slowed down" with respect to the rest of the air stream and require pressure in proportion to the density of the gas, as well as approximately the square of the average air flow (see Fig 28, p. 87).

C. Measurement of Thoracic Gas Volume (V_{TG}) and Airway Resistance (R_{aw}) With the Body Plethysmograph

Thoracic Gas Volume.—For this measurement, the patient is asked to make small inspiratory and expiratory efforts ("pant") against a closed shutter, while keeping the cheeks stiff. Volume changes of the thorax (ΔV) are obtained from recordings of changes in the plethysmograph pressure gauge (P_{BOX}). The sensitivity of P_{BOX} to changes in thoracic volume is calibrated using a motor driven pump that duplicates adiabatic changes in gas pressure and temperature occuring during the patient's respiratory maneuvers. Changes of mouth pressure (ΔP_m) are measured using a separate pressure gauge. Since there is no air flow when the shutter is closed, changes of mouth pressure (ΔP_m) approximate alveolar pressure changes (ΔP_A). In some people whose cheeks bulge or who have a very high airway resistance, the alveolar pressure changes are attenuated before they reach the mouth and esophageal pressure changes (ΔP_{es}) may be a better measure of ΔP_A.

A slope, λ_V, which represents change in mouth (or esophageal or alveolar) pressure (ΔP_m) relative to change in box pressure (ΔP_{BOX}), is measured from the X-Y display on a cathode ray oscillograph and used to calculate thoracic gas volume (V_{TG}) as follows:

$$V_{TG} = \frac{(P_B - 47)}{\lambda_V} \times \frac{\text{Calib. } P_{BOX}}{\text{Calib. } P_m} \qquad (1)$$

This formula is derived from Boyle's law:

$$P_1 V_1 = P_2 V_2 \qquad (2)$$

where: P_1 is the initial (end expiratory) alveolar pressure
P_2 is the end inspiratory alveolar pressure

V_1 and V_2 are the corresponding thoracic gas volumes respectively.

$$\text{Since } P_2 = P_1 + \Delta P \text{ and } V_2 = V_1 + \Delta V \text{, then} \quad P_1 V_1 = (P_1 + \Delta P)(V_1 + \Delta V) \tag{3}$$

Solving for V_1: $V_1 = -P_1(\Delta V/\Delta P) - \Delta V$

For small changes of volume, ΔV approaches zero and

$$V_1 \approx -P_1(\Delta V/\Delta P) \tag{4}$$

Now V_1 is the thoracic gas volume, V_{TG}, in ml BTPS, P_1 is the barometric pressure minus the vapor pressure of water at 37° C, namely (P_B − 47) mm Hg and λ_V is the slope $-\Delta P/\Delta V$.

Airway Resistance.—Airway resistance, R_{aw}, is measured in two steps that require that the person pant through a flow meter with the mouth shutter open, then continue to pant while the shutter is closed to measure V_{TG} as described above. This rapid shallow breathing serves two purposes: it keeps the larynx wide open and it prevents large changes of air temperature, humidity, or CO_2 concentration during breathing.

In the first procedure plethysmographic pressure changes (ΔP_{BOX}), which are proportional to changes in thoracic gas volume (ΔV_{TG}) and airflow ($\dot{V}$) are measured. The slope, $\Delta\dot{V}/\Delta P_{BOX}$ equals λ_R, and is measured between points of 0 flow and 0.5 L/sec of inspiratory flow.

$$\text{Resistance, } R = \frac{P_A}{\dot{V}} \text{ where R is airway plus apparatus resistance.} \tag{5}$$

P_A is measured in this procedure and so equals the driving gradient for airflow. P_A can be calculated from ΔV_{TG}, during step 1, using Eq. 4.

$$P_A = -\frac{\Delta V_{TG}}{V_{TG}} \times P_1 \tag{6}$$

From which

$$R = -\frac{\Delta V_{TG}}{V_{TG}} \times \frac{P_1}{\dot{V}} \tag{7}$$

We can now insert the value of V_{TG} obtained in step 2 into Eq. 7 and solve for R. We then subtract the apparatus resistance to obtain R_{aw}. This can be combined in one step:

$$R_{aw} = \frac{\lambda_V \times \text{calib. } P_m}{\lambda_R \times \text{calib. } \dot{V}} - R_{app} \tag{8}$$

The calibration of P_{BOX} is assumed the same in the first step, the denominator, as in the second step, in the numerator.

It is desirable to know V_{TG} during panting because the resistance of the airways is partly dependent on lung volume. Therefore, R_{aw} should be related to V_{TG}, panting. *Specific airway resistance* is the product of R_{aw} and V_{TG}, and is fairly constant in an individual unless the bronchial tone changes. *Airway conductance* (G_{aw}) is the reciprocal of airway resistance ($G_{aw} = 1/R_{aw}$) and it is generally dependent on thoracic gas volume. Hence, the ratio G_{aw}/V_{TG} is fairly constant in normal people and is called *specific airway conductance.* However, in people with emphysema, G_{aw} approaches zero at their residual volume, which in turn is generally larger than normal. In such people, a line plotted on a graph of G_{aw} vs. V_{TG} has an intercept on the volume axis at a volume indicative of the amount of air that cannot be expelled from the lungs.

D. The Work of Expiration

The work of breathing equals the product of pressure and volume (Fig 24, p. 71). It can be measured as the work performed during inspiration, during expiration or during the whole respiratory cycle. Some of this work is required to move the thorax and some to move the lungs and air. If the transpulmonary pressure is measured by determining intrathoracic or esophageal pressure, the work required to move the lungs and air can be calculated. The work required to move the whole system (thorax + lungs + air) is more difficult to measure because the energy comes from the contraction of the respiratory muscles and there is no direct way of measuring this. However, if the patient's muscular force could be eliminated and a *measurable* force substituted for the contractile force of the muscles, the total work could be measured. This can be accomplished by placing the patient in a body respirator, requesting the patient to relax voluntarily all of his respiratory muscles, and then ventilating the lungs by the action of the respirator. Inspiration must always be accomplished by active work of the respirator pump and bellows, just as inspiration by muscular effort must always be accomplished by active contraction of the inspiratory muscles. Expiration may be "passive" or "active." It is passive if a large valve is opened quickly so that the subatmospheric pressure in the box returns abruptly to atmospheric; this would be analogous to a sudden and complete relaxation of the inspiratory muscles at end-inspiration. Expiration may be "active" if the pump actually produces a positive (greater than atmospheric) pressure in the box; this is analogous to an active contraction of the expiratory muscles. There is a third possibility, namely, that the negative pressure around the thorax is brought back to atmospheric slowly; this is analogous to a continued contraction of some of the inspiratory muscles during part of expiration (i.e., slow relaxation of inspiratory tone).

In order to measure the total work of breathing it is necessary to use the body respirator. When this method is used, it is convenient to think in the following terms:

1. Subatmospheric pressure in box = active contraction of *inspiratory* muscles.
2. Greater than atmospheric pressure in box = active contraction of *expiratory* muscles.
3. Abrupt change from subatmospheric to atmospheric pressure = abrupt relaxation of inspiratory muscles (passive expiration).
4. Slow change from subatmospheric to atmospheric pressure = slow relaxation of inspiratory muscles.

(1) and (2) require mechanical work *and* metabolic work (O_2 consumption); (3) requires neither mechanical work nor metabolic work; (4) does not require mechanical work but does require metabolic work.

Active Expiration.—At the end of inspiration, there is a subatmospheric pressure in the respirator and the lungs and thorax have been inflated to a certain volume; this pressure-volume point is *B* in Figure 70. Potential energy is now stored in the elastic tissues of the lungs and thorax; this is numerically equal to the area of triangle *ABC,* and is sufficient to produce passive expiration. However, when very rapid expiration is required (as in exercise) or when expiration must be completed against obstruction in a limited time, active expiration (greater than atmospheric pressure in the box, or active contraction of the expiratory muscles) is required. This requires new energy (in addition to that represented by area *ABC*), and the pressure-volume points during expiration go outside *ABC* and follow a path such as *BCDA*. The total energy used during expiration is therefore *BCDA,* but of this, *ABC* was potential energy created during inspiration and only *CDA* represents work of the expiratory muscles.

Passive Expiration.—The potential energy stored in the elastic tissues at end-inspiration, *BCA,* is sufficient to cause passive expiration. In these circumstances, the pressure-volume points during expiration may follow the path *BCA* or a path such as *BEA*.

1. Assume that, at end-inspiration, a large valve is opened so as to vent the respirator abruptly; this is equivalent to sudden and complete relaxation of the inspiratory muscles. Before the lungs have any time to change volume, the pressure in the box drops to zero and the pressure-volume point moves from *B* to *C.* Then, as the lungs begin to empty (pressure in the respirator remaining at zero), the pressure-vol-

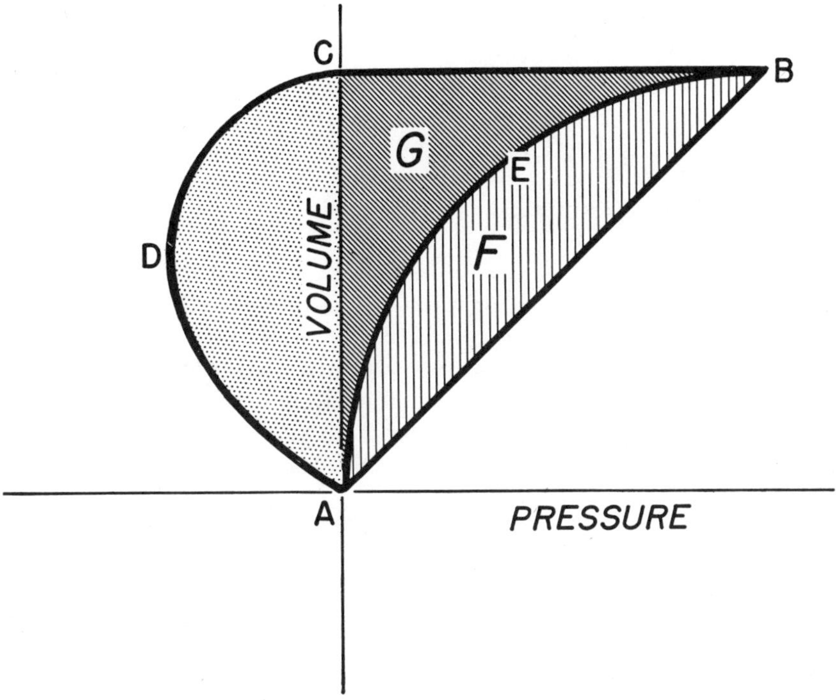

Fig 70.—The work of expiration. Graphic representation of expiratory "pressure-volume loops" as visualized on the cathode ray oscilloscope using the method of DuBois and Ross. The inspiratory portion of the "loop" is omitted. For explanation, see text.

ume points follow the path *CA*. Thus, the expiratory path is *BCA*. The stored end-inspiratory energy was used in producing air flow and overcoming the tissue resistance of the lungs and thorax.

2. The respiratory pattern described above would produce a pneumotachogram in which air flow rose abruptly to a very high value and then decreased in a predictable manner during the remainder of expiration. However, since the *actual* pneumotachogram during "passive" expiration is not of this type, it appears that inspiratory tone does not cease abruptly at end-inspiration but tapers off more gradually. To simulate the latter pattern, it is only necessary to permit the subatmospheric pressure in the body respirator to return gradually to atmospheric pressure. In this case, the volume does not decrease so rapidly

as the pressure (because of resistance to expiration). When the pressure-volume points are plotted during expiration, they move along a path such as *BEA*. At any moment, the pressure represented by the horizontal distance from line *CA* to a point on curve *BEA* is the pressure in the respirator, and the rest of the distance to *BA* is the elastic pressure required to overcome tissue resistance and produce air flow. The *work* in overcoming tissue resistance and airway resistance is equal to area *F*, and the work against the continuing subatmospheric pressure in the body respirator (continuing tone of the inspiratory muscles) is equal to area *G*. The continuing tone of the inspiratory muscles uses O_2 and so constitutes metabolic work but does not produce mechanical work.

Work of Moving the Lungs and Air.—The work of ventilating the lungs alone (without the chest wall) has been measured by determining the transpulmonary pressure, using an intrapleural or esophageal balloon. The P–V diagram for this situation is similar in essentials to that obtained in a body respirator, but the chest wall now assumes the role of the respirator, whereas the lungs alone take the place of the lung-thorax system.

E. Oscillatory Mechanics in the Lung

Rapid frequencies (3 to 10 Hz) of oscillation of air into and out of the lungs have been used either to measure the resistance to breathing or to ventilate the lungs with small volumes of air. A piston pump or a loudspeaker can be used to generate a pressure wave to move air rapidly into and out of an airway tube or to cause rapid pressure fluctuation around the body in a whole body respirator.

If the lungs plus chest wall behaved as if they were a single bellows with elasticity, inertia, and frictional resistance, then the air flow fluctuations into and out of the lungs produced by a given pressure fluctuation across the lungs could be described as a function of frequency by the following equations. At any frequency, the magnitude of the impedance Z, would be:

$$Z = \sqrt{R^2 + \left(2\pi\, fL - \frac{1}{2\pi\, fC}\right)^2} \qquad (1)$$

where Z is mechanical impedance in cm $H_2O \times \text{liters}^{-1} \times \text{sec}$ and is analogous to electrical impedance.

R is resistance in cm $H_2O \times \text{liters}^{-1} \times \text{sec}$.

L is inertance in cm $H_2O \times \text{liters}^{-1} \times \text{sec}^2$ and is analogous to inductance.

C is compliance in liters × cm H_2O^{-1} and is analogous to electrical capacitance.
f is the frequency in hertz, cycles per second.

The second equation describes the phase angle of lag (Ø) of the flow wave with respect to the pressure wave:

$$\text{Tan } \varnothing = \frac{2\pi\, fL - \dfrac{1}{2\pi fC}}{R} \tag{2}$$

The inertial reactance, 2π fL, corresponding to inductive reactance, increases with frequency. The elastic reactance, $\frac{1}{2\pi\, fC}$, or capacitative reactance decreases with increasing frequency. The frequency at which the absolute values of these two reactances are the same is called the *resonant frequency*. According to equation (1), Z becomes equal to resistance at the resonant frequency, which can be calculated from the relation:

$$\text{Resonant frequency} = \frac{1}{2\pi\,\sqrt{LC}} \tag{3}$$

However, the bellows system of the lungs and chest does not behave consistently with frequency as expected of a simple model with single values of inertance, compliance, and resistance as described in the equations above. The diaphragm and abdomen combination resonates at a lower frequency (3 Hz) than do the ribs (7 to 10 Hz). The inertial reactance of air in the tracheobronchial tree becomes significant at 6 Hz or higher. Thus, at "apparent resonance" of the system, the impedance does not equal a pure resistance, but contains an admixture of these other factors.

Sonic frequencies, sound waves, are reflected from branches in the bronchi, which behave somewhat like organ pipes tuned to different pitches, reflecting back echoes of frequencies that happen to be out of tune with the lower bronchus. The reflected waves (echoes) at the mouth tell how far away and how wide are the entrances of the bronchi from which these waves were reflected.

For Chapter 5, Regulation of Respiration

A. Interaction of CO_2 and O_2 in the Regulation of Ventilation

Ventilation is stimulated by elevated CO_2 (or H^+) and decreased O_2. In clinical testing, each can be separately evaluated by maintaining the other constant. Thus, the response to CO_2 is tested using gas mix-

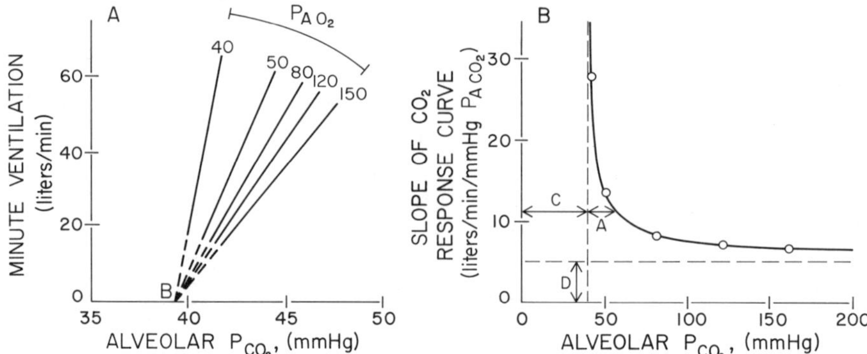

Fig 71.—Response of minute ventilation to changes in alveolar P_{CO_2} and alveolar P_{O_2}. **A,** increase in minute ventilation with increasing alveolar P_{CO_2} at constant alveolar P_{O_2}. **B,** rate of change of minute ventilation/alveolar P_{CO_2} that is the slope of the CO_2 response curve versus alveolar P_{O_2}.

tures with high oxygen in order to avoid an effect of hypoxia. The ventilatory response to hypoxia is likewise tested by maintaining a constant alveolar P_{CO_2} or by performing tests of short duration before the CO_2 effect is manifest. However, more complex but detailed evaluation of the respiratory control system can be obtained by measuring the interaction of CO_2 and O_2.

To perform the test, the response to increased alveolar P_{CO_2} is tested for several different (but constant) alveolar P_{O_2}.* Experimentally, it is found that the CO_2 response curve becomes increasingly steep as the alveolar P_{O_2} is decreased (Fig 71,A). These curves when extrapolated to zero ventilation meet at a common point. This point (termed *B*) has been found experimentally to vary with acid base status of the subject.

As a next step, the slope of the CO_2 response curves is plotted as a function of alveolar P_{O_2} (Fig 71,B). This plot shows a hyperbolic relationship in which one asymptote (designated *C*) indicates the alveolar P_{O_2} at which the slope *(S)* of the CO_2 response curve approaches infinity, while the other asymptote (designated *D*) represents the limit of the slope of the CO_2 response curve at infinite P_{O_2}. The experimental data can be described by an equation of the following form:

$$S = D\left(1 + \frac{A}{P_{A_{O_2}} - C}\right)$$

*A family of CO_2 response curves also can be generated by maintaining constant $P_{A_{CO_2}}$ using a servo control system and varying $P_{A_{O_2}}$. This approach is generally easier and results in more rapid attainment of steady state than the constant $P_{A_{O_2}}$ approach.

Solving for *A* yields:

$$A = \frac{(S - D)(P_{A_{O_2}} - C)}{D}$$

Letting *S* equal 2*D*:

$$A = P_{A_{O_2}} - C$$

Thus, the parameter *A* indicates the difference between *C* and the hyperbolic line at the point where the slope of the CO_2 response curve equals *2D*.

It is also possible to obtain one equation relating the parameters *A*, *B*, *C*, *D* by solving for the slope of the CO_2 response curve:

$$S = \frac{\dot{V}}{(P_{A_{CO_2}} - B)}$$

Substituting into the formula for the hyperbola and rearranging gives the following:

$$\dot{V} = D\,(P_{A_{CO_2}} - B)\left(1 + \frac{A}{P_{A_{O_2}} - C}\right)$$

In physiologic terms, *D* represents the sensitivity to P_{CO_2} in which the effect of O_2 has been eliminated, *C* represents the response to O_2 where the effect of CO_2 has been eliminated, *B* represents the extrapolated threshold of the ventilatory response system for CO_2, and *A* represents the degree of interaction between CO_2 and O_2. The following values for these parameters have been obtained in normal subjects:

A = 10–40 mm Hg $P_{A_{O_2}}$
B = 34–40 mm Hg $P_{A_{CO_2}}$
C = 20–35 mm Hg $P_{A_{O_2}}$
D = 2–6 L/min/mm Hg $P_{A_{CO_2}}$.

For Chapter 6, Pulmonary Circulation

A. Calculation of Pulmonary Blood Flow and Pulmonary Tissue Volume From the Disappearance of Inert Gas From Alveolar Air

A patient who makes a rapid inspiration of a gas mixture containing an insoluble inert gas tracer (helium, about 10%) plus a soluble inert gas tracer (acetylene 7.5%) in a bolus of air, holds this inspiration for several to 20 seconds and expires. The dead space gas is discarded and an alveolar sample is collected and analyzed for helium and acetylene.

It is assumed that inert gases equilibrate practically instantaneously amongst alveolar gas, pulmonary capillary and the parenchymal tissues of the lung. It is also assumed that inert gas equilibration between alveolar and lung tissue occurs before a significant amount of the soluble inert gas is transported out of the lung by the pulmonary capillary blood. Thus, immediately after the inspiration, both the insoluble (helium) and soluble (acetylene) gases will be diluted in alveolar gas to the same proportion, but the acetylene will in addition dissolve in lung tissue reducing its alveolar concentration in relation to helium in the following ratio:

$$\frac{\text{Volume of Acetylene in Alveolar Gas}}{\text{Volume of Acetylene in Alveolar Gas} + \text{Volume of Acetylene in Lung Tissue}}$$

This fractional reduction in alveolar acetylene can be expressed in mathematical symbols as follows:

$$\frac{F_{A_{C_2H_2}} / F_{I_{C_2H_2}}}{F_{A_{He}} / F_{I_{He}}} = \frac{V_A \times F_{A_{C_2H_2}}}{V_A \times F_{A_{C_2H_2}} + \alpha_t \dfrac{P_B - 47}{760} V_t \, F_{A_{C_2H_2}}} \tag{1}$$

$$= \frac{V_A}{V_A + \alpha_t \dfrac{P_B - 47}{760} V_t}$$

where V_A is alveolar volume in ml STPD, $F_{A_{C_2H_2}}$ is the fractional concentration (also a fraction of atmospheric pressure) of acetylene in a dry gas sample; α_t is the solubility of acetylene in tissue in ml gas STPD per milliliter of tissue per atmosphere at 37° C, numerically 0.77. V_t is the volume of lung tissue in milliliters.

The fraction $(P_B - 47)760$ corrects for the fact that $F_{A_{C_2H_2}}$ is measured in dry gas but the actual partial pressure of acetylene of alveolar gas is less because of its dilution by water vapor.

$F_{A_{C_2H_2}}$ obviously will divide out.

After this initial rapid dilution has occurred, acetylene disappears logarithmically (linearly on a semilogarithmic plot, as in Fig 44) as it is carried away from the lungs dissolved in the blood. This process is described in equation 2 below, where the left-hand side of the equation is the rate of change of alveolar acytylene concentration multiplied by the volumes in which this acetylene is stored, alveolar air and pulmonary tissue. The right-hand side represents the rate at which the blood carries away the acetylene, capillary blood volume flow rate times the end capillary acetylene concentration.

$$\frac{dF_{A_{C_2H_2}}}{d_t}\left(V_A + \alpha_t \frac{P_B - 47}{760} V_t\right) = \dot{Q}_C\alpha_B \frac{P_B - 47}{760} F_{A_{C_2H_2}} \qquad (2)$$

Where $\dot{Q}_C$ is the pulmonary capillary blood flow in milliliters per second; α_B is the solubility of acetylene in milliliters of gas STPD per milliliter of blood per atmosphere in blood at 37° C, numerically equal to 0.74.

Equation 2 can be solved by integration giving the exponential equation:

$$\frac{F_{A_{C_2H_2}}}{F_{A_{C_2H_2,O}}} = \exp \frac{-\dot{Q}_C\alpha_B \dfrac{P_B - 47}{760} t}{V_A + \alpha_t \dfrac{P_B - 47}{760} V_t} \qquad (3)$$

$F_{A_{C_2H_2,O}}$ is the alveolar acetylene concentration just after the rapid equilibration of the soluble inert gas among blood, gas, and tissue. This initial alveolar acetylene concentration is given by the following equation:

$$F_{A_{C_2H_2}} = F_{I_{C_2H_2}} \frac{F_{A_{HE}}}{F_{I_{HE}}} \times \frac{V_A}{V_A + \alpha_t \dfrac{P_B - 47}{760} V_t} \qquad (4)$$

where $F_{A_{HE}}$ is the alveolar fractional concentration of helium and $F_{I_{C_2H_2}}$ and $F_{I_{HE}}$ are the inspired concentrations of acetylene and helium, respectively.

The ratio $F_{A_{HE}}/F_{I_{HE}}$ describes the dilution of inspired acetylene in alveolar gas. The ratio furthest on the right, a restatement of equation 1, describes the further reduction of alveolar acetylene by its solution in lung tissue. Equation 4 can be used to calculate lung tissue volume, and the value of lung tissue volume can then be combined with other experimental data to calculate pulmonary blood flow using equation 3.

A sample calculation using the data in Figure 44 from chapter 6 may help explain the procedure. The extrapolated intercept of the acetylene disappearance curve from the ordinate gives a measure of the reduction of alveolar acetylene concentration by solution in lung tissue as described by equation 1 and by the furthest ratio to the right in equation 4.

We can now solve for lung tissue volume but first we need an independent measure of alveolar volume, which in this experiment was 3,468 ml STPD. Thus:

$$0.9 = \frac{3{,}468}{3{,}468 + 0.77 \times \frac{713}{760} V_t}$$

Solving for V_t gives 535 ml.

Next to obtain pulmonary blood flow ($\dot{Q}c$). The alveolar acetylene concentration decreases from 0.9 at time zero to 0.5 at 40 seconds so the exponential constant equals 1/40 Ln_e (0.5/0/9) equals -0.0202 sec^{-1}.

Substituting the experimental data into equation 3, we obtain the following:

$$0.0202 = \frac{\dot{Q}c\ 0.74 \times 713/760}{3468 + 0.77 \times 713 \times 535/760}$$

and

$$\dot{Q}c = 112 \text{ ml/sec or } 6{,}720 \text{ ml/min.}$$

B. Indicator Dilution Method of Measuring Blood Flow and Distribution Space

When a bolus of a nontoxic, nonmetabolized tracer that is not stored in the cells is injected into the blood supply to an organ, all of it must eventually leave by the venous outflow. The total amount of tracer leaving the organ equals the summation of the instantaneous venous tracer concentration times blood flow from the time of injection to infinity (or a relatively long time after injection). In mathematical terms

$$\text{Quantity of tracer} = {}_{\text{time injection}}\int^{\infty} \text{venous tracer concentration} \times \text{blood flow} \times dt \quad (1)$$

The quantity of tracer is in grams, concentration in grams per milliliter, and blood flow in milliliters per second.

The blood flow is considered constant so it can move outside the integral sign, and equation 1 can be rearranged to give the following:

$$\text{Blood flow rate} = \frac{\text{Quantity tracer injected}}{{}_{\text{time injection}}\int^{\infty} \text{venous tracer concentration} \times dt} \quad (2)$$

The integral in the denominator can be conveniently evaluated by plotting venous concentration against time (or recording a continuous record of concentration). A major problem, as shown in Figure 44,A, is that there is often recirculation of the tracer before the venous concentration from the original pulse reaches zero. The accepted way of correcting for this is to consider that the venous concentration falls exponentially with time (see Fig 43,B) and extrapolate the concentration beyond the point where recirculation begins, as shown in Figure 43,A.

Many types of tracers can be used. The only absolute condition is that the tracer must not be metabolized or stored in the cells. If the tracer is not confined to the vascular bed but diffuses out into the surrounding tissue cells, its venous concentration will be reduced to less than that of a label that is confined to the vascular bed (see Fig 47) for the early part of the curve. The concentration of the diffusible tracer in the venous blood will become greater than that of the nondiffusible tracer later in the curve because the diffusible tracer will reenter the blood from the tissue while the nondiffusible tracer is approaching zero. While the integral over time of the venous concentration of the diffusible tracer × blood flow will still equal the quantity of diffusible material injected, there may be great practical difficulties in measuring the very low venous concentrations at the tail of the curve.

It is necessary that all of the blood into which the tracer is injected be delivered to the organ and that the venous outflow sampled represent a mixture of all the venous outflow from the same organ. The method is not invalidated if there are other vessels supplying blood to the organ, but then the blood flow calculated will be that of the total blood flow through the organ and not just that of the vessel into which the injection was made.

Injection of a bolus of cold saline instead of the tracer dye and the measurement of temperature by thermistor or thermocouple in the outflowing blood, rather than concentration, is a convenient, widely used modification of this technique. The measurement can be repeated frequently, and the instrumentation is relatively simple and inexpensive. Heat will diffuse out into the surrounding tissue (it represents the most easily diffusible tracer species possible) which will reduce the venous dilution peak and delay the temperature curve. However, the volume of lung tissue is relatively small in relation to the pulmonary capillary blood, so that this does not produce a prohibitive delay in measuring pulmonary blood flow.

Inspection of the venous concentration curves of a tracer confined intravascularly as compared to those of a diffusible tracer (such as tritiated water) (see Fig 47,A) makes clear that water is diffusing out of the capillary bed and can give an index of the volume into which the diffusible tracer is distributed. This distribution volume can be estimated from the difference in *mean transit* times of the two species. Mean transient time is the summation of the amounts in each differential volume of venous blood weighted by the time that differential volume took to pass through the tissue, all divided by the total amount of tracer passing through the organ. In mathematical terms,

$$\text{Mean transit time} = \frac{\text{Blood flow } {}_{\text{time injection}}\int^{\infty} \text{venous dye concentration} \times \text{time post injection} \times dt}{\text{Blood flow } {}_{\text{time injection}}\int^{\infty} \text{venous dye concentration} \times dt} \tag{3}$$

The volume of distribution of the diffusible tracer then becomes equal to

$$(\text{Mean transit time for diffusible tracer} - \text{mean transit time for the intravascular tracer}) \times \text{blood flow} \tag{4}$$

If an injected substance is removed from the blood (and does not return) the venous dilution curve will be smaller than the venous dilution curve of intravascular indicator, but the peak will not necessarily be delayed. This is shown in Figure 47,B, where the lung takes up 5-hydroxytryptamine in proportion to its concentration in the capillary blood.

For Chapter 7, Distribution of Ventilation and Blood Flow

A. Relationship of Alveolar Ventilation to Pulmonary Blood Flow

This mathematical equation is very helpful in displaying the factors that determine the adequacy of alveolar ventilation. The equation is based on the fact that, in any steady state, the quantity of CO_2 that leaves the venous blood to enter the alveoli must equal the amount of CO_2 that leaves the alveoli to enter the expired gas.

The CO_2 leaving the pulmonary capillary blood each minute equals the pulmonary capillary blood flow in ml/min × the A–V difference in ml of gas/ml of blood.

$$\dot{V}CO_2 = \dot{Q}C\,(C\overline{V}_{CO_2} - C\acute{C}_{CO_2}) \tag{1}$$

where $\dot{Q}C$ is pulmonary capillary blood flow and $C\overline{V}_{CO_2}$ and $C\acute{C}_{CO_2}$ refer to the concentration of CO_2 in mixed venous and end-pulmonary capillary blood, respectively.

The quantity of CO_2 washed out of the alveoli by alveolar ventilation is described by

$$\dot{V}CO_2 = \dot{V}AFA_{CO_2}\ 0.83^* \tag{2}$$

Since equations (1) and (2) are equal,

$$0.83\ \dot{V}AFA_{CO_2} = \dot{Q}C(C\overline{V}_{CO_2} - C\acute{C}_{CO_2}) \tag{3}$$

This can be rearranged to give

$$\frac{\dot{V}A}{\dot{Q}C} = \frac{(C\overline{V}_{CO_2} - C\acute{C}_{CO_2})}{FA_{CO_2}\ 0.83} \tag{4}$$

If it is desired to express FA_{CO_2} as $PA_{CO_2}/713$, equation (4) becomes

$$\frac{\dot{V}A}{\dot{Q}C} = \frac{863\ (C\overline{V}_{CO_2} - C\acute{C}_{CO_2})}{PA_{CO_2}} \tag{5}$$

Substituting normal values (concentrations expressed in ml of CO_2/ml of blood),

$$\frac{\dot{V}A}{\dot{Q}C} = \frac{863\ (0.530 - 0.493)}{40} = 0.8$$

Since in any individual, the mixed venous blood distributed to all the pulmonary capillaries has the same CO_2 concentration, and since end-pulmonary capillary blood has the same PCO_2 as alveolar gas, the alveolar PCO_2 is determined by the ratio $\dot{V}A/\dot{Q}C$.

An analogous equation can be derived for O_2, but is considerably more complex because of the necessity for correcting for the change in volume between inspired tidal volume and expired tidal volume (see p. 268). The *uncorrected* equation for O_2 is

$$\frac{\dot{V}A}{\dot{Q}C} = \frac{(C\acute{C}_{O_2} - C\overline{V}_{O_2})}{(FI_{O_2} - FA_{O_2})}$$

B. Calculation of Quantity of a Venous-to-Arterial Shunt

When a patient has a venous-to-arterial shunt, his arterial blood contains some mixed venous blood that bypassed the lungs and some

*Since $\dot{V}A$ is expressed in ml (BTPS) and $\dot{V}CO_2$ is in ml (STPD)/min, $\dot{V}A$ must be multiplied by $\frac{PB - 47}{PB}$ to convert to a dry gas volume, multiplied by $\frac{PB}{760}$ to convert to standard pressure (760 mm Hg), and multiplied by $\frac{273}{273 + 37}$ to convert to standard temperature (0° C). The combined factor equals

$$\frac{760 - 47}{760} \times \frac{760}{760} \times \frac{273}{310} = 0.83$$

when ambient pressure is sea level (760 mm Hg).

well-oxygenated blood that had passed through the pulmonary capillaries. The equation that expresses this relationship for blood is quite analogous to Bohr's equation for the calculation of respiratory dead space.

$$\text{Amt. of } O_2 \text{ in arterial blood} = \text{amt. of } O_2 \text{ in blood that has traversed the pulmonary capillaries} + \text{amt. of } O_2 \text{ in shunted blood} \qquad (1)$$

Since the amount of $O_2 = C_{O_2} \times \dot{Q}$, therefore

$$Ca_{O_2}\,\dot{Q} = C\acute{c}_{O_2}\,\dot{Q}c + C\bar{v}_{O_2}\,\dot{Q}s \qquad (2)$$

where $\dot{Q}$ = total blood flow, $\dot{Q}c$ = blood flow through pulmonary capillaries, and $\dot{Q}s$ = blood flow (of mixed venous blood) through shunt.

$$\dot{Q}c = \dot{Q} - \dot{Q}s$$

Therefore, equation (2) becomes

$$Ca_{O_2}\dot{Q} = C\acute{c}_{O_2}\,(\dot{Q} - \dot{Q}s) + C\bar{v}_{O_2}\,\dot{Q}s$$

Rearranging

$$\dot{Q}s = \frac{Ca_{O_2} - C\acute{c}_{O_2}}{C\bar{v}_{O_2} - C\acute{c}_{O_2}} \times \dot{Q} \qquad (3)$$

If $\dot{Q}$ has been measured, $\dot{Q}s$ can be calculated in absolute quantities; if not, $\frac{\dot{Q}s}{\dot{Q}}$ can be calculated as the fraction of the total cardiac output that flows through the shunt:

$$\frac{\dot{Q}s}{\dot{Q}} = \frac{Ca_{O_2} - C\acute{c}_{O_2}}{C\bar{v}_{O_2} - C\acute{c}_{O_2}}$$

Arterial and mixed venous blood can be obtained so that Ca_{O_2} and $C\bar{v}_{O_2}$ may be measured. End-pulmonary capillary blood cannot be obtained for direct analysis of $C\acute{c}_{O_2}$ but its P_{O_2} and hence its C_{O_2} can be estimated by the procedure described on page 304. The final value for $\dot{Q}s/\dot{Q}$ is that of the "physiologic shunt," which includes not only anatomic shunts but also a quantity of blood coming from regions with a low ventilation/blood flow ratio. The latter is included because the calculated "end-capillary" P_{O_2} is really a *contrived* end-capillary P_{O_2} that deliberately eliminates any component due to variations in ventilation/blood flow ratios.

The quantity of blood flowing through the anatomic shunt can be revealed by giving the patient 100% O_2 to breathe for a long enough period to wash all of the N_2 from the alveoli. Alveolar P_{O_2} will then be $760 - P_{A_{H_2O}} - P_{A_{CO_2}}$, or approximately 673 mm Hg. With such a high alveolar P_{O_2}, there will be no alveolar to end-capillary gradient and end-capillary blood can be assumed to contain an amount equal to the O_2 capacity of Hb plus 2.0 ml of dissolved O_2/100 ml.

For example, if during inhalation of 100% O_2, O_2 capacity = 20 vol%, O_2 content of end-pulmonary capillary blood = 22 vol%, O_2 content of arterial blood = 21 vol%, and O_2 content of mixed venous blood = 17.5 vol%, then

$$\frac{\dot{Q}s}{\dot{Q}} = \frac{21 - 22}{17.5 - 22} = \frac{-1}{-4.5} = 22\% \text{ shunt}$$

C. The O_2-CO_2 Diagram (Devised by Rahn and Fenn)

A computer appears to be an extremely complicated instrument at first sight, but once one becomes accustomed to using it, one can solve many complex mathematical problems with it without ever knowing how or why the computer works. Similarly, the O_2-CO_2 diagram appears to be formidable at first glance, but with very little practice one can use it to solve quickly many dificult problems dealing with pulmonary gas exchange without knowing how the diagram was constructed.

Two graphs are included: Figure 72 is the basic diagram, and Figure 73 is the same diagram with additional lines, much more complex but also more useful.

How to Use Figure 72

The conventional coordinates are P_{O_2} and P_{CO_2}. On this grid have been placed isopleths for O_2 saturation and CO_2 content (lines of equal O_2 saturation and lines of equal whole blood CO_2 concentration). This graph thus combines all of the O_2 and CO_2 dissociation curves (as these vary with changing P_{CO_2} and O_2 saturation, respectively) in Figures 65 (p. 224) and 70 (p. 238) into one. The O_2 saturation isopleths do not run vertically because of the effect of changing P_{CO_2} (Bohr effect); the CO_2 content isopleths do not run horizontally because of the effect of changing O_2 saturation (Haldane effect).

Example 1.—Alveolar P_{O_2} is 80 mm Hg and alveolar P_{CO_2} is 43 mm Hg. Assuming that no difference exists between P_{O_2} and P_{CO_2} in alveolar gas and in arterial blood, determine arterial O_2 saturation and whole blood CO_2. *A* is the point where P_{O_2} of 80 and P_{CO_2} of 43 meet. This coincides with an arterial O_2 saturation of 95% and CO_2 content of 50 volumes %.

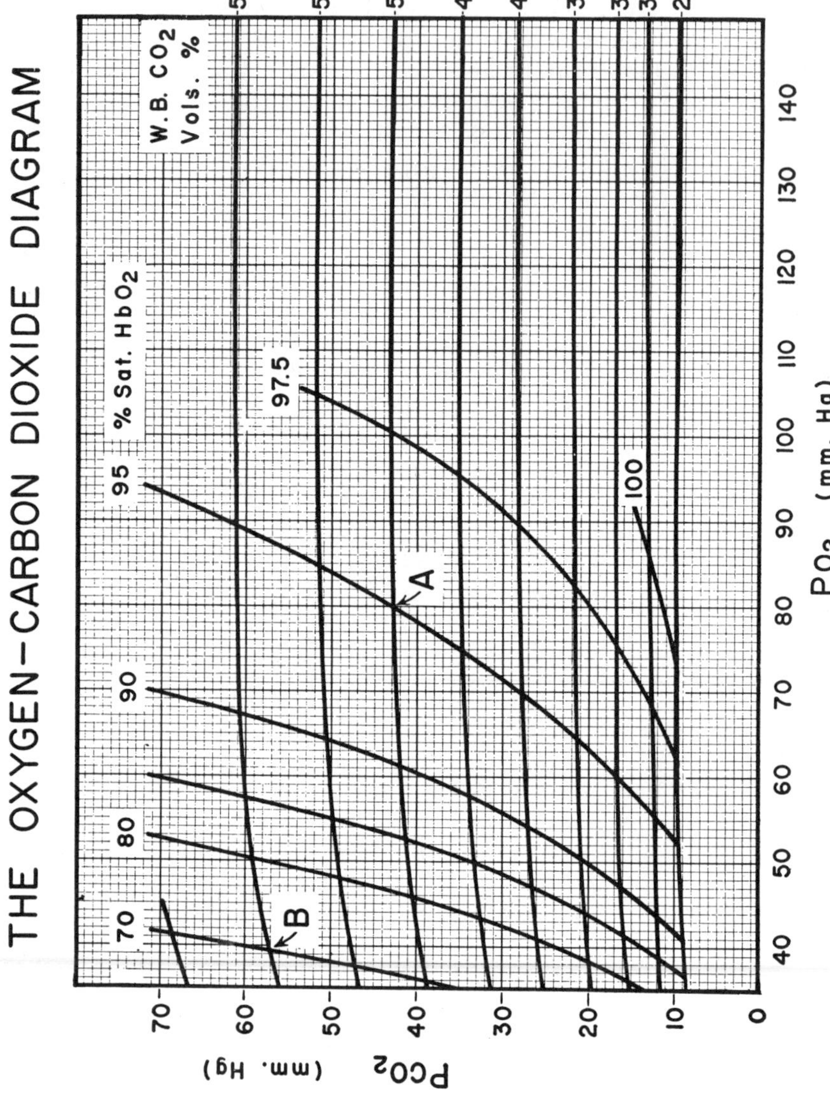

Fig 72.—The O_2-CO_2 diagram of Rahn and Fenn (see text).

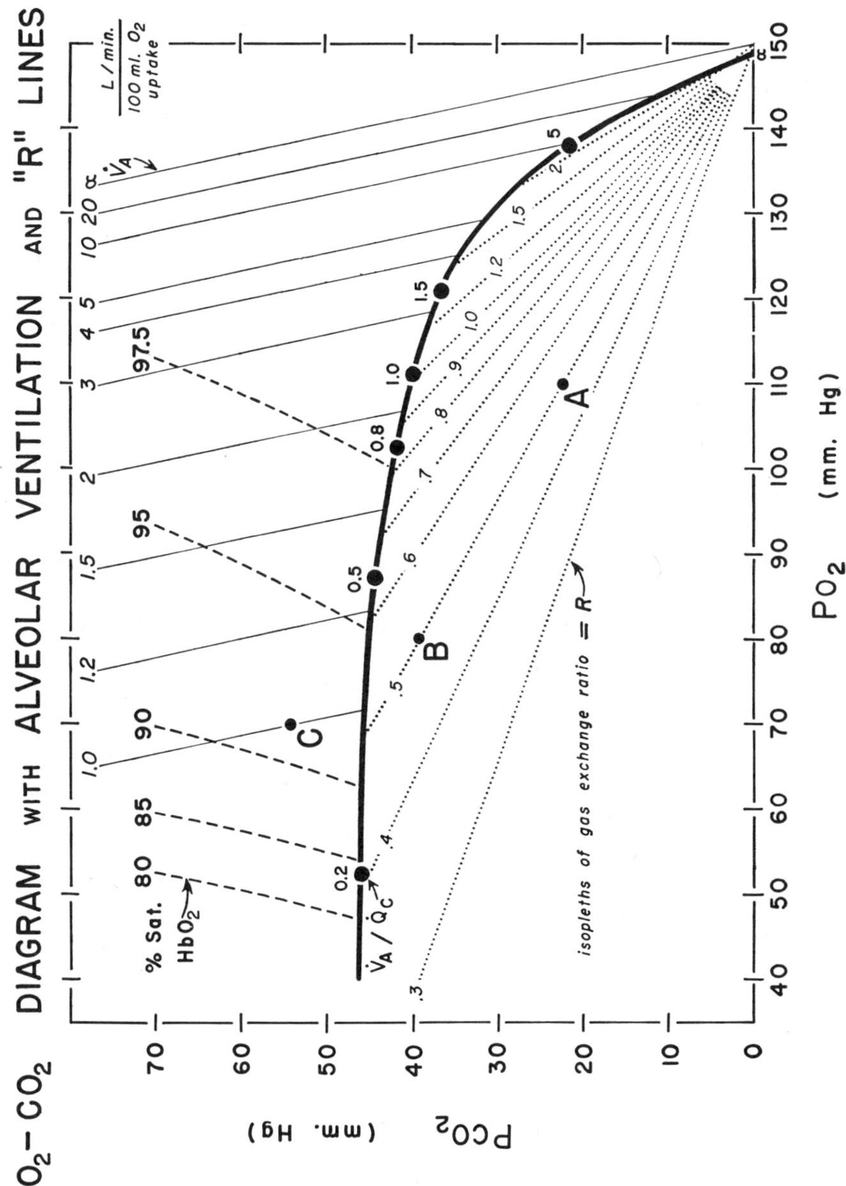

Fig 73. This diagram is identical with Figure 72, and one may be superimposed on the other. It differs in that the graph lines, lower part of the O_2 saturation isopleths and all of the CO_2 isopleths have been omitted to permit inclusion of new lines. The latter are (1) The heavy curved $\dot{V}_A/\dot{Q}_C$ line that originates at the left with mixed venous blood (no ventilation) and passes through ratios labeled 0.2, 0.5, 0.8, 1.0, 1.5, and 5 to infinity at the moist inspired gas point (no pulmonary capillary blood flow). (2) The dotted isopleths of gas exchange ratio (R lines) that radiate from the moist inspired gas point (P_{O_2}, 149 mm Hg; P_{CO_2}, 0 mm Hg); R lines from 0.3 to 2.0 are included on this graph. (3) The alveolar ventilation lines ($\dot{V}_A$), which range from 1.0 to 20 or more L/min for every 100 ml O_2 uptake. For further explanation, see text.

Example 2.—Analysis of arterial blood in a patient with hypoventilation shows that the O_2 saturation is 70% and the whole blood CO_2 is 58 volumes %. What is the equivalent P_{O_2} for this saturation and CO_2 content, and what is the equivalent P_{CO_2} for this CO_2 content and degree of anoxemia? *B* is the point at which saturation = 70% and CO_2 content = 58 volumes %. P_{O_2} = 39.4 mm Hg and P_{CO_2} = 57.5 mm Hg.

How to Use Figure 73

The conventional coordinates are the same as in Figure 71, and again lines of equal O_2 saturation have been placed on this grid; however, the O_2 isopleths (equal volume lines) are incomplete and the CO_2 isopleths are deleted so that additional lines may be clearly visible. The latter include the following:

1. A group of lines of equal R (respiratory exchange ratio) radiating from the moist inspired gas point (P_{O_2} = 149 and P_{CO_2} = 0 mm Hg). These are analogous to lines of equal barometric pressure on a weather map. These were calculated from the alveolar air equation. Every point on any one of these lines could represent an alveolus that is exchanging O_2 and CO_2 in the same *ratio,* although the absolute quantities may be different. Thus, an alveolus at *A* on the 0.5 R line might have a P_{O_2} of 110 and a P_{CO_2} of 22 mm Hg, whereas another alveolus at *B* on the same 0.5 R line might have a P_{O_2} of 80 and a P_{CO_2} of 39 mm Hg. In both, the ratio is the same. These R lines permit ready determination of $P_{A_{CO_2}}$, $P_{A_{O_2}}$, or R if two of the three values are known. If $P_{A_{O_2}}$ = 110 mm Hg and R = 0.7, $P_{A_{CO_2}}$ must be 30 mm Hg. If $P_{A_{CO_2}}$ is 40 and R = 0.8, $P_{A_{O_2}}$ must be 102 mm Hg.

2. A series of parallel lines of alveolar ventilation expressed as L/min of alveolar ventilation for every 100 ml of O_2 consumed.

3. A curved "distribution line" ($\dot{V}_A/\dot{Q}_C$), which represents all of the possible combinations of P_{O_2} and P_{CO_2} that could occur in alveolar gas and pulmonary capillary blood after mixed venous blood has equilibrated with alveolar gas at all possible ventilation/blood flow ratios. This particular line applies only when venous blood and inspired air have the composition indicated at the two extremes of the line.

It will be seen that one end of the distribution line terminates at the inspired gas point and the other terminates at the venous blood point. An alveolus at point 0.8 has an alveolar ventilation of 4 units and pulmonary capillary blood flow of 5 units. An alveolus at point 0.2 has an alveolar ventilation of 1 unit and blood flow of 5 units; this approaches a shunt and is very close to the mixed venous point. An alveolus at point 5.0 has alveolar ventilation of 5 units and blood flow of 1.0 unit; this approaches ventilation of the dead space volume and so is very close to the inspired gas point.

Example.—A patient has an alveolar P_{O_2} of 70 and P_{CO_2} of 54 mm Hg. What is his alveolar ventilation? *C* marks the intersection of $P_{A_{O_2}}$ 70 and $P_{A_{CO_2}}$ 54. This point lies on the $\dot{V}_A$ 1.0 line. Therefore, $\dot{V}_A$ is 1.0 L/min for each 100 ml of O_2 consumed. If there is no impairment of diffusion, arterial O_2 saturation will be 91%.

The same information could be obtained if one knew that $P_{A_{CO_2}}$ was 54 mm Hg and R (determined from analysis of expired gas) was 0.6.

D. Multiple Inert Gas Method for Estimating Distribution of Ventilation-Blood Flow

The technique (described on p. 183) is to infuse saline containing six inert gases of different solubilities at a constant rate into a peripheral vein until a steady state of secretion has been reached in the expired air, at which point arterial and mixed venous blood alveolar and expired gas samples are collected and analyzed for the inert gas concentrations.

Under steady-state conditions the rate of elimination of an inert gas in the expired air must equal the rate of delivery of this gas to lungs by the blood, as described in the following equation:

$$\dot{V}_A \frac{P_{A_{inert}}}{P_B - 47} = \dot{Q}_C\,(C\bar{v} - Cc'_{inert}) \qquad (1)$$

where: $\dot{V}_A$ is alveolar ventilation in milliliters (STPD) per minute. $P_{A_{inert}}$ is the partial pressure of inert gas in alveolar air in mm Hg. $C\bar{v}_{inert}$ and Cc'_{inert} are the concentrations of inert gas in mixed venous and end-capillary blood, respectively, in milliliters of gas STPD per milliliter of blood. $\dot{Q}_C$ is capillary blood flow in milliliters per minute.

In addition, since an inert gas equilibrates in the alveoli, $P_{A_{inert}} = P_{c'_{inert}}$. Therefore,

$$Cc'_{inert} = \frac{P_{A_{inert}}}{P_B - 47}\,\alpha_B \qquad (2)$$

where α_B is the solubility of inert gas in blood in ml gas STPD per milliliter of blood for 1 atmosphere of pressure.

Combining equations 1 and 2 and rearranging, we obtain the important relationship below:

$$\frac{P_{A_{inert}}}{P_{\bar{V}_{inert}}} = \frac{1}{1 + \dfrac{\dot{V}_A}{\alpha_B \dot{Q}_C}} \tag{3}$$

$P_{A_{inert}}$ over $P_{\bar{V}_{inert}}$ is graphed in Figure 56 against $\dot{V}_A/\dot{Q}_C$. For a given solubility as $\dot{V}_A/\dot{Q}_C$ increases $P_{A_{inert}}/P_{\bar{V}_{inert}}$ goes to zero; as $\dot{V}_A/\dot{Q}_C$ decreases, $P_{A_{inert}}/P_{\bar{V}_{inert}}$ approaches unity.

Equation 3 applies to an individual alveolus, but we measure in patients the partial pressures of inert gases in alveolar air from the whole lung and in arterial blood, which is a mixture of all the individual end capillary bloods. Expired alveolar gas partial pressure is the sum of the alveolar gas in each alveolus, weighted by its fractional contribution to the total expired volume. Thus, the partial pressure of the inert gas in the expired alveolar air divided by its partial pressure in mixed venous blood (which is the same for all alveoli), and therefore a convenient reference value is described by the following relationship:

$$\frac{P_{A_{inert}}}{P_{\bar{V}_{inert}}} = \frac{1}{\dot{V}_A} \sum_{i}^{n} \frac{\dot{V}_{A_i}}{1 + \dfrac{\dot{V}_{A_i}}{\alpha_B \dot{Q}_{C_i}}} \tag{4}$$

where $\dot{V}_A$ is total lung alveolar ventilation in milliliters (STPD) per minute, $\dot{V}_{A_i}$ is the alveolar ventilation of one alveolus, the ith, in milliliters (STPD) per minute. $\dot{Q}_{C_i}$ is the capillary blood flow of the ith alveolus in milliliters per minute. Σ indicates that the fractions from each alveolus should be summated for all alveoli from the first to *n*, the last.

A similar equation describes the arterial inert gas partial pressure.

$$\frac{Pa_{inert}}{P_{\bar{V}_{inert}}} = \frac{1}{\dot{Q}_C} \sum_{i}^{n} \frac{\dot{Q}_{C_i}}{1 + \dfrac{V_{A_i}}{\alpha_B \dot{Q}_{C_i}}} \tag{5}$$

where Pa_{inert} is the partial pressure of inert gas in arterial blood in mm Hg. $\dot{Q}_C$ is the total pulmonary blood flow.

Inspection of equations 4 and 5 show that $P_{A_{inert}}/P_{\bar{V}_{inert}}$ is always less than $Pa_{inert}/P_{\bar{V}_{inert}}$ if there is any nonuniformity of ventilation/blood flow. (If there is none, they will be equal.) The argument is as follows. An alveolus with a large $\dot{V}_A/\dot{Q}_C$ will have a relatively low concentration of inert gas. On the average it will have a large alveolar ventilation and contribute more to the expired alveolar gas, lowering $P_{A_{inert}}$ in respect to $P_{\bar{V}_{inert}}$. In contrast, this same alveolus will on the average have a lower capillary blood flow, contributing less to arterial blood, tending to raise its Pa_{inert} in relation to $P_{\bar{V}_{inert}}$.

The values of arterial and expired alveolar P_{inert} vary markedly with solubility (see Fig 56) in a nonlinear fashion so that the proportional differences between Pa_{inert} and PA_{inert} vary with solubility. Therefore, by trial and error (computer) one can vary the distribution of total alveolar ventilation to alveoli with different ventilation/blood flow until the $Pa_{inert}/P\overline{V}_{inert}$ and $PA_{inert}/P\overline{V}_{inert}$ calculated from equations 4 and 5 give the best fit for all six inert gases.

For Chapter 8, Diffusion

A. Diffusion of Gases

The molecules of gas are constantly in motion and moving in random direction. Consequently, if there is a greater concentration of molecules of a particular gas in one region than in another, the laws of statistics permit us to predict the time required to abolish this difference in concentration. The conservation of energy is such that two different gases having an equal number of molecules in an equal volume possess the same molecular energy. Light molecules, since they possess the same molecular energy as heavier molecules, will travel faster, collide more frequently and diffuse faster than heavy molecules.

Graham's Law.—The relative rates of diffusion of gases under the same conditions are inversely proportional to the square root of the densities of those gases.

Henry's Law.—When a gas diffuses between a gaseous phase and a liquid phase, the solubility of the gas in the liquid must also be considered. This is expressed by Henry's law, which states that the weight of a slightly soluble gas that dissolves in a definite weight of a liquid at a given temperature is very nearly directly proportional to the partial pressure of that gas. This holds for gases that do not unite chemically with the solvent. At the surface of the liquid or tissue into which gas is diffusing the gas tension will be equal to that in the gas phase, but immediately below the surface it will be less. The solubility of CO_2 in water is higher than O_2, and therefore its concentration in the surface layer will be higher. Thus, for the diffusion of CO_2 into a liquid or tissue, there will be a large *concentration* gradient between the surface and deeper layers. Since the diffusion rate within a liquid is dependent upon its *concentration* gradient, the greater the solubility of a gas in a liquid, the more rapid its rate of diffusion will be in the liquid.

When the laws of diffusion and solubility are combined, the relative rates of diffusion of two different gases between a gaseous and a liquid phase is found to be proportional to the ratio of solubilities of the gases in the liquid, and inversely proportional to the ratio of the square roots of the molecular weights of the gases. For example,

$$\frac{D_{O_2}}{D_{CO}} = \frac{\text{Sol. } O_2}{\text{Sol. CO}} \times \frac{\sqrt{MW_{CO}}}{\sqrt{MW_{O_2}}} = \frac{0.0244}{0.0185}\sqrt{\frac{28}{32}} = 1.23$$

Another gas, CO_2, is much more soluble than oxygen in water and

$$\frac{D_{CO_2}}{D_{O_2}} = \frac{0.592}{0.0244}\sqrt{\frac{32}{44}} = 20.7$$

There are two types of diffusion that are important in pulmonary physiology.

1. *Diffusion in a gas medium.*—This is the process by which a gas diffuses from one point within an alveolus to another or from an alveolus along the bronchial tree to the mouth (when there is no mass movement of air, i.e., alveolar ventilation). The alveolus is so small that any difference between the partial pressure of a gas at one point and another in the alveolus will be eliminated by gaseous diffusion within a fraction of a second. However, when a gas must diffuse over longer distances, e.g., from an alveolus to the mouth, the rate of diffusion is much too slow to permit any useful gas exchange. This is well illustrated by the accumulation of CO_2 that occurs in the alveoli, blood, and tissues during a period of respiratory arrest. (The process by which arterial O_2 saturation may be maintained for a while by supplying O_2 to the nose and mouth, during a period of complete respiratory arrest, is really not "diffusion respiration"; the saturation is maintained in part by a very high initial P_{O_2} in the alveoli and in part by mass movement of O_2 from mouth to alveoli caused by an R of <1.0, so that the alveolar gas volume shrinks slightly and lowers the total pressure of gases in the alveoli below atmospheric pressure.)

2. *Diffusion across a membrane.*—This has been discussed in chapter 8; certain special problems relating to this process are discussed below.

B. Pulmonary Diffusing Capacity Measured by Single-Breath CO Method

In this technique, starting from residual volume, the subject inspires maximally a gas mixture containing a low concentration (0.3%) of CO and 10% helium. He holds this breath for about 10 seconds, then rapidly expires an alveolar gas sample. If the lung is considered a closed bag of volume V_A (STPD) from which gas CO disappears at a rate proportional to its concentration, the alveolar CO concentration ($F_{A_{CO}}$) at any time is given by the equation of Krogh:

$$F_{A_{CO}} = F_{A_{CO_0}} \text{ exponent}\left(\frac{D_L 713\ t}{V_A\ 60}\right) \tag{1}$$

where $F_{A_{CO_0}}$ is the alveolar CO concentration before any absorption into the blood has occurred, 713 is the total pressure of dry gases, D_L is the diffusing capacity, 60 is the number of seconds in a minute and t is the time in seconds. This can be rearranged to solve for D_L.

$$D_L = \frac{V_A 60}{713\ t} \text{Ln}_e \left[\frac{F_{A_{CO_0}}}{F_{A_{CO}}}\right] \tag{2}$$

$F_{A_{CO}}$ can be measured in the expired sample. t is 10 seconds. V_A is the total alveolar volume which can be calculated from the volume inspired plus the residual volume. The initial alveolar CO concentration $F_{A_{CO}}$ is calculated from the concentration of He in the expired alveolar sample ($F_{A_{He}}$); because He is relatively insoluble, its dilution in the expired sample equals the dilution of the inspired CO *before* any of it had been absorbed by the blood. Therefore,

$$\frac{F_{A_{He}}}{F_{I_{He}}} = \frac{F_{A_{CO}}}{F_{I_{CO}}} \text{ or } F_{A_{CO}} = \frac{F_{A_{He}}}{F_{I_{He}}} F_{I_{CO}} \tag{3}$$

Since inspired CO ($F_{I_{CO}}$) and inspired He ($F_{I_{He}}$) are known, as well as expired alveolar He ($F_{A_{He}}$), the initial alveolar CO ($F_{A_{CO_0}}$) can be calculated. All the unknowns in equation (1) are then available, and D_L can be calculated. In a typical example,

Inspired CO concentration ($F_{I_{CO}}$) = 0.300%
Inspired He concentration ($F_{I_{He}}$) = 10%
Expired alveolar CO ($F_{A_{CO}}$) = 0.159% after 10 sec breath-holding
Expired alveolar He ($F_{A_{He}}$) = 8%

Total alveolar volume during breath-holding equals 4,930 ml STPD; inspired volume is 4,000 ml STPD and residual alveolar volume 930 ml STPD. Substituting in equation (3)

$$F_{A_{CO_0}} = \frac{8\%}{10\%} \times 0.300\% = 0.240\%\text{CO}$$

Substituting in equation (2)

$$D = \frac{4930 \times 60}{713 \times 10} \text{Ln}_e \left(\frac{0.240}{0.159}\right) = 41.4 \times 0.415$$

$$= 17 \text{ ml CO/min/mm Hg pressure difference}$$

The breath-holding time is generally measured from the start of the inspiration of the CO mixture to the start of expiration of the alveolar sample. This is an approximation because inspiration and expiration require a finite time and the CO does not spend all the 'breath-holding' time so calculated in the alveolar gas at the inspired volume.

C. Alveolar CO Tension Calculated for Steady-State Method

The object of this method is to calculate the alveolar P_{CO}, knowing expired CO_2 concentration ($F_{E_{CO_2}}$), expired CO concentration ($F_{E_{CO}}$), arterial P_{CO_2} (Pa_{CO_2}) and inspired CO concentration ($F_{I_{CO}}$) under steady-state conditions, when the patient is breathing a gas mixture containing a low percentage of CO. We can rearrange Bohr's equation to give

$$\frac{V_D}{V_E} = \frac{F_{A_{CO_2}} - F_{E_{CO_2}}}{F_{A_{CO_2}}} \qquad (1)$$

We can calculate V_D/V_E for CO_2, as on page 000. If we rearrange equation (5) under Bohr's equation and consider the unknown gas x to be CO

$$\frac{V_D}{V_E} = \frac{F_{A_{CO}} - F_{E_{CO}}}{F_{A_{CO}} - F_{I_{CO}}} \qquad (2)$$

We assume that V_D/V_E is the same for CO. Therefore we can solve equation (2) for the desired $F_{A_{CO}}$ because we know V_D/V_E, $F_{E_{CO}}$, and $F_{I_{CO}}$. These two operations have been combined into one by Filley by equating (1) and (2).

$$\frac{V_D}{V_E} = \frac{F_{A_{CO_2}} - F_{E_{CO_2}}}{F_{A_{CO_2}}} = \frac{F_{A_{CO}} - F_{E_{CO}}}{F_{A_{CO}} - F_{I_{CO}}} \qquad (3)$$

This is now solved for alveolar CO concentration

$$F_{A_{CO}} = F_{I_{CO}} - \frac{F_{A_{CO_2}}}{F_{E_{CO_2}}}(F_{I_{CO}} - F_{E_{CO}}) \qquad (4)$$

It is of interest to point out that if O_2 were substituted for CO in this equation, it would become another form of the alveolar air equation given on page 267.

In a typical example, arterial P_{CO_2} is 40 mm Hg (40/713 equals 5.6%), expired CO_2 concentration is 3.7%, inspired CO concentration is 0.2%, and expired CO concentration is 0.102%. Substituting in equation (4)

$$F_{A_{CO}} = 0.2 - \frac{5.6}{3.7}[0.2 - 0.102] = 0.2 - 0.148 = .052\%\ CO$$

This value, converted to $P_{A_{CO}}$, can be used to calculate D_{CO}.

D. Calculation of Alveolar Pco in Equilibrium With Alveolar Capillary Blood

The CO equilibrium curve for hemoglobin has the same shape as that for the oxygen equilibrium curve, but the affinity of CO for hemoglobin is 225 to 250 times that for oxygen. If blood is in equilibrium with a mixture of CO and O_2, the concentrations of carbon monoxyhemoglobin (HbCO) and oxyhemoglobin (HbO_2) will be in the ratio 225 times P_{CO}/P_{O_2} as given in the following equation:

$$\frac{HbCO\%}{HbO_2\%} = \frac{M\ P_{CO}}{P_{O_2}} \qquad (1)$$

"M" is known as the Haldane factor, named after the man who first described this phenomenon. The equilibrated P_{CO} can be calculated from this equation knowing the ratio $P_{O_2}/HbO_2\%$ and HbCO%.

If there is a significant concentration of HbCO in the pulmonary capillary blood, this will produce an equilibrated P_{CO} in the red cells ($P_{RBC_{CO}}$) which will decrease the effective diffusing gradient from the alveolar gas to the hemoglobin molecule and if it is not taken into account will decrease the measured value of D_LCO. The correct diffusion gradient is ($Pa_{CO} - P_{RBC_{CO}}$), and this should replace Pa_{CO} in all calculations of D_LCO.

The $P_{RBC_{CO}}$ can be obtained in the patient by first measuring [HbCO] in a sample of venous blood, assuming that the capillary P_{O_2} equals alveolar P_{O_2} and that HbO_2 saturation equals 100% and calculating $P_{RBC_{CO}}$ from equation 1. The arterial-venous difference of CO content in any of the capillary beds is so small under any safe conditions that [HbCO] can be considered the same in any blood sample. At high Pa_{O_2}, that is, at 200 mm Hg or greater, the mean capillary P_{O_2} can be considered equal to Pa_{O_2}, as discussed in section E on D_M and V_C. This will not be true at P_{O_2} around 100 mm Hg, the level for most measurements of D_LCO and use of Pa_{O_2} in equation 1 will lead to an over-estimate of $P_{RBC_{CO}}$. The average $HbO_2\%$ along the capillary will be nearly 100% for high P_{O_2}, but breathing air will range between 75% and 95% saturation.

$P_{RBC_{CO}}$ is normally not important in the single-breath D_LCO measurement. 1% HbCO saturation at a P_{O_2} of 400 mm Hg would produce an equilibrated $P_{RBC_{CO}}$ of 0.009 mm Hg, less than 1% of the alveolar

P_{CO_2} at the end of the normal 10-second period of breath-holding, which is not significant. Whole blood samples have some HbCO (about 0.5%) even in nonsmokers, because 0.4 ml of CO is produced per hour in a normal adult from a metabolism of heme. One molecule of CO is produced for every porphyrin molecule split.

The correction for $P_{RBC_{CO}}$ is much more important for the steady-state $D_{L}CO$ measurement since the alveolar P_{CO} is kept much lower in order to reduce the total amount of CO taken up in the procedure.

Another procedure for the estimation of equilibrated blood P_{CO} is to have the patient rebreathe 100% oxygen from a bag until CO approaches an equilibrium between alveolar gas and pulmonary capillary blood (over 30 seconds), and then measure P_{CO} in the rebreathing bag gas. The equilibrated back pressure, $P_{RBC_{CO}}$, for any particular alveolar P_{O_2} can be obtained simply by multiplying by the ratio Pa_{O_2}/P_{O_2} in the rebreathing bag. This calculation assumes the average capillary HbO_2% saturation is the same.

E. Calculation of D_M and V_C

The exchange path for CO from alveolar air to the hemoglobin molecule inside the red cell in the pulmonary capillary can be divided into two parts (see Fig 58).

1. *The alveolar-capillary membrane.*—From the alveolar gas through the alveolar epithelium, basement membrane and interstitial space and then through a plasma layer to the surface of the red cell.

2. *The red blood cell.*—Including diffusion through a possible stagnant layer at its surface, through the membrane and then transport by simultaneous diffusion and chemical reaction with a high concentration of hemoglobin in the cell interior.

During the measurement of $D_{L}CO$, the flux of CO through each of the two steps above is the same and is proportional to the pressure difference across the two segments of the total path. We can therefore break up the P_{CO} gradient into these steps and divide by the rate of CO uptake as follows:

$$\frac{P_{A_{CO}} - P_{RBC_{CO}}}{\text{CO uptake rate}} = \frac{P_{A_{CO}} - P_{PL_{CO}}}{\text{CO uptake rate}} + \frac{P_{PL_{CO}} - P_{RBC_{CO}}}{\text{CO uptake rate}} \qquad (1)$$

$P_{A_{CO}}$, $P_{PL_{CO}}$, and $P_{RBC_{CO}}$ are the partial pressure of CO in mm Hg in alveolar gas, plasma, and within the red blood cell, respectively. CO uptake rate is in ml STPD/min.

By definition,

$$\frac{P_{A_{CO}} - P_{RBC_{CO}}}{\text{CO uptake rate}} = \frac{1}{D_L} \tag{2}$$

Again by definition,

$$\frac{P_{A_{CO}} - P_{PL_{CO}}}{\text{CO uptake rate}} = 1/D_M \tag{3}$$

D_M is the diffusing capacity of the alveolar-capillary membrane. $P_{A_{CO}} - P_{L_{CO}}$ is the partial pressure difference across that membrane. $(P_{PL_{CO}} - P_{RBC_{CO}})$/CO uptake is by analogy the reciprocal of the diffusing capacity of all the red cells in the pulmonary bed in any instant.

There is no available technique to measure the plasma $P_{CO}(P_{PL_{CO}})$. The partial pressure of CO in the red cell, $P_{RBC_{CO}}$ is the value of P_{CO} in equilibrium with the carbon monoxyhemoglobin present and can either be neglected or its value measured directly (see section D). However, we can measure the rate (ml/min) at which a milliliter of normal whole blood combines with CO in solution at 1 mm Hg partial pressure using a rapid mixing apparatus in vitro. This is the diffusing capacity of 1 ml of whole blood for CO and is customarily symbolized as θ_{CO}. The diffusing capacity of the red cells in the lung capillary bed will equal θ_{CO} times the volume of blood in the capillary bed in milliliters or θV_C.

If we now substitute these three relations in equation 1 we obtain equation 4:

$$\frac{1}{D_L} = \frac{1}{D_M} + \frac{1}{\theta V_C} \tag{4}$$

This derivation assumes that the P_{O_2} (and HbO_2) of alveolar capillary blood is constant along the capillary and equal to alveolar P_{O_2}. This is only true when $P_{A_{O_2}}$ is high, over 200 mm Hg.

Theta (θ) depends on the rate of the chemical reaction of CO with hemoglobin within the red cell plus diffusion through the cell substance. The chemical reaction rate is proportional to the concentration of CO times the concentration of unliganded hemoglobin (with neither CO or O_2 attached). As P_{O_2} increases, the concentration of unliganded hemoglobin decreases almost precisely proportional to $1/P_{O_2}$ once the P_{O_2} is over 200 mm Hg. This alone should cause θ also to decrease proportionally to $1/P_{O_2}$.

The reason for this is as follows. There are four Fe^{++} atoms on each hemoglobin tetramer, and as each CO (or O_2) molecule binds to the protein the reaction velocities for the succeeding bindings are altered; the actual reaction velocity constant increases. However, above 200 mm Hg there are practically no molecules with more than one remaining unliganded position, so the reaction velocity constant does not increase further with increasing P_{O_2} and the chemical reaction rate is proportional to $1/P_{O_2}$.

In the red blood cell there is a complicated interaction between the diffusion and chemical reaction processes so that the rate of uptake of CO by the red blood cell is considerably less than the corresponding reaction rate in free solution. However, at high P_{O_2} the overall CO exchange slows down so much that intracellular diffusion becomes less important and the reciprocal relationship of θ with P_{O_2} holds.

In summary, above an alveolar P_{O_2} of 150 to 200 mm Hg, we can assume that θ for the cells in the pulmonary capillary bed varies proportionally to $1/P_{O_2}$. The most extensive data fit the relation

$$\frac{1}{\theta} = 0.0049 + 1.98 \; P_{O_2} \text{ in mm Hg}$$

If we now measure D_LCO in a patient at different alveolar P_{O_2} values and plot the measured values of $1/D_L$ against the value of $1/\theta$ for that alveolar P_{O_2}, we obtain a graphical solution of equation 4. The intercept on the ordinate, the $1/D_L$ axis, equals $1/D_M$. The slope equals $1/V_C$.

Theta depends on the number of red cells present, or the hemoglobin concentration, and the CO diffusing capacity of the individual red cells. We assume that the hematocrit, or O_2 (or CO) capacity of the blood in the pulmonary capillary bed is the same as that in the peripheral venous blood, although this is probably not strictly true. Variations in peripheral hematocrit such as the decrease seen in anemia, will decrease θ_{CO} and therefore decrease D_LCO. No significant variation in θ_{CO} for the same volume of red blood cells among individuals has been reported.

Theta$_{CO}$ for a patient with an abnormal hemoglobin concentration can be calculated from θ_{CO} at normal hemoglobin concentration (15 gm/100 ml), given by the regression above, using the relation

$$\theta_{CO} \text{ for X gm/100 ml} = \theta_{CO} \text{ for 15 gm/100 ml} \times X/15$$

The equation for $1/D_LCO$ on p. 299 can be used to calculate the D_LCO corrected for the abnormal hemoglobin concentration as follows:

$$D_LCO \text{ corrected} = D_LCO,X \; \frac{1 + 1/(\theta_{CO,X} V_C/D_M)}{1 + 1/(\theta_{CO,15} \; V_C/D_M)}$$

D_LCO,X is measured in the patient with a hemoglobin concentration of X gm/100 ml. V_C/D_M must be measured, or assumed to be normal, about 1.5.

When D_LCO is measured at altitude the lower $P_{A_{O_2}}$ will increase

θ_{CO} and thus increase D_LCO. $Theta_{CO}$ for the particular PA_{O_2} can be calculated from the regression equation above. The D_LCO corrected to the normal alveolar PO_2 of 100 mm Hg can then be computed from the relation above where the subscript X refers to values at the abnormal alveolar PO_2.

F. Bohr's Integration Procedure for Calculation of Mean PO_2 of Pulmonary Capillary Blood

In measurements of pulmonary diffusing capacity, it is necessary to know the mean pressure gradient driving O_2 across the alveolar-capillary membranes. Under certain conditions (see lower part of Fig 62, p. 210), the mean gradient is very close to the (initial gradient-final gradient)/2, but it is often far removed from the latter value (see upper part of Fig 62). The mean gradient can be determined precisely only if the PO_2 gradient from gas to blood is known at every instant along the pulmonary capillary. This can be determined by Bohr's integration procedure, which requires knowledge of (1) alveolar PO_2, (2) mixed venous PO_2, (3) end-pulmonary capillary PO_2, and (4) the interrelationship between blood PO_2 and O_2 saturation (the oxyhemoglobin dissociation curve).

Table 22 shows each step in the integration procedure. The subject is a normal man breathing 14% O_2. Alveolar PO_2 is calculated to be 57 mm Hg. The PO_2 of his mixed venous blood is 32 mm Hg and the O_2 saturation is 58%; the PO_2 of end-pulmonary capillary blood is 51 mm Hg (obtained by the "trial and error" procedure), and the O_2 saturation is 84%. In column *A* is listed each 1% increase in HbO_2 saturation between mixed venous blood (58%) and end-pulmonary capillary blood (84%). In column *B* is listed the blood PO_2 that corresponds to each saturation value.

Although this presents all the increments in PO_2 and O_2 saturation that the blood must experience in changing from venous to arterialized blood, it gives no information as to the *time* that is required for each of these unit changes in saturation. When the saturation (SO_2) is 60% (see Table 22) and the driving pressure is 24 mm Hg, O_2 diffuses across the alveolar-capillary membranes twice as fast as when the saturation has risen to 79% and the driving pressure is only 12 mm Hg. Thus, it takes twice as long for the saturation to rise from 79% to 80% as it does to rise from 60% to 61%. The relative time *(t)* required for each increment in SO_2 (Δ SO_2) can be determined as follows:

$$\text{Rate of diffusion of } O_2 = \text{change in } O_2 \text{ saturation/time}$$

$$\therefore \text{Rate of diffusion of } O_2 = \frac{\Delta\ SO_2}{t}$$

TABLE 22.—Calculation of the Oxygen Tension Along the Pulmonary Capillary in a Normal Man Breathing 14% O_2

	A PUL. CAP. HBO_2 % SAT. SO_2	B PUL. CAP. O_2 TENSION FC_{O_2} MM HG	C ALV.-CAP. GRADIENT AT EACH POINT $57 - PC_{O_2}$ MM HG	D RECIPROCAL OF EACH GRADIENT $\frac{1}{57 - PC_{O_2}}$	E SUM OF RECIPROCALS TO EACH POINT $\sum \frac{1}{57 - PC_{O_2}}$	F % OF TOTAL (1.7661) TO EACH POINT	G TIME (SEC) TO EACH POINT
Mixed venous blood →	58	32			0.000	0.0	0.0
	59	32.5	24.5	0.0409	0.0409	2.3	0.017
	60	33	24	0.0416	0.0825	4.7	0.035
	61	33.5	23.5	0.0425	0.1250	7.1	0.053
	62	34	23	0.0435	0.1685	9.6	0.072
	63	34.5	22.5	0.0445	0.2130	12.0	0.090
	64	35	22	0.0455	0.2585	14.6	0.110
	65	35.5	21.5	0.0465	0.3050	17.3	0.130
	66	36.0	21	0.0475	0.3525	20.0	0.150
	67	37	20	0.0500	0.4025	22.8	0.172
	68	37.5	19.5	0.0513	0.4538	25.7	0.194
	69	38	19	0.0526	0.5064	28.7	0.215
	70	38.5	18.5	0.0540	0.5604	31.8	0.237
	71	39	18	0.0556	0.6160	35.0	0.263
	72	40	17	0.0588	0.6748	38.2	0.287
	73	40.5	16.6	0.0606	0.7354	41.6	0.313
	74	41.5	15.5	0.0645	0.7999	45.4	0.340
	75	42	15	0.0666	0.8665	49.0	0.367
	76	43	14	0.0715	0.9380	53.2	0.400
	77	43.5	13.5	0.0740	1.0120	57.2	0.430
	78	44	13	0.0770	1.0890	61.6	0.462
	79	45	12	0.0834	1.1724	66.3	0.496
	80	46	11	0.0910	1.2634	71.4	0.535
	81	47	10	0.1000	1.3634	77.0	0.577
	82	48	9	0.1110	1.4744	83.5	0.626
	83	49	8	0.1250	1.5994	90.5	0.680
End-pulmonary capillary blood →	84	51	6	0.1667	1.7661	100.0	0.750

This rate is proportional to the Po_2 gradient between alveolar gas and pulmonary capillary blood.

$$\therefore \frac{\Delta\ So_2}{t} \propto (P_{A_{O_2}} - P_{C_{O_2}})$$

or

$$\frac{\Delta\ So_2}{t} = K\ (P_{A_{O_2}} - P_{C_{O_2}})$$

The time required for each increment in So_2 then becomes

$$t = \frac{\Delta\ So_2}{K\ (P_{A_{O_2}} - P_{C_{O_2}})}$$

Since, in our example (Table 22), each increment in So_2 is constant (1%) and since K is a constant, the time required for each increment to occur is proportional to the reciprocal of the Po_2 gradient. Thus,

$$t \propto \frac{1}{P_{A_{O_2}} - P_{C_{O_2}}}$$

$\frac{1}{P_{A_{O_2}} - P_{C_{O_2}}}$ is the reciprocal of the O_2 pressure gradient at each point along the pulmonary capillary and provides an index of time required to achieve each ΔO_2 saturation.

Column *C* is a tabulation of each ($P_{A_{O_2}} - P_{C_{O_2}}$*), or the alveolar capillary pressure gradient. Column *D* lists the reciprocal of each alveolar-capillary pressure gradient in column *C;* each reciprocal is proportional to the time needed to produce each 1% increase in saturation. Each figure in column *E* is the total of the reciprocals up to each point, and each is therefore proportional to the time needed to increase the blood O_2 saturation from the mixed venous value to the saturation at that point. The last number in column *E* (1.766) is proportional to the total time the capillary blood took to increase from the mixed venous saturation to the end-capillary saturation. Column *F* shows the percentage of the total time required for the transfer of O_2 to each point. The total time required for the blood to traverse the pulmonary capillary in a resting normal subject is about 0.75 sec. Using this value, column *G* shows the actual time required for the transfer of each unit of O_2 in the pulmonary capillary. In Figure 62 the capillary Po_2 values (column *B*) are plotted against time (column *G*).

*The Po_2 of pulmonary capillary blood at the *end* of each stepwise increase of saturation is used instead of the average. Actually, this procedure is inexact unless a very large number of steps is used.

Calculation of Mean Capillary P_{O_2}.—Once the capillary P_{O_2} is plotted as in Figure 62, the mean capillary P_{O_2} can be obtained graphically, by finding the value of P_{O_2}, which is as often above as below the actual capillary P_{O_2}. This mean capillary P_{O_2} (42 mm Hg) is shown as a dotted line in Figure 62; the two shaded areas between the mean capillary P_{O_2} and the actual capillary P_{O_2} must be equal.

If alveolar P_{O_2}, mixed venous P_{O_2}, and end-pulmonary capillary P_{O_2} are known, the mean capillary P_{O_2} can be determined. In fact, if any three of these four figures are known, the fourth can be determined without further measurement.

*G. Trial-and-Error Estimation of Diffusing Capacity of Lungs for Oxygen**

$$D_{L}O_2 = \frac{\dot{V}O_2}{\overline{P}A_{O_2} - \overline{P}C_{O_2}}$$

Where $D_{L}O_2$ = diffusing capacity of the lungs for O_2; $\dot{V}O_2$ = O_2 consumption/min; $\overline{P}A_{O_2}$ = mean alveolar O_2 pressure (calculated) and $\overline{P}C_{O_2}$ = mean pulmonary capillary O_2 pressure. $\overline{P}C_{O_2}$ requires knowledge of the *end*-pulmonary capillary P_{O_2} ($P\acute{C}_{O_2}$). This cannot be measured directly but can be estimated by a trial-and-error method of Riley as follows:

Step 1: Patient breathing air

MEASURE	ESTIMATE	CALCULATE
1. Arterial P_{O_2} and O_2 content 2. Mixed venous P_{O_2} and O_2 content 3. Mean alveolar P_{O_2} 4. O_2 consumption/min	5. End-pulmonary capillary P_{O_2} (see Fig 61) and O_2 content	6. Physiologic shunt ($\dot{Q}s$) (from 1, 2, and 5 using the shunt equation) $\frac{\dot{Q}s}{\dot{Q}} = \frac{Ca_{O_2} - C\acute{c}_{O_2}}{C\overline{v}_{O_2} - C\acute{c}_{O_2}}$

Step 2: Patient breathing 14% O_2

MEASURE	ASSUME	CALCULATE

*See page 211.

7. Arterial PO_2 and O_2 content	11. Physiologic shunt (=6, above)	12. *End*-pulmonary capillary *O_2 content* (from 7, 8, 11, and shunt equation) and corresponding PO_2 (from O_2 dissociation curve)
8. Mixed venous PO_2 and O_2 content		13. *Mean* capillary PO_2 (from 8, 9, 12 using Bohr's integration procedure)
9. Mean alveolar PO_2		14. DO_2 (from 10, 9, and 13)
10. O_2 consumption/min		

Step 3: Patient breathing air

MEASURE	ASSUME	CALCULATE
15. Use measured values 1, 2, 3, and 4 (above)	16. DO_2 (=14, above)	17. *Mean* pulmonary capillary PO_2 (from 16, 4, and 3)
		18. *End*-pulmonary capillary PO_2 (from 17, 2, and 3)

Steps 1 and 18 all depend on the accuracy of No. 5 (estimated value of end-pulmonary capillary PO_2), since No. 5 is used to calculate the physiologic shunt and the latter is necessary to calculate DO_2 (No. 14).

This value for DO_2 is the *true* one *only* if, when used with the *measured* values 2 and 3, it yields the estimated value for end-pulmonary capillary pressure. If it does not, the "trial" was in "error" and a new estimate of No. 5 must be made until compatible values are found that fit the values obtained both during the breathing of air and of 14% O_2. The process of trial and error is facilitated by the use of graphs prepared by Riley.

The method depends on the assumptions that the physiologic shunt and the DO_2 do not change when the patient breathes 12% to 14% O_2 instead of air.

The trial-and-error method interprets experimental measurements of alveolar and arterial PO_2 breathing low O_2 concentrations (about 14%) and air, in terms of a uniform lung of single D_LO_2 plus a right-to-left venous-to-arterial shunt across the pulmonary capillary bed. It is accepted that the shunt is in part a result of nonuniform alveolar ventilation/blood flow.

Briscoe and King have developed a more realistic model, which considers the lung as made up of two different phases, or spaces, with two different alveolar volumes and ventilations, pulmonary blood flows, and diffusing capacities for O_2, plus a true right-to-left shunt across the pulmonary capillary bed. Arterial and expired P_{O_2} and P_{CO_2} and minute ventilation are measured under steady-state conditions during the inspiration of three different O_2 concentrations: low (about 20.9%, or air), medium (about 25%), and high (about 30%). Blood flow through the right-to-left shunt is obtained from values of arterial P_{O_2} and alveolar P_{O_2} while breathing 100% O_2 (according to equation 3 on p. 286). The volumes and alveolar ventilation of the two phases of the lung are obtained from analysis of the nitrogen washout curves (chapter 3).

The remaining unknowns are the two $D_{L}O_2$ values for the two lung spaces and the pulmonary blood flow through one space (pulmonary blood flow through the second space is calculated by subtraction from the total blood flow, which is known), for which we have three sets of data, essentially ($P_{A_{O_2}} - P_{a_{O_2}}$), at three different $P_{I_{O_2}}$. The solution is simplified by development of graphical techniques, plotting the HbO_2% saturation against P_{O_2} for the following:

1. Blood oxygen equilibrium curve

2. Lines for constant ventilation alveolar ventilation/blood flow, which approximates $(S_{c_{O_2}} - S_{\bar{v}_{O_2}})/(P_{I_{O_2}} - P_{A_{O_2}})$ at each inspired oxygen concentration where $S_{c_{O_2}}$ and $S_{\bar{v}_{O_2}}$ are the HbO% saturation in capillary blood at any point and mixed venous blood respectively. This line is approximately straight and decreases with increasing P_{O_2}.

3. Lines for constant $D_{L}O_2/\dot{Q}c$ (Bohr isopleths), which equal:

$$\int_{S_{\bar{v}_{O_2}}}^{S_{c'_{O_2}}} \frac{d\,S_{c_{O_2}}}{P_{A_{O_2}} - P_{c_{O_2}}}$$

where $S_{c'_{O_2}}$ is the HbO_2% saturation in end capillary blood. These lines are also approximately linear, but *increase* as P_{O_2} increases.

This method is particularly suitable for patients with severe lung disease where $(P_{A_{O_2}} - P_{c'_{O_2}})$ is large, even at inspired oxygen concentrations greater than air. Results in patients with severe chronic obstructive lung disease show that the poorly ventilated space of the lung is much larger than the better ventilated space and may have a remarkably low $D_{L}O_2$.

Bibliography

General

Macklin C.C.: The musculature of the bronchi and lungs. *Physiol. Rev.* 9:1–60, 1929.

Miller W.S.: *The Lung,* ed. 2. Springfield, Ill., Charles C Thomas, Publisher, 1947.

Baldwin E.deF., Cournand A., Richards D.W. Jr.: Pulmonary insufficiency. *Medicine* 27:243–278, 1948; 28:1–25, 1949; 28:201–237, 1949.

Comroe J.H. Jr. (ed.): Pulmonary function tests, in *Methods in Medical Research.* Chicago, Year Book Medical Publishers, 1950, vol. 2, pp. 74–244.

Comroe J.H. Jr.: The functions of the lung. *Harvey Lect.* 48:110–144, 1952–53.

Dittmer D.S., Grebe R.M. (eds.): *Handbook of Respiration.* Philadelphia, W.B. Saunders Co., 1958.

Bartels H., et al.: *Lungenfuntionsprufungen.* Berlin, Springer Verlag, 1959.

Gordon B. (ed.): *Clinical Cardiopulmonary Physiology,* ed. 2. New York, Grune & Stratton, 1960.

Rossier P.H., Buhlmann A.A., Wiesinger K.: *Respiration: Physiologic Principles and Their Clinical Application,* Luchsinger P.C., Moser K.M. (trans.). St. Louis, C.V. Mosby Co., 1960.

deReuck A.V.S., O'Connor M. (eds.): *Pulmonary Structure and Function: Ciba Foundation Symposium.* London, Churchill Ltd., 1962.

Cunningham D.J.C., Lloyd B.B. (eds.): *J.S. Haldane Symposium.* Oxford, Blackwell Scientific Publications Ltd., 1962.

Bates D.V., Macklem P.T., Christie R.V.: *Respiratory Function in Disease,* ed. 2. Philadelphia, W.B. Saunders Co., 1971.

Comroe J.H. Jr.: *Physiology of Respiration,* ed. 2. Chicago, Year Book Medical Publishers, 1974.

Nunn J.F.: *Applied Respiratory Physiology,* ed. 2. London, Butterworths, 1977.

Cotes J.E.: *Lung Function Assessment and Application in Medicine,* ed. 4. Oxford, Blackwell Scientific Publications, 1979.

West J.B.: *Respiration Physiology: The Essentials,* ed. 2. Baltimore, Williams & Wilkins, 1979.

Laslo G., Sudlow M.F.: *Measurement in Clinical Respiratory Physiology,* Medical Physics Series. London, Academic Press Inc., 1983.

Morris A.H., Kanner R.E., Crapo R.O., et al.: *Clinical Pulmonary Function Testing,* ed. 2. Salt Lake City, Intermountain Thoracic Society, 1984.

Fishman A.P. (ed.): The Respiratory System, Section 3, in *Handbook of Physiology*. Bethesda, American Physiological Society, Vol. 1, 1985; vol. 2, 1986.

Lung Volumes

Davy H.: *Researches, Chemical and Philosophical, Chiefly Concerning Nitrous Oxide or Dephologisticated Air and Its Respiration,* ed. 2. London, A. Waldie, 1840.

Hutchinson J.: Lecture on vital statistics, embracing an account of a new instrument for detecting the presence of disease in the system. *Lancet* 1:567–570, 594–596, 1844.

Christie R.V.: Lung volume and its subdivisions. *J. Clin. Invest.* 11:1099–1118, 1932.

McMichael J.: A rapid method for determining lung capacity. *Clin. Sci.* 4:167–173, 1939.

Darling R.C., Cournand A., Richards D.W. Jr.: Studies on the intrapulmonary mixture of gases: III. An open circuit for measuring residual air. *J. Clin. Invest.* 19:609–618, 1940.

Gilson J.G., Hugh-Jones P.: Measurement of total lung volume and breathing capacity. *Clin. Sci.* 7:185–216, 1949.

Meneely G.R., Kaltreider N.L.: Volume of the lung determined by helium dilution. *J. Clin. Invest.* 28:129–139, 1949.

Rahn H., Fenn W.O., Otis A.B.: Daily variations of vital capacity, residual air and expiratory reserve including a study of the residual air methods. *J. Appl. Physiol.* 1:725–736, 1949.

Whitefield A.G., Waterhouse J.A.H., Arnott W.M.: Subdivisions of lung volume: Normal standards. *Br. J. Soc. Med.* 4:1–25, 1950.

Hickman J.B., Blair E., Frayser R.: An open-circuit helium method for measuring functional residual capacity and defective intrapulmonary gas mixing. *J. Clin. Invest.* 33:1277–1286, 1954.

DuBois A.B., Botelho S.Y., Bedell G.N., et al.: A rapid plethysmographic method for measuring thoracic gas volume: A comparison with a nitrogen washout method for measuring functional residual capacity in normal subjects. *J. Clin. Invest.* 35:322–326, 1956.

Helliesen P.J., Cook C.D., Friedlander L., et al.: Mechanics of respiration and lung volumes in 85 normal children 5 to 17 years of age. *Pediatrics* 22:80–93, 1958.

Polgar G., Promadhat V.: *Pulmonary Function Testing in Children: Techniques and Standards.* Philadelphia, W.B. Saunders Co., 1971.

Pulmonary Ventilation

Henderson Y., Chillingworth F.P., Whitney J.L.: Respiratory dead space. *Am. J. Physiol.* 38:1–19, 1915.

Krogh A., Lindhard J.: The volume of dead space in breathing and the mixing of gases in the lungs of man. *J. Physiol.* 51:59–90, 1917.

Cournand A., et al.: Studies on intrapulmonary mixture of gases: IV. Significance of pulmonary emptying rate. *J. Clin. Invest.* 20:681–689, 1941.

Darling R.C., Cournand A., Richards D.W. Jr.: Studies on intrapulmonary mixture of gases: V. Forms of inadequate ventilation in normal and emphysematous lungs, analyzed by means by breathing pure oxygen. *J. Clin. Invest.* 23:55–67, 1944.

Rauwerda P.E.: *Unequal Ventilation of Different Parts of the Lung,* thesis, University of Groningen, Holland, 1946.

Riley R.L., Lilienthal J.L., Proemmel D.D., et al.: On the determination of the physiologically effective pressures of O_2 and CO_2 in alveolar air. *Am. J. Physiol.* 147:191–198, 1946.

Fenn W.O., Rahn H., Otis A.B.: A theoretical study of the composition of the alveolar air at altitude. *Am. J. Physiol.* 146:637–653, 1946.

Fowler W.S.: The respiratory dead space. *Am. J. Physiol.* 154:405–416, 1948.

Fowler W.S.: Uneven pulmonary ventilation. *J. Appl. Physiol.* 2:283–299, 1949.

Bates D.V., Christie R.V.: Intrapulmonary mixing of helium in health and in emphysema. *Clin. Sci.* 9:17–29, 1950.

Comroe J.H. Jr., Fowler W.S.: Detection of uneven ventilation during a single breath of O_2. *Am. J. Med.* 10:408–413, 1951.

Briscoe W.A.: Further studies on the intrapulmonary mixing of helium in normal and emphysematous subjects. *Clin. Sci.* 11:45–58, 1952.

Fowler W.S.: Intrapulmonary distribution of inspired gas. *Physiol. Rev.* 32:1–20, 1952.

Fowler W.S., Cornish E.R., Kety S.S.: Analysis of alveolar ventilation by pulmonary N_2 clearance curves. *J. Clin. Invest.* 31:40–50, 1952.

Briscoe W.A., Forster R.E., Comroe J.H. Jr.: Alveolar ventilation at very low tidal volumes. *J. Appl. Physiol.* 7:27–30, 1954.

Radford E.P. Jr.: Ventilation standards for use in artificial respiration. *J. Appl. Physiol.* 7:451–460, 1955.

Rossier P.H., Buhlmann A.: The respiratory dead space. *Physiol. Rev.* 35:860–876, 1955.

Otis A.B., et al.: Mechanical factors in distribution of pulmonary ventilation. *J. Appl. Physiol.* 8:427–443, 1956.

Severinghaus J.W., Stupfel M.: Alveolar dead space as an index of distribution of blood flow in pulmonary capillaries. *J. Appl. Physiol.* 10:335–348, 1957.

Shepard R.H., Campbell E.J.M., Martin H.B., et al.: Factors affecting the pulmonary dead space as determined by single breath analysis. *J. Appl. Physiol.* 11:241–244, 1957.

Griggs W.A., Hackney J.D., Collier C.R., et al.: The rapid diagnosis of ventilatory failure with the CO_2 analyzer. *Am. J. Med.* 25:31–36, 1958.

Bouhuys A., Lundin G.: Distribution of inspired gas in the lungs. *Physiol. Rev.* 39:731–750, 1959.

Milic-Emili J., Henderson J.A.M., Dolovich M.B., et al.: Regional distribution of inspired gas in the lung. *J. Appl. Physiol.* 21:749–759, 1966.

Macklem P.T.: Airway obstruction and collateral ventilation. *Physiol. Rev.* 51:368–436, 1971.

Mechanics

Rohrer F.: Der Strömungswiderstand in den menschlichen Atemwegen und der Einfluss der unregelmassigen Verzweigung des Bronchialsystems auf den Atumungsverlauf verscheidenen Lungenbezirken. *Arch. Ges. Physiol.* 162:225–299, 1915.

Neergaard K., Wirz K.: Uber eine Methode zur Messung der Lungenelastizitat am lebenden Menschen, insbesondere beim Emphysem. *Ztschr. Klin. Med.* 105:35–51, 1927.

Christie R.V., MacIntosh C.A.: The measurement of the intrapleural pressure in man and its significance. *J. Clin. Invest.* 13:279–294, 1934.

Bayliss L.E., Robertson G.W.: The visco-elastic properties of the lungs. *Q. J. Exp. Physiol.* 29:27–47, 1939.

Dean R.B., Visscher M.B.: The kinetics of lung ventilation. *Am. J. Physiol.* 134:450–468, 1941.

Vuilleumier P.: Uber eine Methode zur Messung des intra-alveolaren Druckes und der Strömungswiderstande in den Atemwegen des Mensches. *Ztschr. Klin. Med.* 143:698–717, 1944.

Rahn H., et al.: The pressure-volume diagram of the lung and thorax. *Am. J. Physiol.* 146:161–178, 1946.

Buytendijk H.J.: *Intraesophageal Pressure and Lung Elasticity,* thesis, University of Groningen, Holland (Electrische Drukkerij I. Oppenheim N.V.), 1949.

Otis A.B., Fenn W.O., Rahn H.: Mechanics of breathing in man. *J. Appl. Physiol.* 2:592–607, 1950.

DuBois A.B., Ross B.B.: A new method for studying mechanics of breathing using a cathode ray oscillograph. *Proc. Soc. Exp. Biol. Med.* 78:546–549, 1951.

Gaensler E.A.: Analysis of the ventilatory defect by timed capacity measurement. *Am. Rev. Tuberc.* 64:256–278, 1951.

Fenn W.O.: Mechanics of respiration. *Am. J. Med.* 10:77–99, 1951.

Dayman H.: Mechanics of airflow in health and emphysema. *J. Clin. Invest.* 30:1175–1190, 1951.

Fry D.L., et al.: The mechanics of pulmonary ventilation in normal subjects and in patients with emphysema. *Am. J. Med.* 16:80–96, 1954.

Otis A.B.: The work of breathing. *Physiol. Rev.* 34:449–458, 1954.

Pattle R.E.: Properties, function and origin of the alveolar lining layer. *Nature* 175:1125–1126, 1955.

DuBois A.B., et al.: Oscillation mechanics of lungs and chest in man. *J. Appl. Physiol.* 8:587–594, 1956.

DuBois A.B., Botelho S.Y., Comroe J.H. Jr.: A new method for measuring airway resistance in man using a body plethysmograph: Values in normal subjects and in patients with respiratory disease. *J. Clin. Invest.* 35:327–335, 1956.

Marshall R., DuBois A.B.: Measurement of the viscous resistance of the lung tissues in normal man. *Clin. Sci.* 15:161–170, 1956.

Briscoe W.A., DuBois A.B.: Relationship between airway resistance, airway conductance and lung volume in subjects of different age and body size. *J. Clin. Invest.* 37:1279–1285, 1958.

Hyatt R.E., Schilder D.P., Fry D.L.: Relationship between maximum expiratory flow and degree of lung inflation. *J. Appl. Physiol.* 13:331–336, 1958.

Agostoni E., Fenn W.O.: Velocity of muscle shortening as a limiting factor in respiratory air flow. *J. Appl. Physiol.* 15:349–353, 1960.

Fry D.L., Hyatt R.E.: Pulmonary mechanics. *Am. J. Med.* 29:672–689, 1960.

Von Hayek H.: *The Human Lung,* Krahl V.E. (trans.). New York, Hafner Publications, 1960.

Mead J.: Mechanical properties of lungs. *Physiol. Rev.* 41:281–330, 1961.

Clements J.: Studies of surface phenomena in relation to pulmonary function. *Physiologist* 5:11–28, 1962.

Nadel J.A., Colebatch M.J.M., Olsen C.R.: Location and mechanism of airway constriction after barium sulfate microembolism. *J. Appl. Physiol.* 19:387–394, 1964.

Mead J., Turner S.M., Macklem P.T., et al.: Significance of the relationship between lung recoil and maximum expiratory flow. *J. Appl. Physiol.* 22:95–108, 1967.

Macklem P.T., Mead J.: Resistance of central and peripheral airways measured by a retrograde catheter. *J. Appl. Physiol.* 22:395–401, 1967.

Woolcock A.J., Vincent N.J., Macklem P.T.: Frequency dependence of compliance as a test for obstruction in the small airways. *J. Clin. Invest.* 48:1097–1106, 1969.

Mead J., Takashima T., Leith D.: Stress distribution in lungs: A model of pulmonary elasticity. *J. Appl. Physiol.* 28:596–608, 1970.

Macklem P.T.: Airway obstruction and collateral ventilation. *Physiol. Rev.* 51:368–436, 1971.

McCarthy D.S., Spencer R., Green R., et al.: Measurement of 'closing volume' as a simple and sensitive test for early detection of small airway disease. *Am. J. Med.* 52:747–753, 1972.

Menkes H., Gamsu G., Schroter R., et al.: Interdependence of lung units in isolated dog lungs. *J. Appl. Physiol.* 32:675–680, 1972.

Menkes H., Lindsay D., Wood L., et al.: Interdependence of lung units in intact dog lungs. *J. Appl. Physiol.* 32:681–686, 1972.

Mead J.: Respiration: Pulmonary mechanics. *Ann. Rev. Physiol.* 35:169–192, 1973.

Bouhuys A.: Flow volume curve, in *Breathing.* New York, Grune & Stratton, 1974, chap. 9, pp. 174–204.

Gluck L., Kulivoch M.V., Borer R.C., et al.: The interpretation and significance of the lecithin/sphingomyelin ratio in amniotic fluid. *Am. J. Obstet. Gynecol.* 120:142–155, 1974.

Wood L.D.H., Engel L.A., Griffin P., et al.: Effect of gas physical properties and flow on lower pulmonary resistance. *J. Appl. Physiol.* 41:234–244, 1975.

Drazen J.M., Loring S.H., Ingraham R.H., Jr.: Distribution of pulmonary resistance: Effects of gas density, viscosity, and flow rate. *J. Appl. Physiol.* 41:388–395, 1976.

Roussos C.S., Macklem P.T.: Diaphragmatic fatigue in man. *J. Appl. Physiol.* 43:189–197, 1977.

West J.B.: Bioengineering aspects of the lung, in *Lung Biology in Health and Disease.* New York, Marcel Dekker, vol. 3, 1977.

Goldstein D., Slutsky A.S., Ingram R.H. Jr., et al.: CO_2 elimination by high frequency ventilation (4 to 10 Hz) in normal subjects. *Am. Rev. Respir. Dis.* 123:251–255, 1981.

Knudson R.J.: Detection of early airway dysfunction, in Loepsky J.A., Riedesel M.L. (eds.): *Oxygen Transport to Human Tissues.* New York, Elsevier Holland, 1982, pp. 319–333.

Tsao F.H., Gulyas B.J., Hodgen G.D.: Prenatal assessment of fetal lung maturation: A critical review of amniotic fluid phospholipid test, in Farrell P. (ed.): *Lung Development: Biological and Clinical Perspectives,* vol. 2, *Neonatal Respiratory Distress.* New York, Academic Press, 1982, pp. 167–203.

West J.B.: *Pulmonary Pathophysiology,* ed. 2. Baltimore, Williams & Wilkins Co., 1982.

Katyal S.L., Singh G.: An enzyme-linked immunoassay of surfactant apoproteins: Its application to the study of fetal lung development in the rat. *Pediatr. Res.* 17:439–443, 1983.

Laszlo G.: Standardized lung function testing, editorial. *Thorax* 37:881–886, 1984.

Regulation of Respiration

Haldane J.S., Priestley J.G.: *Respiration.* London, Oxford University Press, 1935.

Comroe J.H. Jr.: The hyperpnea of muscular exercise. *Physiol. Rev.* 24:319–339, 1944.

Rahn H., Otis A.B.: Alveolar air during simulated flights to high altitudes. *Am. J. Physiol.* 150:202–221, 1947.

Heymans C., Neil E.: *Reflexogenic Areas of Cardiovascular System.* Boston, Little, Brown & Co., 1958.

Robin E.D., et al.: Alveolar gas tensions, pulmonary ventilation and blood pH during physiologic sleep in normal subjects. *J. Clin. Invest.* 37:981–989, 1958.

Brodovsky D., MacDonell J.A., Cherniack R.M.: The respiratory response to carbon dioxide in health and in emphysema. *J. Clin. Invest.* 39:724–729, 1960.

Cunningham D.J.C., Shaw D.G., Lahiri S., et al.: The effect of maintained ammonium chloride acidosis on the relation between pulmonary ventilation and alveolar oxygen and carbon dioxide in man. *Q. J. Exp. Physiol.* 46:323–334, 1961.

Paintal A.S.: The mechanism of excitation of type J receptors, and the J reflex, in Porter R. (ed.): *Breathing*, Hering-Breuer Centenary Symposium. London, Churchill, 1970, pp. 59–71.

Lourenco R.V. (ed.): Clinical methods for the study of regulation of breathing. *Chest* 70:109–195, 1976.

Remmers J.E., de Groot W.J., Sauerland E.K., et al.: Pathogenesis of upper airway occlusion during sleep. *J. Appl. Physiol.* 44:931–938, 1978.

Hornbein T.F. (ed.): *Regulation of Breathing*. New York, Marcel Dekker, 1981.

Richter D.W.: Generation and maintenance of respiratory rhythm. *J. Exp. Biol.* 100:93–107, 1982.

von Euler C.: On the central pattern generator for the basic breathing rythmicity. *J. Appl. Physiol.* 55:1647–1659, 1983.

Pulmonary Circulation

Roughton F.J.W.: The average time spent by the blood in the human lung capillary. *Am. J. Physiol.* 143:621–633, 1945.

Riley R.L., et al.: Studies of the pulmonary circulation at rest and during exercise in normal individuals and in patients with chronic pulmonary disease. *Am. J. Physiol.* 152:372–382, 1948.

Hellems H.K., Haynes F.W., Dexter L.: Pulmonary 'capillary' pressure in man. *J. Appl. Physiol.* 2:24–29, 1949.

Cournand A.: Some aspects of the pulmonary circulation in normal man and in chronic cardiopulmonary diseases. *Circulation* 2:641–657, 1950.

Donald K.W., et al.: The effect of exercise on the cardiac output and circulatory dynamics of normal subjects. *Clin. Sci.* 14:37–73, 1955.

Lee G., DuBois A.B.: Pulmonary capillary blood flow in man. *J. Clin. Invest.* 34:1380–1390, 1955.

Cander L., Forster R.E.: Determination of pulmonary parenchymal tissue volume and pulmonary capillary blood flow in man. *J. Appl. Physiol.* 14:541–551, 1959.

Fishman A.P.: Respiratory gases in the regulation of the pulmonary circulation. *Physiol. Rev.* 41:214–280, 1961.

Permutt S., et al.: Effect of lung inflation on static pressure-volume characteristics of pulmonary vessels. *J. Appl. Physiol.* 16:64–70, 1961.

Anthonisen N.R., Milic-Emili J.: Distribution of pulmonary perfusion in erect man. *J. Appl. Physiol.* 21:760–766, 1966.

Gillis C.N., Cronau L.H., Mandel S., et al.: Indicator dilution measurement of 5-hydroxytryptamine clearance by human lung. *J. Appl. Physiol.* 46:1178–1183, 1979.

Lassen N.A., Perl W.: *Tracer Kinetic Methods in Medical Physiology*. New York, Raven Press, 1979.

Rickaby D.A., Dawson C.A., Linehan J.H.: Influence of blood and plasma flow rate on kinetics of serotonin uptake by lungs. *J. Appl. Physiol.* 53:677–684, 1982.

Distribution of Ventilation and Blood Flow

Riley R.L., Cournand A.: 'Ideal' alveolar air and the analysis of ventilation-perfusion relationships in the lungs. *J. Appl. Physiol.* 1:825–847, 1949.

Rahn H.: A concept of mean alveolar air and the ventilation-blood flow relationships during pulmonary gas exchange. *Am. J. Physiol.* 158:21–30, 1949.

Riley R.L., Cournand A.: Analysis of factors affecting partial pressures of O_2 and CO_2 in gas and blood of lungs: Methods. *J. Appl. Physiol.* 4:102–120, 1951.

Riley R.L.: Pulmonary gas exchange. *Am. J. Med.* 10:210–220, 1951.

Rahn H., Fenn W.O.: *A Graphical Analysis of the Respiratory Gas Exchange: The O_2-CO_2 Diagram.* Washington, D.C., American Physiological Society, 1955.

Fahri L.E., Rahn H.: A theoretical analysis of the alveolo-arterial O_2 difference with special reference to the distribution effect. *J. Appl. Physiol.* 7:699–703, 1955.

West J.B., et al.: Measurement of the ventilation-perfusion ratio inequality in the lung by the analysis of a single expirate. *Clin. Sci.* 16:529–547, 1957.

Briscoe W.A.: A method for dealing with data concerning uneven ventilation of the lung and its effect on blood gas transfer. *J. Appl. Physiol.* 14:291–298, 1959.

Colldahl J., Alväger T., Uhler J.: A comparison between pulmonary elimination capacity of acetylene and radioactive argon and xenon injected intravenously dissolved in saline. *Acta Allerg.* 15:406–416, 1960.

Severinghaus J.W., et al.: Unilateral hypoventilation produced in dogs by occluding one pulmonary artery. *J. Appl. Physiol.* 16:53–60, 1961.

Swenson E.W., Finley T.N., Guzman S.V.: Unilateral hypoventilation in man during temporary occlusion of one pulmonary artery. *J. Clin. Invest.* 40:828–835, 1961.

West J.B., Dollery C.T., Hugh-Jones P.: The use of radioactive CO_2 to measure regional blood flow in the lungs of patients with pulmonary disease. *J. Clin. Invest.* 40:1–12, 1961.

Ball W.C., et al.: Regional pulmonary function studied with xenon. *J. Clin. Invest.* 41:519–531, 1962.

Kaneko K., Milic-Emili J., Dolovich M.B., et al.: Regional distribution of ventilation and perfusion as a function of body position. *J. Appl. Physiol.* 21:767–777, 1966.

Wagner P.D., Saltzman H.A., West J.B.: Measurement of continuous distributions of ventilation-perfusion ratio: Theory. *J. Appl. Physiol.* 36:588–599, 1974.

Diffusion

Krogh M.: Diffusion of gases through the lungs of man. *J. Physiol.* 49:271–300, 1914–15.

Barcroft J.: *The Respiratory Function of the Blood: I. The Diffusion of O_2 Through Pulmonary Epithelium.* Cambridge, England, Cambridge University Press, 1925, vol. 1, pp. 63–74.

Lilienthal J.L., et al.: An experimental analysis in man of the O_2 pressure gradient from alveolar air to arterial blood. *Am. J. Physiol.* 147:199–216, 1946.

Kety S.S.: Pulmonary diffusion coefficient, in Comroe J.H. Jr. (ed.): *Methods in Medical Research.* Chicago, Year Book Medical Publishers, 1950, vol. 2, pp. 234–242.

Riley R.L., Cournand A.: Analysis of factors affecting partial pressures of O_2 and CO_2 in gas and blood of lungs: Theory. *J. Appl. Physiol.* 4:77–101, 1951.

Riley R.L., Cournand A., Donald K.W.: Analysis of factors affecting partial pressures of O_2 and CO_2 in gas and blood of lungs: Methods. *J. Appl. Physiol.* 4:102–120, 1951.

Bates D.V.: Uptake of CO in health and emphysema. *Clin. Sci.* 11:21–32, 1952.

Filley G.F., MacIntosh D.J., Wright G.W.: Carbon monoxide uptake and pulmonary diffusing capacity in normal subjects at rest and during exercise. *J. Clin. Invest.* 33:530–539, 1954.

Forster R.E., et al.: The absorption of CO by the lungs during breath-holding. *J. Clin. Invest.* 33:1135–1145, 1954.

Riley R.L., et al.: Maximal diffusing capacity of the lungs. *J. Appl. Physiol.* 6:573–587, 1954.

Kruhøffer P.: Studies on the lung diffusion coefficient for carbon monoxide in normal subjects by means of $C^{14}O$. *Acta Physiol. Scand.* 32:106–123, 1954.

Forster R.E.: Exchange of gases between alveolar air and pulmonary capillary blood: Pulmonary diffusion capacity. *Physiol. Rev.* 37:391–452, 1957.

Marks A., et al.: Clinical determination of the diffusion capacity of the lungs: Comparison of methods in normal subjects and patients with alveolar-capillary block syndrome. *Am. J. Med.* 22:51–73, 1957.

Ogilvie C.M., et al.: A standardized breath holding technique for the clinical measurement of the diffusing capacity of the lung for carbon monoxide. *J. Clin. Invest.* 36:1–7, 1957.

Forster R.E., et al.: Apparent pulmonary diffusing capacity for CO at varying alveolar O_2 tensions. *J. Appl. Physiol.* 11:277–289, 1957.

McNeill R.S., Rankin J., Forster R.E.: The diffusing capacity of the pulmonary membrane and the pulmonary capillary blood volume in cardiopulmonary disease. *Clin. Sci.* 17:465–482, 1958.

Rankin J., McNeill R.S., Forster R.E.: Influence of increased alveolar CO_2 tension on pulmonary diffusing capacity for CO in man. *J. Appl. Physiol.* 15:543–549, 1960.

King T.K.C., Briscoe W.A.: Bohr integral isopleths in the study of blood gas exchange in the lung. *J. Appl. Physiol.* 22:59–674, 1967.

Power G.: Gaseous diffusion between airways and alveoli in the human lung. *J. Appl. Physiol.* 27:701–709, 1969.

Arndt H., King T.K.C., Briscoe W.A.: Diffusing capacities and ventilation perfusion in patients with the clinical syndrome of alveolar capillary block. *J. Clin. Invest.* 49:408–421, 1970.

Menkes H.A., Sera K., Rogers R., et al.: Pulsatile uptake of CO in the human lung. *J. Clin. Invest.* 49:335–345, 1970.

Weibel E.R.: Morphological basis of alveolar-capillary gas exchange. *Physiol. Rev.* 53:419–495, 1973.

Crapo R.O., Morris A.H.: Standardized single breath normal values for carbon monoxide diffusing capacity. *Am. Rev. Respir. Dis.* 123:185–189, 1981.

Crapo J.D., Crapo R.O.: Comparison of total lung diffusion capacity and the membrane component of diffusion capacity as determined by physiologic and morphometric techniques. *Resp. Physiol.* 51:181–194, 1983.

Forster R.E., Ogilvie C.: The single-breath carbon monoxide transfer test 25 years on: A reappraisal. *Thorax* 38:1–9, 1983.

Graham B.L., Mink J.T., Cotton D.J.: Overestimation of the single breath CO diffusing capacity in patients with airflow obstruction. *Am. Rev. Respir. Dis.* 129:403–408, 1984.

Blood O_2, CO_2 and pH

Van Slyke D.D., Neill J.M.: Determination of gases in blood and other solutions by vacuum extraction and manometric measurement. *J. Biol. Chem.* 61:523–573, 1924.

Van Slyke D.D., Sendroy J., Jr.: Line charts for graphic calculations by Henderson-Hasselbalch equation for calculating plasma CO_2 content from whole blood content. *J. Biol. Chem.* 79:781–798, 1928.

Roughton F.J.W.: The transport of carbon dioxide by the blood. *Harvey Lect.* 39:96–142, 1943–44.

Roughton F.J.W., Darling R.D., Root W.S.: Factors affecting the determination of oxygen capacity, content and pressure in human arterial blood. *Am. J. Physiol.* 142:708–720, 1944.

Drabkin D.L., Schmidt C.F.: Spectrophotometric studies: Direct determination of the saturation of hemoglobin in arterial blood. *J. Biol. Chem.* 157:69–83, 1945.

Riley R.L., Proemmel D.D., Franke R.E.: Direct method for determination of O_2 and CO_2 tension in blood. *J. Biol. Chem.* 161:621–633, 1945.

Comroe J.H. Jr., Botelho S.: The unreliability of cyanosis in the recognition of arterial anoxemia. *Am. J. Med. Sci.* 214:1–6, 1947.

Singer R.B., Hastings A.B.: Improved clinical method for estimation of disturbances of acid base balance of human blood. *Medicine* 27:223–242, 1948.

Davenport H.: *The ABC of Acid Base Chemistry,* ed. 5. Chicago, University of Chicago Press, 1969.

Astrup P.: A simple electrometric technique for the determination of carbon dioxide tension in blood and plasma, total content of carbon dioxide in plasma, and bicarbonate content in 'separated' plasma at a fixed carbon dioxide tension (40 mm Hg). *Scand. J. Clin. Lab. Invest.* 8:33–43, 1956.

Riley R.L., Campbell E.J.M., Shepard R.H.: A bubble method for estimation of PCO_2 and PO_2 in whole blood. *J. Appl. Physiol.* 11:245–249, 1957.

Kreuzer F., Watson T.R. Jr., Ball J.M.: Comparative measurements with a new procedure for measuring the blood oxygen tension in vitro. *J. Appl. Physiol.* 12:65–70, 1958.

Hackney J.D., Sears C.H., Collier C.R.: Estimation of arterial CO_2 tension by rebreathing technique. *J. Appl. Physiol.* 12:425–430, 1958.

Severinghaus J.W., Bradley A.F.: Electrodes for blood PO_2 and PCO_2 determination. *J. Appl. Physiol.* 13:515–520, 1958.

Forster R.E.: Buffering in blood with emphasis on kinetics, in Seldin D.W.,

Giebisch G. (eds.): *The Kidney: Physiology and Pathophysiology*. New York, Raven Press, chap. 7, 1985.

Woodbury J.W.: Body acid-base state and its regulation, in Ruch T.C., Patton H.D. (eds.): *Physiology and Biophysics*, ed. 20. Philadelphia, W.B. Saunders Co., 1974, chap. 27.

Shapiro B.A., Harrison R.A., Walton J.R.: *Clinical Application of Blood Gases*, ed. 2. Chicago, Year Book Medical Publishers, 1977.

Index

C

D

E

F

G

H

I

L

N

O

P

R

S

T

U

V